State of the Young Child in India

This Report is one of the first comprehensive studies on young children in India. It focuses on children under 6 years of age and presents key aspects of their well-being and development. With the highest number of neonatal, infant and under-5 deaths in the world, there is an urgent need to address issues that continue to affect the young child in India.

This volume:

- Introduces two young child indices aggregating selected indicators to separately track child outcomes and child circumstances.
- Provides an account of the current situation of the young child in terms of physical and cognitive development, access to care, disadvantaged children and major issues that have led to the continued neglect of this age group.
- Explores the policy and legal framework, fiscal space and the role and obligations of key stakeholders, including the state, private sector, civil society, media and the family.
- Highlights key recommendations and action points that can help to improve the ecosystem for early childhood care and development.

Drawing on specially commissioned technical background papers, supplemented by extensive field experience of Mobile Creches in childcare, this Report will be of interest to practitioners, policymakers and influencers, think tanks and researchers of public policy, development studies, human rights, sociology and social anthropology, as well as general readers.

Mobile Creches (MC) is a leading organisation for Early Childhood Development (ECD) in India. Headquartered in New Delhi, it works at the grassroots level for young children under 6 years across the country, with a focus on the most vulnerable – in particular children of migrant families and slum dwellers. It has also developed appropriate training resources to enable a cadre of early childhood care workers across government and non-government settings. As a knowledge organisation, MC presents this Report, which draws upon its decades of working with young children and their families and its engagement with local communities, businesses, practitioners, advocates and policymakers.

With the support of

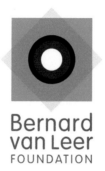

Bernard
van Leer
FOUNDATION

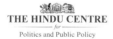
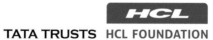
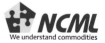

State of the Young Child in India

Mobile Creches

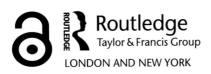

Routledge
Taylor & Francis Group
LONDON AND NEW YORK

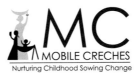

MC
MOBILE CRECHES
Nurturing Childhood Sowing Change

First published 2020 by Routledge

2 Park Square, Milton Park, Abingdon, Oxon OX14 4RN
605 Third Avenue, New York, NY 10017

Routledge is an imprint of the Taylor & Francis Group, an informa business

First issued in paperback 2021

Publisher's Note

The publisher has gone to great lengths to ensure the quality of this reprint
but points out that some imperfections in the original copies may be apparent.

British Library Cataloguing-in-Publication Data
A catalogue record for this book is available from the British Library

Library of Congress Cataloging-in-Publication Data
Names: Mobile Creches (Organization : Mumbai, India), corporate
    author.
Title: State of the young child in India / Mobile Creches.
Description: 1. | New York : Taylor & Francis Group, 2020. |
    Includes bibliographical references and index.
Identifiers: LCCN 2019056991 (print) | LCCN 2019056992 (ebook)
Subjects: LCSH: Children—India—Social conditions—21st century. |
    Children—India—21st century. | Child development—India.
Classification: LCC HQ792.I5 S665 2020 (print) | LCC HQ792.I5
    (ebook) | DDC 305.230954—dc23
LC record available at https://lccn.loc.gov/2019056991
LC ebook record available at https://lccn.loc.gov/2019056992

ISBN: 978-0-367-46018-1 (hbk)
ISBN: 978-1-03-217380-1 (pbk)
DOI: 10.4324/9781003026488

Typeset in Sabon
by Apex CoVantage, LLC

State of the Young Child in India team

Core team

Anuradha Rajivan, Lead Technical Advisor
Sanjay Kaul
Sumitra Mishra
V. S. Sambandan
Samreen Mushtaq

Editor

Neelam Singh

Young Child indices

Pronab Sen, Technical Advisor

Technical background paper contributors

Mridula Bajaj
Nandita Chaudhary
Ranjana Kesarwani
Ranjani Murthy
Renu Singh
Venkatesan Ramani
Vimala Ramachandran

Contents

Figures

Tables

Annexure tables

Boxes

Foreword

This inaugural issue of the *State of the Young Child in India* brings to the fore the pressing and urgent need to provide primary focus for policy and programme action to this most vulnerable and critical stage of human development. It is prepared with the aim to place the young child at the centre of policy dialogue, borne out of the conviction that each child has an inalienable right to opportunities to develop her full potential. The first six years are the foundation of human life. The young child needs nutritious food to survive and grow, mental and physical stimulation, safe and hygienic environment, timely access to basic services and, above all, love, care and dignity.

There is widespread consensus on the vital importance of Early Childhood Development (ECD) but the neglect of this sector by various stakeholders has led to the denial of rightful opportunities for physical and cognitive development and emotional security to the young child in India. This Report recognises that structural inequities, neglect and injustice keep many young children (and their families) disadvantaged, invisible and excluded. It highlights the inextricable linkages between issues affecting children, women, parents and childcare providers, the interconnected socioeconomic environment including inequities and the ultimate role and responsibility of the State in addressing the challenges that the young child faces. The commitment of the State has been piecemeal, fragmented and half-hearted despite a fair amount of policy work in addressing the multitude of issues concerning the young child.

This Report was compiled and completed before the Covid-19 pandemic set in. The pandemic, and the subsequent lockdown, has had an unprecedented adverse impact on the social and economic fabric of the country. Its scale and magnitude has exposed multiple fault lines and vulnerabilities, especially in the informal sector and the rural economy. The effects on families and children have been devastating. In this context, the rights perspective and economic imperative to focus on the young child assumes even more importance and urgency. A key objective of the Report is to enable policy makers to identify and bring about both short-term as well as long-term policy measures for addressing the deprivations that confront the young child and mitigate the ill effects of such a crisis in the future.

Over the past five decades, Mobile Creches (MC) has emerged as India's leading organisation for ECD through its long work at the grassroots level for young children under 6 years. It has focussed on the most vulnerable children, especially children of migrant families and slum dwellers and has used its evidence based experience to work with local communities, governments, businesses, practitioners, advocates, programme implementers and policymakers. It has harnessed this knowledge in the form of this Report.

The Report introduces two "Young Child Indices," which facilitate inter-state comparisons, and are an important component of the Report. An outcome based "Young Child Outcomes Index" (YCOI) uses indicators of physical well-being and cognitive development and captures trends over the years. The "Young Child Environment Index" (YCEI) uses process and input indicators that are critical to the child's well-being and growth. In the process of identifying indicators for these indices, the Report also identified serious data gaps that hinder a holistic understanding of challenges. These need to be addressed by the country's decision makers to ensure that the status of the young child is properly depicted – a *sine quo non* for effective and durable policy interventions on behalf of the child. In addition to presenting the current status, the Young Child Indices aim to trigger policy discussions on a holistic view of the child, and the environmental enablers during early childhood that can have a transformative effect on building inclusive and equitable societies.

The Report also recognises the biological role in caregiving and its influence on the young child's physical and emotional development. Drawing upon MC's grassroots work in early childhood period, it advocates professionalisation of childcare services and the unmet need for quality crèches and day-care services. It also challenges the traditional gender stereotyping due to an overemphasis on the 'mother' in the primary caregiving role and highlights the importance of parenting and outside care. It addresses both traditional persisting issues such as under-nutrition, gender-based discrimination, the burden on women, as well as emerging challenges in a rapidly changing India which include need for day-care, climate change issues, exposure to digital technology and increasing reports of violence.

The objective of this Report is to identify solutions for the chronic obstacles to the fulfilment of the potential that lies in India's children by studying the approaches, policy constraints, measurement metrics, legislation, programmatic interventions and investment of human, technical and financial resources.

The Executive Summary collates the most significant issues and challenges related to ECD in India. The chapters provide in-depth accounts of the current situation of the young child in terms of their physical and cognitive development, access to care and the multitude of factors that enhance their vulnerabilities and deprivations. The imperative that no child should be left behind guided the analyses of the state of the young child, gaps in programme implementation, desirable practices and recommendations.

Positioned as the most authoritative and latest resource for policymakers, child advocates, development practitioners, elected representatives, the media, human rights campaigners, education, health and nutrition activists, poverty alleviation architects and many other co-travellers, this Report also places before its readers the unheard voice for the young child in India that cries out for informed collective action on multiple fronts. As an important reference for strategic and policy decisions required for securing the rights and entitlements of the youngest citizens of India, the Report not only critiques the government policies and systems but also suggests the ways forward. It is now up to the readers to respond and galvanise action within their spheres of influence to address all the impediments that hamper the well-being and all-round development of the young child.

Amrita Jain
Chairperson
Mobile Creches, New Delhi
March 2020

Acknowledgements

The *State of the Young Child in India* situates the young child within a set of integrated rights at the foundational age and its inextricable linkages with issues related to women, work and socio-economic inequities. It analyses relevant policies and their implementation, identifies gaps, barriers and bottlenecks, highlights some good practices, compares performance of states against relevant indicators and makes key recommendations. It offers a 'solutions oriented' analysis of government policies and systems and suggests a way forward.

Above all, the Report draws its inspiration and knowledge from the founding team of Mobile Creches (MC), General Body members, hundreds of co-travellers, young children and their overburdened families, tireless crèche workers, who have walked the long path of ensuring a just and caring world for the most vulnerable young children of India. This Report is a tribute to their love, dedication and hard work.

It gives me great pleasure to introduce this Report produced in collaboration with like-minded partners, including Bernard van Leer Foundation, The Hindu Centre for Politics and Public Policy, Tata Trusts, HCL Foundation and National Collateral Management Services Limited (NCML). We remain deeply grateful for your financial support in producing this Report. Most importantly, for sharing our vision of creating a nurturing environment for young children where they can grow to achieve their full potential.

MC acknowledges and appreciates the contributors of Technical Background Papers, whose work shaped the content of the Report – Mridula Bajaj, Nandita Chaudhary, Ranjana Kesarwani, Ranjani Murthy, Renu Singh, Venkatesan Ramani and Vimala Ramachandran. They played the vital role in translating the vision behind the Report to a technically sound publication.

The Report was brought to fruition by a core team, led by Anuradha Rajivan, a former civil servant and development economist who provided technical guidance on all aspects of the Report. Sanjay Kaul, a former civil servant with several years of grassroots level experience in the social sector, contributed to the Report from conceptualisation to its final production. V. S. Sambandan, of The Hindu Centre for Politics and Public Policy, remained engaged and made meaningful contributions through the process. Samreen Mushtaq, research associate, held the Report very close to the scientific process and her heart, as she navigated competing opinions and deadlines to ensure that you have a good publication in your hands.

We remain grateful to Neelam Singh, Editor of the Report, for her meticulous, organised and enthusiastic handling of the content to make it accessible to our audiences.

We are grateful to Pronab Sen, former Chief Statistician of India, for his guidance on developing the two Young Child Indices created for this Report and the indexing process. The support of the knowledge management team at NCML for their timely statistical support in preparing these Young Child Indices has been invaluable.

We appreciate the valuable technical contributions of Sachin Tiwari, Tarishi Khanna, Ratanpriya Agarwal and Radhika Sharma throughout the process of preparing this Report.

Last, but certainly not the least, I remain deeply grateful to the entire team at MC, without whose direct and indirect efforts, this journey would not have been as momentous as it turned out to be.

Sumitra Mishra
Executive Director
Mobile Creches, New Delhi
March 2020

Acronyms

AAM	Action Against Malnutrition
AERC	Applied Economics Research Centre
ANC	Ante natal care
ANM	Auxiliary Nurse Midwife
ART	Assisted Reproductive Technology
ASER	Annual Status of Education Report
ASHA	Accredited Social Health Activist
AWC	*Anganwadi* Centre
AWH	*Anganwadi* Helper
AWW	*Anganwadi* Worker
BCG	Bacillus Calmette-Guérin
BMI	Body Mass Index
BOCWA	Building and Other Construction Workers Act
BvLF	Bernard van Leer Foundation
CABE	Central Advisory Board of Education
CARA	Central Adoption Resource Agency
CARINGS	Child Adoption Resource Information and Guidance System
CBGA	Centre for Budget and Governance Accountability
CBO	Community Based Organisation
CCI	Child Care Institutions
CDPO	Child Development Project Officer
CECED	Centre for Early Childhood Education and Development
CLR	Centre for Learning Resources
CMAM	Community-based Management of Acute Malnutrition
CNNS	Comprehensive National Nutrition Survey
CPAP	Country Programme Action Plans
CRC	Convention on the Rights of the Child
CRPD	Convention on the Rights of Persons with Disabilities
CSO	Civil Society Organisation
CSR	Child Sex Ratio
DCPU	District Child Protection Unit
DIET	District Institute of Education and Training
DISE	District Information System for Education

DoH	Department of Health
DPT	Diptheria, Pertussis (whooping cough), and Tetanus
DWCD	Department of Women and Child Development
EAG	Empowered Action Group
ECCE	Early Childhood Care and Education
ECD	Early Childhood Development
ECE	Early Childhood Education
EdCIL	Educational Consultants of India Limited
FFRC	Food Fortification Resource Centre
FOCUS	Focus On Children Under 6
FSSAI	Food Safety and Standards Authority of India
GDP	Gross Domestic Product
GEI	Gender Equality Index
GER	Gross Enrolment Ratio
GIS	Geographic Information System
GoI	Government of India
GPRS	General Packet Radio Service
HDI	Human Development Index
ICDS	Integrated Child Development Services
ICMR	Indian Council of Medical Research
ICPS	Integrated Child Protection Services
ICT	Information and Communications Technology
IECEI	India Early Childhood Education Impact
IFPRI	International Food Policy Research Institute
IMR	Infant Mortality Rate
IPCC	Intergovernmental Panel on Climate Change
IT	Information Technology
IUGR	Intra Uterine Growth Retardation
IYCF	Infant and Young Child Feeding
JSY	*Janani Suraksha Yojana*
LBW	Low Birth Weight
MC	Mobile Creches
MCAFPD	Ministry of Consumer Affairs, Food and Public Distribution
MCTS	Mother & Child Tracking System
MDM	Mid-Day Meal Scheme
MDWS	Ministry of Drinking Water and Sanitation
MoHFW	Ministry of Health and Family Welfare
MHRD	Ministry of Human Resource Development
MMR	Maternal Mortality Rate
MNREGA	Mahatma Gandhi National Rural Employment Guarantee Act
MoHFW	Ministry of Health and Family Welfare
MoSPI	Ministry of Statistics and Programme Implementation
MPR	Monthly Progress Report
MWCD	Ministry of Women and Child Development
NCERT	National Council of Educational Research and Training

NCPCR	National Commission for Protection of Child Rights
NCRB	National Crime Records Bureau
NCS	National Crèche Scheme
NCTE	National Council of Technical Education
NER	Net Enrolment Ratio
NFHS	National Family Health Survey
NGO	Non-Governmental Organisation
NHM	National Health Mission
NIPCCD	National Institute of Public Cooperation and Child Development
NIUA	National Institute of Urban Affairs
NMR	Neonatal Mortality Rate
NMS	Nutrition Monitoring System
NNM	National Nutrition Mission
NNS	National Nutrition Strategy
NPAC	National Plan of Action for Children
NPAN	National Plan of Action on Nutrition
NRC	National Register of Citizens
NRHM	National Rural Health Mission
NSSO	National Sample Survey Office
OBC	Other Backward Class
ODF	Open Defecation Free
PALM	Pregnant and Lactating Mothers
PCPNDT	Pre-Conception and Prenatal Diagnostic Techniques
PDS	Public Distribution System
PHC	Primary Health Centre
PNC	Postnatal Care
PNDT	Prenatal Diagnostic Techniques
PNMR	Post Neonatal Mortality
POCSO	The Protection of Children from Sexual Offences
POCUS	Progress of Children Under 6
PRI	*Panchayati Raj* Institutions
PWD	Persons with Disability
RBI	Reserve Bank of India
RCH	Reproductive and Child Health
RMSA	*Rashtriya Madhyamik Shiksha Abhiyan*
RSOC	Rapid Survey On Children
RTE	Right to Education
RWA	Resident Welfare Association
SAM	Severe and Acute Malnutrition
SBM	*Swachh Bharat* Mission
SC	Scheduled Caste
SCERT	State Council of Educational Research and Training
SD	Standard Deviation
SDG	Sustainable Development Goals

SEWA	Self Employed Women's Association
SHG	Self Help Group
SIE	State Institute of Education
SNP	Supplementary Nutrition Programme
SOP	Standard Operating Procedure
SRB	Sex Ratio at Birth
SRS	Sample Registration System
SSA	*Sarva Shiksha Abhiyan*
SSA	*Samagra Shiksha Abhiyan*
SSE	Social Sector Expenditure
ST	Scheduled Tribe
TE	Teacher Education
THR	Take Home Rations
TSG	Technical Support Group
TT	Tetanus Toxoid
U5	Under 5 Years of Age
U5MR	Under 5 Mortality Rate
U6	Under 6 Years of Age
UID	Unique Identification number
UNDESA	United Nations Department of Economic and Social Affairs
UNDP	United Nations Development Programme
UNESCO	United Nations Educational Scientific and Cultural Organisation
UNICEF	United Nations Children's Fund
VNR	Voluntary National Review
WHO	World Health Organization
YCEI	Young Child Environment Index
YCOI	Young Child Outcomes Index

Executive summary

The young child in India

The Indian Constitution, sectoral policy frameworks and legislation entitle every child to basic rights. India is a State Party to the Convention on the Rights of the Child and is committed to achieving the Sustainable Development Goals (SDGs) by 2030, which necessitates actions addressing the young child. However, the situation of India's children aged under 6 years of age is grim. Of the 159 million children in this age group, 21% are undernourished, 36 percent are underweight and 38 percent do not receive full immunisation.[1] While the disadvantaged child remains further relegated to the margins, impacted by socio-cultural beliefs and gender relations and neglect, young child abuse has also emerged as a serious concern that is not confined to any specific social group.

There is insurmountable evidence of the huge returns on investment in Early Childhood Development (ECD) at the individual, household and country levels. Proper nutrition, stimulation and care during the first 1,000 days of life (from conception to the second birthday) has a profound impact on the child's ability to grow, learn and rise out of poverty, and in the process shape society's long term stability and prosperity. Indeed, early childhood is a period which offers the highest returns on investment, leading to economic growth and sustained human development of a country.

Early childhood is a phase of life when significant human growth takes place. All that is required is a nurturing ecosystem – health, nutrition, stimulation and early education, responsive parenting – together with intersections of maternal health, care and protection, to enable the youngest rights' holders to realise their full potential. Several interconnected factors cutting across development sectors determine outcomes for the young child. Although there has been some focus on survival, physical and cognitive development of the young child, nurturing childcare which is critical for holistic ECD has remained largely neglected.

The eight states of Assam, Meghalaya, Rajasthan, Chhattisgarh, Madhya Pradesh, Jharkhand, Uttar Pradesh and Bihar lag behind as their ranking and values on the Young Child Outcome Index (YCOI) show, scoring even below the national average. Kerala, Goa, Tripura and Tamil Nadu are among the top performers. Most of the states that perform poorly in the YCOI are also poor performers in the Young Child Environment Index.

The role of the State is crucial for creating conditions to enable families in ensuring the well-being of the young child. But budgetary commitments have been inadequate and the implementation of policies and programmes has been mixed. In addition, civil society and the corporate sector have a vital complementary role to play, which is yet to be fully leveraged.

Advancing physical well-being

India contributes the highest number of neonatal, infant and under 5 deaths in the world notwithstanding the significant decline in Infant Mortality Rate (IMR) in the last two decades. Globally, 20 million infants are born every year with low birth weight, out of which an estimated 7.5 million births occur in India.[2] Many are born with congenital defects and disabilities, and many are vulnerable to infections. Poor nutrition, inadequate immunisation, low access to safe drinking water and well-maintained sanitation facilities and overall environmental hygiene exacerbate the situation.

Persistently adverse child sex ratio indicates deep-rooted gender bias and neglect of the girl child. The health and nutrition status of mother is intricately linked to preterm birth and impacts the health and nutrition status of infants and young children.

In addition to an adequate supply of nutritious food, the presence of an adult caregiver who can feed the child at regular intervals, maintain hygiene and provide adequate care, is equally important for early childhood nutrition.

Economic status of the households influences the availability, accessibility and utilisation of basic health, nutrition and social development services. Sub-optimal functioning of government systems, flagship programmes and schemes in many states subject the very poor and marginalised to greater distress and further compound inequality in wealth.

A holistic approach to development, including public awareness and parental education, improved living conditions with access to clean drinking water, proper sanitation and a reliable primary healthcare service, is critical for making a difference to the health and nutritional standards among children.

Malnutrition reduction needs to be addressed with urgency by coordinating implementation of measures. The *Poshan Abhiyaan* targets are ambitious but with political and administrative commitment they offer an opportunity for galvanising national efforts to reduce child malnutrition and achieve the SDG targets.

The two national flagship programmes, *Swachh Bharat* and *Poshan Abhiyaan*, provide strategic windows of opportunities for sustained nationwide campaigns and parental education programmes. Parental and family coun-selling could provide opportunities for promoting early and exclusive breast-feeding, timely complementary feeding, full immunisation, water handling, hygiene and use of improved toilets. School-based health and nutrition pro-grammes could enable regular check-ups of young children, to initiate them to healthy food habits, regular intake of water, proper handwashing and hygienic practices, and to enrol those who have been identified as malnour-ished or have other health issues for special interventions.

Promoting early learning

There is substantial evidence that learning begins at birth. The holistic needs of health, nutrition, protection and stimulation during the early years of life facilitate cognitive and psycho-social development of children. The limited understanding of the holistic nature of Early Childhood Care and Educa-tion (ECCE) among parents, who tend to prioritise formal schooling, results in a cumulative burden that a child carries through schooling years into adulthood.

Unregulated pre-schools and day-care centres that pressure children to read and write way ahead of their developmental readiness have mush-roomed, while the integrated elements of care, health, nutrition and love take a backseat. The regulation by the State is nonexistent in the absence of uniform norms and minimum standards for ECCE services.

Although India has the world's largest programme for young children, viz., the Integrated Child Development Services (ICDS), it has faced relative neglect of ECCE since its inception and has been constrained by resource and capacity deficits. There are rural-urban differences, social category dif-ferences and wealth index differences in participation in the *Anganwadi* Centres (AWCs) and private pre-school education centres.

Various non-governmental organisations (NGOs) offer ECCE services to children who are unreachable by the services provided by the Government or the private sector, yet universalisation of ECCE services is still a distant dream. Many innovations on the ground are valuable but limited in their reach and impact, necessitating an urgent need for public systems and struc-tures to ensure quality ECCE to all, especially the most excluded children.

More investment in policy, legislation and planning, less so in monitor-ing and evaluation, and hardly any in implementation and quality enhance-ment, has led to the lack of a comprehensive perspective for good quality early education services.

Policy and practice need to situate ECCE within a comprehensive ECD framework in order to optimise outcomes for young children. The exten-sion of the Right to Education to early childhood age group is important for according priority to ECD on the policy agenda, programmes and inter-ventions and securing increased budgetary allocation for quality ECCE. Development of capacities and competencies of ECCE teachers for early education could help in improving the delivery of quality services. But ultimately the ECCE workforce needs to be professionalised for universalised quality service provision.

The disadvantaged young child

Threats to early childhood development tend to cluster together, often in conjunction with poverty, social status, exclusion and gendered inequality. Exposure to one risk commonly means exposure to multiple risks and varied crisis in the family tend to contribute to widespread neglect of young children during their critical and formative years.

Disadvantaged children deserve urgent and extra attention. This would have to include children who fare poorly in terms of development indicators (e.g., extreme poor, young girls, Scheduled Caste and Scheduled Tribes), the marginalised (e.g., children with disabilities, children living in urban slums, homeless and street children) and the invisible child (e.g., children of migrants, children in the care of older children or with siblings on street, children in institutions and in single-headed households).

While the number of young children living in the poorest and richest households varies tremendously across states, about 25 percent of children under the age of five in India live in households belonging to the poorest quintile, and only 14.7 percent live in households in the richest quintile.

Unequal distribution of income, goods and services pushes children born into Scheduled Tribe and Scheduled Caste households in the category of most disadvantaged.

Children with disabilities are more vulnerable to neglect, violence, abuse and exploitation. Access to high quality early intervention services is critical to assist these children to reach their potential; however, available services are not ready to respond effectively and provide accessible and equitable services to such children from early childhood.

Despite multiple legislations, policy frameworks, campaigns and schemes, there continues to be a deficit in gender and socially transformative parenting of the young child. When parents are subjected to intersections of discrimination and disempowerment at various levels, they are not exposed to positive parenting practices, nor do they find the resources or the time and interest to spend on such parenting.

Childcare and the childcare worker

The significance of environmental inputs, stimulation and interaction influencing the overall growth and well-being of infants and young children has been strongly iterated by neuroscientific research. However, even as childcare is central to the holistic conception of ECD, multi-sectoral policies and programmes and multi-disciplinary research has for long neglected it in India.

The dominant narratives position the family as the best place for a young child to grow up in, relegating the perspectives on the young child within the political leadership and policymakers to the background as it is primarily seen to be the responsibility of the family, mainly mothers, with a minimal role to be played by the State.

Diverse challenges, especially women working in the unorganised sector for long hours, without adequate social protection support, result in the family being unable to provide an optimal caring environment for the holistic development of the child, necessitating assistance and support from the State in the form of crèches and day-care services.

Despite the centrality of the role of *Anganwadi* Workers (AWWs) in the machinery meant to provide services to mothers and children, they have never got their due in terms of recognition, appreciation or remuneration. ICDS has, de facto, treated AWWs as part-time, 'honorary' workers and provided them with compensation well below the minimum wage in most states. This lack of recognition has severely undermined the overall perception of childcare.

Fiscal allocations and expenditure for child development

Public investment in education, nutrition, healthcare and protection sectors, which comprise the childcare ecosystem in India, is critical for strengthening the nurturing and comprehensive development of the young child. Analysis of budgetary allocation and expenditure shows consistent inadequacy of financial resources for interventions in the interests of the young child as well as under-utilisation of allocated resources. A major funding gap is seen in the spending per child in India.

The ICDS must assume universal application of the services under the umbrella, and therefore even at the current cost norm, the ICDS will need to enhance its spending to INR 800 billion. The overall budget and the budget for the training component of just the *anganwadi* workers need to increase significantly to cover training cost and material cost annually. The additional budget requirement for learning material and AWCs is estimated at INR 4.2 billion per annum, while for training the additional requirement is estimated at INR 10 billion per annum.

A sum of INR 167.76 billion would be required annually to pay the proposed monthly salary of INR 10,000 for about 1,400,000 sanctioned positions of AWW and INR 8,000 for about 900,000 sanctioned positions of Accredited Social Health Activist (ASHA) workers.

INR 30.36 billion would be required annually to support 100,000 *anganwadi*-cum-crèches, which would benefit children belonging to poor urban and rural households and have multiplier beneficial impact on the economy.

Effective implementation of direct interventions in these sectors for child development together with the performance of other interconnected sectors and issues can impact the outcomes for children positively. However, the interventions of the Central and state governments have been ad-hoc. The widest intervention is made in nutrition, whereas reproductive and child health remain poorly targeted, as seen by the low utilisation rate of allocated budgets.

Key recommendations

The deprivations, exclusion, vulnerabilities, inaccessibility and how they impact the young child as this Report highlights, have clearly emerged as the fault lines of the COVID pandemic. The Report has presented the stark denial of the rights of the young child and the capacities of especially poor families to fulfill their needs and requirements. The crisis that this pandemic has set in further necessitates urgent actions. The recommendations also need to be seen in this changed context.

> **ECD as a national priority:** The State must assume greater responsibility and create an enabling environment by prioritising and investing in ECD to ensure the well-being of the young child. However, the multi-dimensional nature of ECD necessitates multiple stakeholders, with varied expertise, to come together for equitable, effective, efficient and synergistic delivery of a wide range of services.
>
> **Increased allocations for ECD to expand outreach and the quality of services:** The budgetary outlays for ECD need to be quadrupled for meeting the holistic needs and entitlements of the young child and achieving SDGs. The child budget would be INR 1.25 trillion annually (20 percent of the social sector outlay), if it is to enable minimum allocations set out for providing a 'childcare ecosystem service' per child.
>
> Eight states (viz., Madhya Pradesh, Bihar, Rajasthan, Uttar Pradesh, Jharkhand, Chhattisgarh, Assam and Meghalaya) fare poorly on the young child indices. Geographies within some states (e.g., Maharashtra, Gujarat, Karnataka, Andhra Pradesh and Telangana) have also languished behind. Along with higher budgetary support, these states also need support to improve their implementation capacity and address their governance deficit.
>
> **Decentralisation and comprehensive actions to overhaul ICDS services:** ICDS needs to be restructured and recalibrated to reach the most marginalised. Various service packages delivered under the ICDS need to be complementary and convergent for meeting the holistic needs of the young child. However, early learning and care, which have been weak in ICDS, need to be strengthened, owing to their criticality for ECD. Decentralised governance and community engagement through support committees with clearly demarcated accountability structures, *panchayat* upwards, could improve services, address area-specific challenges and promote accountability.

Crèche services and complementary childcare services as the backbone of ECD: Setting up of well-equipped crèches under the ICDS, which follow the required minimum standards, could help in providing psychosocial support and care to children under 3 years of age at scale. They could help address the childcare deficit and enable women, especially those in the unorganised sector, to attend work without neglecting the care of their young ones. The capacities of *anganwadi* as well as ASHA workers will have to be enhanced manifold to enable them to engage with households, work for gender and socially transformative change in parenting.

Phased conversion of *anganwadis* into *anganwadi*-cum-crèches: A phased process of conversion is recommended to provide holistic care, stimulation and protection services to children of women working in the unorganised sector with priority given to backward districts and urban slums with a high presence of working mothers and poor child indicators.

Universalisation of quality ECCE: All children in the 3–6 years age group must have a right to quality ECCE, irrespective of their location and access to types of services. The Right to Education Act, 2009, amended to include the 3–6 years age group, could create conditions for intensive training of AWWs, development of appropriate curriculum and learning tools and appropriate training of pre-school teachers who can then deliver equitable quality ECCE for children in the 3–6 age group, across settings.

Professionalisation of the ECD workforce: Towards recognising AWWs as professional cadre, systems for training and accreditation need to be operationalised and remuneration enhanced in line with full-time professional role and the intensive community engagement envisaged for these workers. The creation and strengthening of a cadre of childcare professionals (including AWWs), would require considerable investment in ECD but with commensurate outcomes.

Urgent response to violence against the young child: A support-group structure led by properly trained frontline workers needs to be mobilised to strengthen the protective, caring and inclusive environment of the young child, and reinforce parenting skills and closely monitor the child's well-being and caregiving environment.

Fundamental revamping of child database and monitoring systems: In order to address the serious paucity of credible data that hampers evidence-based policy and programme interventions, credible multi-dimensional disaggregated data on children district level upwards as well as financial allocation and expenditure needs to be generated and made available in the public domain.

The State and other stakeholders are obligated to be cognisant of the fact that the young child is a holder of rights, while undertaking all possible measures to create an ecosystem for early childhood development. In offering a solutions oriented critique of government policies and systems, the primary aim of this Report discussing the situation of the young child in India is to suggest a way forward in terms of approaches, policy parameters, legislation, programmatic interventions and investment of human, technical and financial resources.

Notes

1 NFHS 4 (2015–16).
2 Balarajan et al., 2013.

1   The young child in India

Early childhood, the age group from birth to the age of 6 or 8 years, is the first and arguably the most important stage in human development. Research in neurosciences has bolstered the claim of child development experts that early childhood establishes the foundation for a healthy, well-integrated individual, gives the next generation a better start and contributes to economic growth and sustainable development.[1]

This chapter initiates an enquiry into the status of the young child in India and the major issues that have led to the persistent neglect of this age group. In this context, it explores the policy and legal framework, approaches and programmes and the role and obligations of key stakeholders, including the state, civil society, media, private sector, communities and the family. In order to develop deeper understanding into the various measures of young child well-being and the kind of variance across states, the chapter introduces the **Young Child Outcomes Index** (YCOI) and the **Young Child Environment Index** (YCEI) for children under 6. The indexing, including the outcome indicators for measurement and the process indicators that look into the circumstances in which a young child grows, allow this Report to understand the nuances in significant differences in performances across states and regions.

While the continuum from conception to the age of eight years is important for early childhood development, this Report narrows the focus on the young child from birth until the age of 6, which marks the beginning of formal education in primary school and has been referred to in Indian policies.

1.1 Focus on the young child is long overdue

A child has been defined by the United Nations Convention of the Rights of the Child (UNCRC) as a person from birth to the age of 18 years. **The development discourse and policy often side-line the exceptional vulnerability of the young child** due to age, in combination with aggravating factors such as gender, caste, class, abilities and residence. Infants, toddlers and pre-schoolers are subsumed together with school-going age children and adolescents within the broader category of children.

Children under 6 years of age formed 13.1 percent (158.79 million) of India's total population in 2011.[2] The neglect of this age group is evident in the country's weak performance in ensuring child survival, optimal care and development, and protection. In 2015–2016, 21% children below age 5 in India were undernourished,[3] 91.4 percent of children aged 6–23 months did not receive an adequate diet,[4] one in three (38 percent) of children under 5 years of age were stunted, one in five (21 percent) of the children were wasted, 36 percent were underweight, 58 percent of children between 6 months–5 years were anaemic and 38 percent had not received full immunisation.[5]

Early Childhood Development (ECD) is an integrated concept that cuts across multiple sectors – including health and nutrition, education and social protection – and refers to the physical, cognitive, linguistic and socio-emotional development of the young child. It deserves greater policy attention for a variety of reasons – tapping development opportunities to provide the young child with a solid foundation for life, empowering women, developing human resources and raising standards of living. Above all, ECD is focussed on realising the rights of the young child encapsulated in the UNCRC and entitlements in accordance with the Indian Constitution, policies and legislation.

1.1.1 Early childhood development is a process that commences at conception

The process of ECD begins with conception and continues up to the age of 6 to 8 years. Children develop motor, cognitive, linguistic and socio-emotional skills during early childhood when the foundational architecture of the brain is laid. Although general patterns of child development are similar, each child is a unique entity with an independent trajectory of growth. Early caring and nurturing environment, timely nutrition and healthcare, clean and safe living environment are among the factors that shape their experiences and establish the foundation for life. Accordingly, ECD as an approach is comprehensive and involves the entire gamut of people who interact with the young child – parents, caregivers and communities from birth through entry into school.

As the thrust of policies and programmes in the interest of young children has been sectoral and thematic, ECD has been defined and described in ways that reflect the priorities they serve for the young children. Early Childhood Education (ECE) programmes have been pre-school education-focussed and aim at 3–6-year olds (as seen in nurseries, kindergartens and preparatory schools. These are often part of a primary school. Early Childhood Care and Education (ECCE) retains the same educational thrust but enlarges its scope to include the care component (including care and early stimulation from birth to the age of 3 years through crèches and home-based parent education).[6]

ECD and Early Childhood Care and Development (ECCD) constitute a still more holistic and integrated concept of programming, which aligns itself with that of the synergistic and interdependent relationship between health, nutrition and psychosocial development or education, and addresses the all-round development of the child. Programmes of ECCD or ECD normally take a life-cycle approach, as in the Integrated Child Development Services (ICDS) in India, and target, in addition to the child, pregnant and lactating mothers and even adolescent girls.[7]

This Report uses both the terms ECD and ECCE, often interchangeably. While ECD is the preferred term due to its comprehensive connotation and perspective, ECCE is more commonly used in the policy and programme documents.

1.1.2 Early childhood provides unique developmental opportunities

Children during early childhood experience the most rapid period of growth and change in terms of their maturing bodies and nervous systems, increasing mobility, communication skills and intellectual capacities and rapid shifts in their interests and abilities. **Child development experts have over the last few decades consistently highlighted the importance of early childhood when remarkable physical, cognitive, socio-emotional and language development takes place.** Ongoing neuroscientific research, discussed in some detail in Chapter 5 of this Report, shows that brain development is at its peak during this stage and early stimulation and caregiving promote neural connections that are considered to be at the core of human potential.

Severe malnutrition and micronutrient deficiencies in the early years heighten the risk of illnesses and cognitive impairment among children, which in turn can lead to poor attainments and reduced or incomplete schooling. Educational deficit later in life limits their access to employment opportunities and thereby earning capacity. Furthermore, studies have associated Vitamin A deficiency and anaemia with reduced productivity levels and lower adult height, partly due to childhood undernutrition, with reduced earnings as an adult. Low per capita productivity eventually contributes to poor economic growth. This cycle of deprivation and missed opportunities clearly needs to be disrupted through investment in ECD towards addressing many challenges faced by children, their families and communities. Box 1.1 details the criticality of early childhood as a window of opportunity.

Isolating the key factors that improve or worsen key child development indicators is difficult because several interconnected factors, in various permutations and combinations, determine the outcomes for the young child. For instance, maternal health, nutrition and education determine their access to nutritious food, timely healthcare and education up to or beyond secondary school. Equally important is the availability and utilisation of safe drinking water, proper sanitation and hygienic practices, which deter

---

Box 1.1   Early childhood is a window of opportunity[8]

Public health experts deem the first 1,000 days of a child as critical for his or her optimal development. The first 270 days in the womb require adequate nutrition and overall well-being of the mother while the remaining 730 days entail timely immunisation, proper infant and young child feeding (including breastfeeding and supplementary feeding), stimulation and early childhood care and education. As brain development occurs at a very fast pace by the age of 3, poor nutrition at this stage can be detrimental to long-term cognitive ability.

The 1,000 days between a woman's pregnancy and her child's second birthday offer a unique window of opportunity to shape healthier and more prosperous future. The right nutrition and care during this 1,000 days' window can have a profound impact on a child's ability to grow, learn and rise out of poverty, and in the process also shape a society's long-term health, stability and prosperity. It entails raising awareness about the importance of the first 1,000 days in a child's life, ultimately reducing the maternal and child mortality through improved health and nutritional status of adolescents, pregnant and lactating women as well as young children.

(Bhatia et al., 2013)

---

communicable diseases and contribute to cognitive development by improving their nutritional intake and reducing worm infestation.

Early childhood initiates the formation of identities and values as the young child picks up cues from her surroundings by observing activities, signs and signals. These surrounds help form early beliefs about who they are and how they see others in terms of markers such as gender, abilities, caste, religion, class and ethnicity. At this stage, the seeds of discriminatory norms are also planted. In India, persistent gender-based discrimination, evident from birth to pre-school, begins to manifest itself even before the girl child is born, through practices of sex-selective abortions. Declining sex ratio at birth and child sex ratio are possibly the worst reflection of patriarchal societal norms and mindsets working in conjunction with modern technologies that facilitate sex determination. Nonetheless, there is immense potential for positive and progressive values through gender and social transformative parenting, which has been discussed in Chapters 3 and 5.

Levels of abject poverty, together with a variety of vulnerability factors that marginalise many households, and access of households to Public Distribution System (PDS), Integrated Child Development Scheme (ICDS) and other government programmes also influence outcomes for the young child.

Chapter 4 discusses the categories of the young child who deserve urgent attention because of consistently poor performance in terms of development indicators, social marginalisation and invisibility.

During early childhood, children form strong emotional bonds with their parents and other caregivers, from whom they seek and require nurturing, care, guidance and protection, in ways that are respectful of their individuality and growing capacities. They actively make sense of the physical, social and cultural dimensions of the world they inhabit, learning progressively from their activities and interactions with other children and adults. They establish important relationships with their peers as well as with younger and older children, which enable them to learn to negotiate and coordinate shared activities, resolve conflicts, keep agreements and accept responsibility for others.

However, a large number of Indian households are not able to provide the nurturing and quality care to their young ones because of the difficult economic circumstances that they are in. **Children belonging to such households need the State as the primary duty-bearer to step in as the families lack resources to provide adequate care.** But the aspect of nurturing and care is a major area of neglect in the wide gamut of measures that currently characterise ECD in India. The weakest link in the overall perspective on childcare is the childcare worker, whose role has not been sufficiently recognised. Chapter 5 situates the enquiry into the issues of childcare, nurture and protection within the ecosystem comprising of various childcare providers and arrangements.

The missed opportunities for the child's physical and mental health, emotional security, cultural and personal identity, and developing competencies during early years are difficult to overcome later. UNICEF had alerted member-states on the criticality of designing programmes for the young child in its flagship *The State of the World's Children* report in 2001. It had warned that it may be too late if states do not take cognizance of the latest advances in neuroscience.

> before many adults even realise what is happening, the brain cells of a new infant proliferate, synapses crackle and the patterns of a lifetime are established. . . . Choices made and actions taken on behalf of children during this critical period affect not only how a child develops but also how a country progresses.[9]

1.1.3 Rights and entitlements address vulnerabilities and optimise potential

The human rights discourse, within which child rights are embedded, deems every child – even an infant – to be a person who has the right to life and development with dignity, protection and participation, a principle which needs to be recognised and respected universally at all times. It calls for additional provision of special measures commensurate with their vulnerability.

The Constitution of India, laws and policies entitle every child to certain basic rights. Furthermore, India as a State Party to the UNCRC is obligated to take all possible measures for realising child rights. And now, having expressed its commitment to achieving Sustainable Development Goals (SDGs) by 2030, it is duty bound to improve its performance on several indicators that determine the status of the young child. The young child is a rights holder, as Box 1.2 notes, who enjoys rights simply by virtue of her existence as a human being.

Box 1.2   Young children are rights holders

A person's a person no matter how small.

– Dr Seuss[10]

The global community of nations recognised children's rights as a distinct sub-set of human rights when the Convention on the Rights of the Child (CRC) came into effect in 1989. This treaty has the unique distinction of being ratified by almost all countries, including India.

The rights-based argument for attention to the early years is grounded squarely in the CRC. The rights framework necessitates the recognition of young children as rights holders and social actors and calls for respect for their agency – as a participant in family, community and society. They are entitled to all rights in the CRC and to special protection measures, and in accordance with their evolving capacities, the progressive exercise of their rights. The notion that young children are individuals who would in due course have their own concerns, interests and points of view based on their experiences is indeed path breaking. In order to exercise their rights, they require in particular physical nurturance, emotional care and sensitive guidance, as well as time and space for social play, exploration and learning.

Its basic principles are articulated by Articles 2 (non-discrimination), 3 (the best interests of the child), 6 (inherent right to life, survival and development) and 12 (participation of the child). Article 12.1 of the UNCRC entails that as holders of rights, even the youngest children are entitled to express their views, which should be "given due weight in accordance with the age and maturity of the child" (art. 12.1). The Committee on the Rights of the Child had clarified that "young children are acutely sensitive to their surroundings and very rapidly acquire understanding of the people, places and routines in their lives, along with awareness of their own unique identity. They make choices and communicate their feelings, ideas and wishes in numerous ways, long before they are able to communicate through the conventions of spoken or written language."

The CRC and the General Comments of the Committee on the Rights of the Child mention young children specifically in terms of survival, health and malnutrition, and birth registration. In addition, the provisions of the CRC specifically relevant to young children are Article 5 (evolving capacities of the child), Article 24 (health and social services), Article 27 (standard of living), Article 28 (education), Article 29 (aims of education) and Article 31 (leisure, recreation and cultural activities). The right to survival and development can be realized if appropriate measures for respecting and supporting the responsibilities of parents and the provision of assistance and quality services (arts. 5 and 18) are also in place.

The rights-based argument is further supported by commitments made by governments at the World Conference on Education for All, in Jomtien, Thailand, in 1990. Article 5 of the Declaration states that "Learning begins at birth. This calls for early childhood care and initial education. These can be provided through arrangements involving families, communities, or institutional programs, as appropriate." The first of the adopted goals at a follow-up meeting in Dakar in 2000 [was]: "Expanding and improving comprehensive early childhood care and education, especially for the most vulnerable and disadvantaged children."

(UNICEF, 2006)

Children's physical growth, cognitive development, vulnerabilities and resilience vary according to their individual nature, social norms and external factors such as living conditions, family organisation, care arrangements and education systems. Respecting the distinctive interests, experiences and challenges facing every young child is the starting point for realising their rights during this crucial phase of their lives.[11]

According to the *Global Report on Ending Violence in Childhood* in 2017, 1.3 billion children around the world experience harsh discipline at the hands of caregivers. Corporal punishment is the most commonly experienced form of abuse by children, starting as early as age 1. In early childhood, children are exposed to direct abuse by primary caregivers and other family members, and they can also be hurt inadvertently in incidents of domestic violence between parents.[12]

The evolving child protection agenda in India has, as yet, not recognised the vulnerabilities and threats of wilful neglect, violence, abuse and exploitation of the young child. India-centric research on child protection issues related to the young child has not been undertaken yet. But increasing media reports, several anecdotal accounts and a few empirical studies indicate that exposure to violence in childhood starts early and is widespread. Adverse sex ratio at birth, neglect, physical punishment, sexual abuse and shaking child syndrome are some of the manifestations of violence against the young child. Chapters 2 and 4 in the discussions on survival and childcare explore in-depth issues related to young child protection.

1.1.4 Early childhood lays the edifice for human development and economic growth

Early childhood is the critical preparatory stage for middle childhood and adolescence, which lays the foundation for life. Putting in place appropriate activities based on the young child's developmental needs and learning patterns has for long been recognised for facilitating their entry and participation in school. Improved health and education standards are crucial for ensuring that the working age population is highly skilled, adaptable and efficient for a competitive market economy. Improvement in overall quality of the young child and her family enhances the quality of their community and society and contributes human capital for national development.

Human development is the most compelling argument for devoting resources to early childhood. India was placed in the medium human development category and ranked 130 on the Human Development Index (HDI), 2018. Among the countries that ranked higher were Sri Lanka (76), Brazil (79), China (86), Maldives (101), Indonesia and Vietnam (116) and the Philippines and South Africa (113).[13] There is significant scope for improvement in India's position through investment in the rights and well-being of the young child.

Early childcare arrangements (e.g., crèches, day-care centres, playschools and nursery) of good quality are necessitated by a child's right to survive and thrive and the Sustainable Development Goals' (SDGs) motto of *leaving no one behind*. They also facilitate unfettered labour participation of women in the organised and unorganised sectors. When their employment potential is unlocked, increased productivity, higher earnings and empowerment are likely to follow. When the older siblings are released from childcare responsibilities, their access to education and developmental opportunities are bound to increase. The positive impact on the young child, the girl child and the woman holds promise for the present and potential productivity of generations and disruption of the cycle of poverty.

Economists point to the prospects of India benefiting from its youthful population composition through 'demographic dividend.' The country has the potential of overtaking many economies, including China, which are currently ahead on the HDI. These economies have begun showing signs of ageing and economic slowdown while India is still in demographic transition, a key factor for economic growth.

Having passed through the early transitional stage of demographic transition, characterised by decline in death rates, India is currently in the middle transitional stage, characterised by a decline in birth rates and continuing decline in death rates, from where it is poised to enter the late transitional stage, due to continuing decline in birth rates and slowdown in the fall in death rates. In principle, the spurt in economic growth usually occurs late in the demographic transition with the increase in the ratio of the more productive working age population (15–64 years) to the 'dependent' population (under 15 years of age and above 65 years) when the fertility rate falls and the youth dependency rate declines.

Though most major economies will witness a decline in working age population, the average Indian will be only 29 years of age in 2020, compared with 37 in China and the United States, 45 in Western Europe and 48 in Japan in 2020. Moreover, by 2030, India will have the youngest median age of 31.2 years in comparison with China's 42.5 years. The demographic dividend would be possible till 2040, after which the Indian population would also begin ageing.

Over the next two decades effective policies can facilitate economic growth and human development in India resulting from the significant rise in the working age population. It could gain from potential outsourcing of jobs from other countries with declining working age population. According to the International Monetary Fund, India's continuing demographic dividend if harnessed well can add about 2 percent to the annual rate of economic growth. Conversely, the failure to ensure developmental opportunities early will be detrimental.

Since 2001, the size of the under 4 and 5–9 age groups has shown clear signs of shrinking within the overall population due to a decline in both birth and death rates. According to the national Census, there was a 3.1 percent decline from 163.84 million in 2001 to 158.79 million in 2011 in the under 6 years age group.[14] The young child holds the key to reaping the benefits of demographic dividend. She will be a valuable asset in national development only if she enters middle childhood, adolescence and the working age, with strong fundamentals in terms of capacities and competencies. Investment in ECD, especially universalisation of basic services for the young child, is a robust approach for the creation of human capital, and thereby sustainable economic growth.

1.2 Policy and legal framework have not delivered consistent results

1.2.1 *There are fairly robust constitutional and legal provisions, but they remain unfulfilled*

The Indian Constitution guarantees fundamental rights to all children in the country and empowers the State to make special provisions for children. It has recognised this period as requiring particular attention and support through many of its statutes as the child needs adult support for an extended period of time.

The Directive Principles of State Policy specifically refer to the responsibility of the State to protect children from abuse and ensure that children receive opportunities and facilities to develop in a healthy manner in conditions of freedom and dignity (Article 39). Article 15(3) empowers the government to promote and practice positive discrimination and affirmative action in favour of socially and economically disadvantaged or vulnerable communities, which should include children under 6. Article 45 urges the State to endeavour to provide early childhood care and education for all children until the age of 6.

Articles 21 (Protection of life and personal liberty), Article 21 A (Free and compulsory education, subsequently amended in 2009 under the Right to Education Act) and Article 23 (Prohibition of traffic in human beings and forced labour) apply to children as much as to adults. Article 47 enjoins the State to work towards raising nutrition and living standards of all people, which includes children below the age of 6. Article 39 (e and f) recognises children's rights and their protection against all forms of abuse and exploitation.

It is noteworthy that a report of the Law Commission in 2015 took cognizance of the Constitution's welfare approach towards children, wherein the child under 6 is to be provided a safe and healthy environment for full growth and development to its human potential, and acknowledged that the promise remains unfulfilled. It advocated for a progressive realisation of the right in favour of children under 6 by translating these principles into justiciable rights. In particular, it suggested that every child under 6 should have an unconditional right to crèche and day-care provided, regulated and operated by the State. The provision of the crèche should be the responsibility of the State rather than the employer, especially in the unorganised sector.[15]

The thrust of the first **National Policy for Children (NPC), 1974**, was on the delivery of services deemed essential for young children. It stated that

> it shall be the policy of the State to provide adequate services to children, both before and after birth and through the period of growth to ensure their full physical, mental and social development. The State shall progressively increase the scope of such services so that within a reasonable time all children in the country enjoy optimum conditions for their balanced growth.[16]

The Integrated Child Development Scheme, one of the Government of India's flagship programmes, was inaugurated in 1975, in partial fulfilment of the obligations cast by Article 39(f) of the Constitution of India, following the adoption of the National Policy for Children, 1974. It is currently the world's most ambitious child health, nutrition and pre-school education programme for children under 6. It targets pregnant and lactating women along with the to-be-born and newborn children. Adolescent girls were included in the list of beneficiaries in recognition of their concerns being acute and crucial for improving outcomes for women and children. Annexure 1 lists the package of services provided under the ICDS.

However, design, delivery and promise of ICDS have come under increasing scrutiny due to continuing high levels of malnutrition, sub-par immunisation rates and poor state of its pre-school component. Several studies have identified major limitations and deficiencies of the ICDS, including the focus on expanding coverage and neglect of the quality of services.

There is relative neglect in the delivery of services to children below the age of three years, who are the most vulnerable and can benefit the most from a carefully calibrated package of interventions. For instance, the interventions to improve feeding and childcare practices may also entail counselling and home visits to advise parents on matters related to Ante-natal Care (ANC), breastfeeding, timely immunisation and regular weighing. The 'take home' facility has had limited results for the young child as the rations are either shared or fed to the cattle.[17]

Research repeatedly reinforces that the most effective ECD programmes are of longer duration, high quality and high intensity, and they are integrated with family support, health, nutrition or educational systems and services, and they target in particular younger and disadvantaged children through direct learning experiences.[18] Such strategies help to promote child development and to prevent or ameliorate the loss of developmental potential.

Supplementary nutrition has occupied the pride of place among the range of tasks required to provide an impetus to ECD for under-3 age group. Aspects such as safe water, sanitation and hygiene practices have not received the kind of attention in the ECD programmes that they deserve while early stimulation comprising of conversations, games and stories have generally been placed on the back burner.

Indeed, the positive developmental outcomes for young children are largely determined by simultaneity of inputs. The divisions into health, nutrition, early learning and childcare in the national policies and programmes have arguably been a stumbling block to achieving the impact of a range of interventions. It may assist with sectoral nature of planning, but weak links undermine the potential outcomes.

The language of children's rights was gaining currency when **the National Charter for Children, 2003,** was framed. It sought

> to secure for every child its inherent right to be a child and enjoy a healthy and happy childhood, to address the root causes that negate the healthy growth and development of children, and to awaken the conscience of the community in the wider societal context to protect children from all forms of abuse, while strengthening the family, society and the nation.[19]

The National Plan of Action for Children (NPAC), 2005, for the first time in the history of planning for children, defined the child as a person up to the age of 18 years and declared that all rights apply to all age groups, including before birth. Most of its 12 priorities sought to address concerns associated with the young child. In addition to abolition of female foeticide and infanticide, reduction in Infant Mortality Rate (IMR) and Maternal Mortality Rate (MMR), malnutrition and civil registration, it prioritised universalisation of early childhood care and development and quality education for all children, achieving 100 percent access and retention in schools, including pre-schools. Although no formal evaluation of NPAC 2005 was undertaken, many of its goals remained unfulfilled. It has been replaced by the NPAC 2016, which will take into account the key priority areas for children listed in the National Policy for Children (2013), to ensure the implementation and monitoring of national constitutional and policy commitments and the CRC.

The Right to Education (RTE) Act, 2009, made free and compulsory education a fundamental right but the right to pre-school education remains a directive principle, which cannot be enforced in the court of law. Article 45, a non-justiciable provision, reads "The state shall endeavour to provide early childhood care and education for all children until they complete the age of six years." The exclusion of the young child from the ambit of the RTE Act has been a major bone of contention with civil society organisations and activists. It has been discussed in Chapter 3.

The 12th National Five Year Plan listed the issues that frame the rights of children in India. In addition to the issues related to survival, health and nutrition, it identified socio-economic disparities, depravations, livelihood insecurity, migration, violence and HIV/AIDS as some of the impediments to child rights. The working group report of the Plan had noted the role of disparities and poverty in undermining access of young children to pre-school education and other basic services. It recognised the multiple deprivations of children of new migrants and urban poor communities, including denial of an identity, violence, abuse and exploitation and, in particular, the vulnerability to neglect and exposure of violence of young children of mothers working in the informal sector (e.g., construction, domestic labour, other forms of daily wage labour, sex work and so on), which harms them physically, emotionally and psychologically.

The **National Policy on Early Childhood Care and Education (ECCE),** 2013,[20] seeks to promote inclusive, equitable and contextualised opportunities for the optimal development of all children below the age of 6. Recognising that ICDS covered only 48.2 percent of children in the under 6 age group and unregulated private sector and the Civil Society Organisations (CSOs), and some more, it seeks universal access, equity and quality in ECCE, capacity development of service providers and strengthening of parent and community outreach programmes.

It refers to the need to eradicate discrimination in early childhood on the basis of gender, social identity, disability and other exclusionary attributes.

While progressive overall, the policy does not refer to promoting the removal of stereotypes about gender and marginalised groups in early childhood education, school curriculum, and parenting practices. It leaves it to career counselling and vocational guidance to address issues like gender and career choices.

The **National Early Childhood Care and Education (ECCE) Policy, 2013,** and **the National Curriculum Framework and Quality Standards, 2014,** recommended institutionalisation of a regulatory and accreditation framework for quality, especially in the private sector.

Several state governments formulated policies for children subsequently with nuances and/or wider scope for action. For instance, the **Kerala State Policy for Child, 2016,** referred specifically to the need to reduce anaemia (lower levels of haemoglobin in the blood) among children between 6 and 59 months of age, promote gender equity and social justice through education curriculum at all levels, and children's participation through *bala sabhas* (children's councils) and *bala panchayats* (children's local government institutions). Importantly, unlike the National Policy on Children, 2013, it identified transgender children and children of transgender persons as rights holders. It also recognises that children in coastal areas need special attention, protection and development.

The National Plan of Action, 2016, which followed the National Policy for Children (NPC), 2013, is more of a critique rather than a roadmap for addressing the impediments to progress in securing children's rights. Nonetheless, it lists several measures in the interest of the young child. It highlights the need to ensure the availability of essential services, supports and provisions for nutritive attainment using a life-cycle approach. Accordingly, it has prioritised provision of locally available, adequate and affordable nutritious food, promotion of gardening of fruits and vegetables in households, government and aided schools, *Anganwadi* Centres (AWCs) and childcare institutions (CCIs) for consumption by children and nutritious diets based on local and low-cost recipes and practices for mothers, infants and young children. Importantly, it recognised the 1,000 day window of opportunity.

Noting the importance of early childhood for holistic learning and growth, it refers to the need for an ECCE programme determined by children's developmental and cultural needs, which provides more need-based inputs and an enabling environment. It acknowledges the inability of a common 'curriculum' to promote such an individualised approach and of available ECCE services to serve the developmental needs of the young child. Yet, it states that the vacuum created by a lack of curriculum framework is being filled with either a minimalist programme or the downward extension of the primary stage curriculum, which overburdens the child and undermines his or her learning potential.

To ensure optimal development for all children, it calls for the creation of a planned curriculum framework, encompassing developmentally appropriate knowledge and skills, with flexibility for contextualisation and to cater to the diverse needs of young children. Instead of a common curriculum, it advocates a curriculum framework to ensure that important learning areas are covered, taking care of all the developmental needs of the young child within his or her specific context and a common pedagogical approach to ensure a certain level of commonality and quality across all ECCE programmes in India.[21]

The young child also features in several sectoral policies and action plans. **The National Policy on Education, 1986,** first recognised pre-school education albeit as a "feeder and support programme for primary education and a support service for working women."[22] The **draft National Education Policy (NEP) 2019,** recognises that learning begins from birth and excellent care, nurture, nutrition, physical activity, psycho-social environment and cognitive and emotional stimulation during a child's first six years are extremely critical for ensuring proper brain development and, consequently, desired learning curves over a person's lifetime. The draft policy recommends "investing in accessible and quality ECCE that has the potential to give all young children such access in an engaging and holistic way, thereby allowing all children to participate and flourish in the educational system throughout their lives." It further recognises that "ECCE is perhaps the greatest and most powerful equalizer."[23]

The **National Nutrition Policy, 1993,** prioritised children below 6 years while recognising them as a 'high-risk' group. The National Plan of Action on Nutrition (NPAN), 1995, updated the targets, strategies and interventions using World Health Organisation (WHO) child health standards for assessing and reviewing programmes.[24] More recently, the National Nutrition Strategy (NNS), 2017, has sought to reduce child malnutrition in India by focussing on those states, districts and specific pockets that fare poorly in terms of nutrition indicators. The NITI Aayog and the Ministry of Women and Child Development (MWCD) plan to use a new Nutrition Monitoring System (NMS) to identify states/districts/blocks that are performing well and those that are lagging for focussed intervention.

India's policy framework had always focussed on child survival and development and to a lesser extent childcare but a spate of laws in the last two decades have dealt with child protection. The Commission for the Protection of Child Rights Act, 2005, led to the creation of national and state level commissions to monitor child rights situation in the country, conduct inspection of institutions for children, undertake enquiries into cases of violation of their rights and research and advise the government on remedial measures and effective implementation of legislation. The Act also provided for Children's Courts for a speedy trial of offences against children and violation of child rights.

The Juvenile Justice (care and protection of children) Act, 2000, amended subsequently in 2006, 2011 and 2015, and the Central Model Rules under the Act, spelt out measures to protect children, including in situations related to adoption, foster care and sponsorship. It addresses concerns related to Children in Need of Care and Protection (CNCP) and children in conflict with law. The Protection of Children from Sexual Offences (POCSO), Act, 2012, provides for the protection of children from sexual assault, sexual harassment and pornography while safeguarding their interests at every stage of the judicial process by incorporating child-friendly mechanisms and procedures for reporting, recording of evidence, investigation and speedy trial and stringent punishment per the gravity of the offence.[25] When a child below the age of 12 is sexually assaulted, Section 5 (m) of the Act deems it as an aggravated act and provides for additional protection.

1.2.2 *Weak implementation persists in policies and programmes for the young child*

The Constitutional provisions, especially those calling for proactive policies to improve the lives of children from vulnerable communities, regions and situations, have neither been implemented in letter nor in spirit. Civil society organisations and activists hold the view that it is due to weak political and administrative will to implement government's own stated policies and programmes, that serious issues related to the young child have persisted for more than seven decades after India's independence.

The first specific programme for the young child was conceptualised and rolled out three decades after the Constitution came into existence. **The ICDS, the nationwide programme, continues to suffer from issues related to its design, delivery mechanisms and sub-par performance.** The delivery of limited services in a mission and time-bound manner (e.g., pulse polio campaign to eradicate polio) has been successful but continuous and consistent basic service delivery through efficient systems is still to be achieved. While specific vertical missions for a specific issue take precedence on the governance agenda, the delivery of routine services for young children needs a major overhaul.

The National Family Health Survey (NFHS) and Sample Registration System (SRS) data shows that mortality rate among neonates, infants and young children has been declining but, as discussed in Chapter 2, it is still unacceptably high. High maternal mortality often due to early and risky pregnancies, inadequate immunisation coverage, difficulties in access to health services and public health challenges of stunting and wasting, a large population without safe drinking water and safe sanitation indicate that India has not been able to deliver on its commitment to the young child.

Lack of political will, administrative priorities and capacities to implement government's stated policies and programmes, public awareness and demand for basic services in the interests of the young child have often been cited as impediments to effective public policy. Available legal provisions are rarely adhered to, and the inability to ensure ground level convergence of health, education, nutrition, water and sanitation and pre-school education services impairs the outcomes of programmes meant for children. Several policies seek the well-being of young child, but their recommendations tend to be repetitive and evidence of their effective implementation is not usually available.

When the Constitution of India was adopted in 1950, issues of child mortality, malnutrition, poor healthcare services and non-existent pre-school education were major concerns, especially among the very poor in rural areas, tribal areas, and remote desert and mountainous regions with poor infrastructure, accessibility and outreach services. About 20 states and Union Territories (UTs) had over one million children in the under 6 years age group, and many of them are among the poorest. About 52 percent of the under 6s reside in the states of Uttar Pradesh (29.7 million), Bihar (18.6 million), Maharashtra (12.8 million), Madhya Pradesh (10.5 million) and Rajasthan (10.5 million). Quantitative and qualitative research in the last three decades has established direct correlation between poverty and child health. Poverty is a thread that runs across all states and all communities in India. Yet, there are wide variations in population distribution and socio-economic development across states and among various districts and sub-districts within states.

Data deficit has for long undermined planning, monitoring, and evaluation processes in development programming, and ECD is no exception. Successive Five-Year plan working groups and mid-term appraisals point to both data gaps to ascertain the impact of government policies and programmes and also absence of ground level monitoring processes that could enable to government to realise its own goals. For example, the mid-term appraisal of the 11th Plan found

> glaring gaps and inconsistencies on nutrition as against the promise made in the Plan. While examining the interventions for better nutritional status, the Mid-term Appraisal referring to different surveys and reports indicate that the progress in addressing undernutrition has been almost negligible.[26]

Even though India has emerged as a leading economy, social protection has not evolved beyond a basic conceptualisation of the idea. Several schemes of the Central and state governments for socio-economic development have not been able to mitigate livelihood insecurity and deprivation experienced by countless Indian households in rural and urban areas.

An overwhelming majority of poor rural and urban women are engaged in paid and unpaid work. Many of them either leave their infants and young children in the care of family members or neighbours or take them along to work. Young children left alone near construction sites, in rural roads related work and near factories are a common sight. Meanwhile, the plethora of legislation and programmes that provide for crèches and day-care services are rarely or poorly implemented.

Children of parents affected by HIV/AIDS and children themselves affected by HIV/AIDS face multiple challenges in society and their ability to go to childcare centres or pre-schools is highly compromised. Insecure environment, especially in areas exposed to conflict, exacerbates their vulnerabilities.

1.2.3 Regions and states show inconsistent performance

India's emergence as an economic power may have helped in reducing poverty – a critical determinant of the well-being of the young child – but its benefits have not percolated evenly. In many pockets of acute poverty and inequity, the condition of the young child remains poor. The impact of poverty on the health and well-being of infants and small children is well known – yet the ability of the very poor and marginalised (especially those belonging to the most disadvantaged social groups) to access public services (rations, healthcare, nutrition supplement) remains tardy.

While some regions of the country and some states seem to handle this better than others, **the lack of attention to detail in programme implementation has affected poorer states like Madhya Pradesh, Uttar Pradesh, Bihar, Jharkhand, Odisha and so on.** A child born in a remote rural area or an urban slum does not have the same chance of survival as a child born in a rich household. Needless to say, the picture varies across different states, rural and urban areas, economic groups, caste and religion-based social groups, gender and household education levels.

The varied performance of states in a country of the size of India could be attributed to the socio-cultural milieu, geography, political environment, historical factors, policy and governance. The interface between gender discriminatory social norms and advances in female education and empowerment has differed across and within different states and among different social groups. Some states have benefited from prolonged experience of progressive social policies and investment in social protection. Demand and utilisation of basic services and development infrastructure is high with greater public awareness. But many of the poor performing states have not been able to utilise the Public Distribution System (PDS), ICDS and other pro-poor programmes to mitigate the distress of the very poor and marginalised households and communities.

1.2.4 Construction of the Young Child Index

This Report presents two child indices, viz., the Young Child Outcomes Index and the Young Child Environment Index, to facilitate comparison of the performance of Indian states and UTs in terms of indicators related to the rights and well-being of infants and young children. Two indices were deemed necessary for making a distinction between the measurement of well-being of the young child (outcome indicators) from the policy and environment enablers and the eco system in which the child is cared for and nurtured (process indicators).

A group of technical experts identified key components of child development (both outcomes and environment) and created a dashboard of relevant indicators under each component to capture the well-being of the young child in India. They identified the most relevant indicators under each component from this data mart and captured the indices for each state. In the construction of the Index, they also took into account the SDGs most relevant to the young child, notably SDG 1 (End poverty in all its forms), SDG 2 (Ending hunger), SDG 3 (Ensure healthy lives), SDG 4 (Ensure inclusive and equitable quality education), SDG 5 (Achieve gender equality), SDG 6 (Ensure availability and sustainable management of water and sanitation for all) and SDG 8 (Promote sustained and inclusive economic growth). Annexure 2 details the methodology used for the selection of these indicators. The Indexing exercise was severely constrained by the lack of credible, disaggregated state-level data.

Young Child Outcomes Index: selection of indicators

Borrowing from the components used in the literature, three major components have been considered for constructing the Young Child Outcomes Index, viz., health, nutrition and cognitive growth and the respective indicators selected are IMR, stunting and net attendance at the primary school level.

The YCOI has been constructed for two time periods 2005–2006 and 2015–2016 while the YCEI has been constructed for 2015–2016. Table 1.1 presents the result of the YCOI.

As may be seen, eight states have scores below the country average. These are Assam, Meghalaya, Rajasthan, Chhattisgarh, Madhya Pradesh, Jharkhand, Uttar Pradesh and Bihar. While each of these states have made progress between 2005–2006 and 2015–2016, they continue to be below the country average and need focussed attention.

Young Child Environment Index

The YCEI has been constructed for 2015–2016 only due to limitations of data availability. Apart from inter-state comparisons, the YCEI also shows that all the eight states that have a below country average score on the Young Child Outcomes Index also fare poorly on the YCEI. This establishes that the five identified policy enablers – to alleviate poverty, strengthen primary health care, improve education levels, augment safe water supply and promote gender equity – all have a bearing on child well-being outcomes.

For the poverty index, the poverty rate using the Tendulkar formula has been used. Immunisation coverage has been selected as the indicator to measure of the efficacy of the public health system. Among the many indicators, female literacy rate has been identified as the most relevant for

Table 1.1 The Young Child Outcomes Index

Rank	State	Young Child Outcomes Index 2005–2006	Young Child Outcomes Index 2015–2016	Change
1	Kerala	0.796	0.858	0.062
2	Goa	0.757	0.817	0.060
3	Tripura	0.582	0.761	0.179
4	Tamil Nadu	0.659	0.731	0.071
5	Mizoram	0.632	0.719	0.088
6	Himachal Pradesh	0.601	0.719	0.118
7	Manipur	0.615	0.712	0.097
8	Punjab	0.581	0.708	0.126
9	Sikkim	0.581	0.700	0.119
10	Nagaland	0.562	0.699	0.137
11	Delhi	0.578	0.692	0.114
12	Maharashtra	0.528	0.679	0.151
13	West Bengal	0.503	0.665	0.163
14	Jammu & Kashmir	0.532	0.660	0.127
15	Telangana	0.536	0.659	0.123
16	Arunachal Pradesh	0.442	0.657	0.215
17	Haryana	0.501	0.643	0.142
18	Uttarakhand	0.524	0.642	0.118
19	Karnataka	0.513	0.634	0.121
20	Andhra Pradesh	0.523	0.624	0.101
21	Odisha	0.450	0.617	0.167
22	Gujarat	0.426	0.615	0.189
	INDIA	**0.443**	**0.585**	**0.142**
23	Assam	0.436	0.583	0.147
24	Meghalaya	0.369	0.562	0.193
25	Rajasthan	0.452	0.556	0.104
26	Chhattisgarh	0.366	0.555	0.189
27	Madhya Pradesh	0.397	0.526	0.129
28	Jharkhand	0.371	0.500	0.129
29	Uttar Pradesh	0.290	0.460	0.170
30	Bihar	0.298	0.452	0.155

the education index and sex ratio for the gender index. The percentage of households with protected water supply source has been used for the water supply index. While child safety index is a relevant indicator, the data does not appear to be credible, making it difficult to draw up the index. Among the correlates, female literacy, immunisation and poverty showed higher associations.

Table 1.2 provides the ranking of states with their values for the YCEI.

In addition to the eight states, Gujarat, Nagaland, Manipur and Arunachal Pradesh also have poor scores. Annexure 2 details the indexing methodology, sources of data and limitations.

Table 1.2 The Young Child Environment Index

Rank	State	Gender Index	Poverty Index	Health Index	Safe Water Supply Index	Educa- tion Index	Child Environment Index
1	Kerala	0.732	0.934	0.787	0.936	0.907	0.855
2	Goa	0.687	0.966	0.862	0.958	0.790	0.846
3	Sikkim	0.714	0.916	0.798	0.973	0.726	0.819
4	Punjab	0.601	0.914	0.870	0.990	0.667	0.794
5	Himachal Pradesh	0.671	0.918	0.637	0.943	0.728	0.769
6	West Bengal	0.721	0.725	0.814	0.939	0.665	0.767
7	Tamil Nadu	0.717	0.866	0.639	0.894	0.696	0.756
8	Delhi	0.624	0.889	0.600	0.775	0.780	0.726
9	Tripura	0.725	0.822	0.458	0.857	0.804	0.716
10	Mizoram	0.746	0.719	0.411	0.903	0.877	0.705
11	Jammu & Kashmir	0.616	0.882	0.704	0.879	0.512	0.703
12	Uttarakhand	0.647	0.866	0.496	0.920	0.659	0.700
13	Telangana	0.713	0.900	0.620	0.752	0.532	0.692
14	Karnataka	0.713	0.711	0.555	0.880	0.629	0.689
15	Haryana	0.583	0.868	0.550	0.907	0.614	0.689
16	Meghalaya	0.745	0.856	0.542	0.639	0.695	0.687
17	Maharashtra	0.644	0.767	0.480	0.904	0.715	0.687
18	Odisha	0.703	0.522	0.745	0.874	0.586	0.675
19	Andhra Pradesh	0.713	0.900	0.587	0.693	0.530	0.673
	INDIA	0.680	0.695	0.548	0.887	0.598	0.672
20	Gujarat	0.647	0.780	0.410	0.898	0.660	0.657
21	Chhattisgarh	0.738	0.404	0.719	0.900	0.540	0.636
22	Rajasthan	0.644	0.811	0.462	0.837	0.450	0.619
23	Bihar	0.702	0.504	0.544	0.980	0.460	0.613
24	Uttar Pradesh	0.662	0.574	0.418	0.960	0.526	0.604
25	Assam	0.729	0.532	0.370	0.818	0.620	0.592
26	Madhya Pradesh	0.677	0.538	0.448	0.828	0.535	0.591
27	Nagaland	0.714	0.743	0.235	0.782	0.729	0.589
28	Jharkhand	0.713	0.451	0.546	0.751	0.491	0.578
29	Manipur	0.703	0.452	0.593	0.344	0.690	0.537
30	Arunachal Pradesh	0.733	0.488	0.264	0.860	0.530	0.533

1.2.5 Social norms undermine legalistic and programmatic approaches

Social justice and inclusion are fairly and squarely part of political debates, policy discussions and social concerns, but the disadvantaged young child remains relegated to the margins. There is general consensus that legislation alone cannot change patriarchal social norms that determine peoples' thought processes, attitudes and behaviours. Their strict enforcement in letter and spirit together with a social movement may alter deeply entrenched prejudices and practices.

The young child is highly influenced by surrounding people and immediate environment. Various markers of identity such as gender, abilities, caste, religion, class and ethnicity play an important role in influencing the young child's immediate social environment that shapes her early experiences. Along with the previous information, the young child observes, experiences and normalises the discriminatory social norms from the immediate environment.

Children belonging to Scheduled Castes carry the burden of regressive social norms, and when they are girls and/or disabled and/or placed in situations such as migration or fragile ecosystem, their vulnerabilities do not add up but multiply. Marginalisation and exclusion have proved difficult to address because they emerge from a multitude of vulnerabilities in a dynamic socio-economic and political context. **Interconnected and synergistic approaches are particularly crucial for ensuring the entitlements of the disadvantaged child.**

Socio-cultural beliefs powerfully shape perceptions of needs and experiences and manifest in the way the vulnerable children are treated and socialised. However, gender relations and gender issues differ across different states and social groups based on caste and religion and evolve through an interface between traditional norms and modernisation. If, for instance, son preference was more prevalent among the landed communities and the rich, it is catching on in urban areas and among more prosperous communities that are able to access and afford modern technologies. Even those communities that have traditionally been relatively gender equal (for instance, the Scheduled Tribes) have begun showing signs of adverse sex ratios.

1.3 Sustainable development goals pose challenges but also opportunities for India

India was among the 193 countries that came together to adopt the SDGs in September 2015 at the United Nations. India played an important role in shaping the SDGs which "has meant that the country's development goals are mirrored in the SDGs."[27] Sustainable development also embeds within it the idea of *leaving no one behind* across all its dimensions. The SDGs provide a shared global radar requiring that the economic, social and environmental dimensions of development are *durable* as well as *inclusive*. Annexure 3 gives the exhaustive list of SDG Goals and Targets.

The SDGs are an ambitious set of 17 Goals to be achieved by 2030, applicable to developed and developing countries, being monitored through 169 specific targets and corresponding indicators, with countries adapting them to local circumstances. They provide a shared blueprint for a better long-term future for people and the planet.

While all 17 goals are essential for humanity, across countries, genders, age groups, other social and economic markers, some of them more directly impact the young child or intersect with each other to influence the circumstances in which he or she grows and develops. These include ending poverty, achieving food security and zero hunger, ensuring healthy lives, ensuring inclusive and equitable quality education, achieving gender equality and promoting peaceful and inclusive societies.

The consensus is that aggregate progress without an explicit focus on the most vulnerable and disadvantaged, or one that prioritises the present generation alone, is not good enough. Thus, children must be central to achieving the SDGs, more so those in their earliest years, when irreversible damage can take place, proving difficult to counter later. Country leadership and international cooperation need to ensure that by 2030 all people, including the children, live in a safer, cleaner, more prosperous and less unequal world.

The Government of India has endorsed the SDGs wholeheartedly, but later chapters in this Report indicate that the country may not achieve several corresponding targets, especially those related to child mortality, nutrition, pre-primary education, safety and security. Increased and prudent investment in ECD can accelerate progress and would entail adequate budgetary provisions at every level. Unless there is a concerted effort to conceptualise ECD holistically with clarity regarding multi-sectoral action by multiple stakeholders, it is difficult to see positive outcomes emerging from the sustained investments.

Countries have been sharing their experiences on SDG progress officially at the UN's High Level Political Forum since 2016 through the platform of Voluntary National Reviews (VNRs). India's VNR highlights several child-relevant aspects – broader ones like growth in rural sanitation facilities, electrification of villages, the public distribution system, and affordable food grains on the one hand, as well as specific ones like the ICDS, mid-day meals, increased institutional deliveries, maternity benefits and initiatives to save and educate the girl child. A decline in poverty across all population groups and a reduction in stunted and underweight children are noted as important outcomes at the national level. Aggregates, however, need to be supplemented by location and population-group specific levels and trends for a fuller picture.

1.4 State is the primary duty bearer to ensure adequate care

Traditionally, the responsibility for childcare, provision of basic needs and upbringing has been vested with parents and families. Within the family, cultural traditions, situational constraints and personal disposition guide the care of the child. In the Indian context, with acute poverty and inequity across several states and regions of the country, millions of households because of their circumstances are unable to adequately care for and nurture their children. In this context, **the State must play the primary role to provide an enabling environment for childcare and well-being of the young child.** Along with the State, civil society, the media and markets have an influential role in childcare, as they define and shape the environment within which families and communities are located.

The State secures the enabling conditions through policies, legislation, programmes and the institutional edifice for effective and efficient delivery of quality ECD services to all children, without discrimination on any grounds. While the Central government lays down the policy, legal and fiscal framework, and determines the overall budgetary outlays in India, the state governments are largely responsible for the implementation of policies and programmes related to ECD. Indeed, their role is critical as they are better placed for mounting responses to issues related to regional differences, diversity and inequality. They can initiate processes of change moving on right up to local self-government institutions.

Furthermore, the Indian Constitution has clearly articulated a distribution of power between the Union and the states. In addition, the *Panchayati Raj* Institutions (PRIs) and urban local bodies have been vested with an important role in the planning, implementation and management oversight of programmes targeting young children, their families and communities. As discussed earlier, the role of the Indian State in working in the interest of the young child has at best been lackadaisical if not indifferent.

Civil society is an underrated but important repository of values and progressive ideas, a watchdog, champion and enabler of policy and practices for public good. Various NGOs, networks and activists have pioneered and championed the cause of ECD. They highlight the issues in the public and policy domains and have influenced legislation and programmes. They have considerable experience, knowledge and skills that can be useful in taking ECD to scale. They have received valuable support from international organisations, which have experiences in the promotion of ECD accruing from their global outreach, and others have developed the knowledge base by investing in practice, research and knowledge management.

Media is no longer a channel of information but also a creator of public opinion as burgeoning social media has revolutionised interpersonal and mass communication. It has highlighted cases of deprivation by corroborating findings of surveys and studies with reports from the ground and human interest stories. It has also brought into public domain instances of violence, abuse and exploitation of children, especially young children, and implications of issues such as surrogacy, which are difficult to be captured by quantitative and qualitative research. Its ability to create a narrative is arguably its strength, which could be channelled in a campaign for the rights and entitlements of the young child.

Businesses, especially the corporate sector, have gained visibility due to their role in provision of food supplies for infant and young children, healthcare, day-care and pre-school services. The conflict of commercial interests with the best interest of the young child, and corporate social responsibility are areas that need further scrutiny.

1.5 A renewed policy focus on the young child is critical

There is clearly a strong case for strengthening the policy and legal framework for the young child and increased investment in interconnected sectors and thematic areas related to child survival, maternal and child health, childcare and early learning and the enabling environment. An enquiry into the current situation of young children, their families and communities in terms of their access to enabling conditions and relevant services of good quality is important for identifying and addressing impediments to improved outcomes. Also crucial is an assessment of the implications in terms of human resources and finances for expanding the access and utilisation of quality ECD services.

Chapter 2 of this Report explores the key factors that impact the physical health and overall well-being of the young child. It analyses multiple determinants of well-being to highlight the significant variances across various states, initiates a discussion on the role of frontline workers in delivering quality services and supporting parents and families for ECD and the effectiveness of, and lacunae in, policy and practices that have limited the coverage, access and quality of ECD services.

As Chapter 3 discusses, the family, available services – notably the AWCs under the ICDS, and pre-schools, in addition to aspects of play, early stimulation and social spaces outside the home, all have a role in ensuring the wherewithal for holistic development and early childhood education for the young child. It highlights the role of frontline workers, especially the *anganwadi* workers (AWWs) and pre-school teachers, in improving the developmental outcomes for the young child, and their capacities and competencies.

The young child is undoubtedly vulnerable, owing to tender age, but, as Chapter 4 shows, there are various categories within this age group that deserve urgent and extra attention for consistently faring poorly in terms of development indicators. Nurturing childcare and protection, as Chapter 5 argues, require an environment that encourages gender transformative parenting and inclusion for the well-being of the young child during his or her foundational period of growth and development. The Chapter further recognises the crucial role of parents and caregivers during this period and argues for the recognition and professionalisation of a cadre of ECD workers.

The patterns of budgetary allocations and expenditure provide insights into the thrust of current policies and programmes. Chapter 6 reviews the available data in order to highlight the key gaps in the current set of provisions for young children and maps out the resources required for improving the overall systems for delivery of ECD services, especially to the most vulnerable young child.

Chapter 7, which presents a way forward, calls for increasing the focus on the young child in the policy and legal frameworks, and programmatic interventions through a 'solutions oriented' critique of government policies and systems.

Many of the things we need can wait. The child cannot. Right now is the time his bones are being formed, his blood is being made and his senses are being developed. To him we cannot answer "Tomorrow", his name is today.

(Gabriela Mistral, 1948)

Key messages

- Persistent neglect of children aged under 6 years of age has led to their grim situation. Of the 159 million children in this age group, 21 percent are malnourished, 36 percent are underweight and 38 percent do not receive full immunisation.
- The right nutrition and care during the first 1,000 days between a woman's pregnancy and the child's second birthday has profound impact on the child's ability to grow, learn and rise out of poverty and, in the process, shape society's long-term stability and prosperity.
- Several interconnected factors cutting across development sectors determine outcomes for the young child. There has been some focus on survival, physical and cognitive development of the young child but childcare and nurturing, which is critical for holistic ECD, has remained largely neglected.
- India's policy framework and legislation entitle every child to basic rights. India is also committed to achieving the SDGs by 2030, in which the child is a central piece. However, this has not converted into positive outcomes for the young child.
- Effective investment in early childhood, with due accountability, is critical for children's rights and entitlements and human capital formation.
- India is well positioned to take full advantage of the demographic dividend if it can ensure adequate care of the young child.
- Inconsistent performance across regions and states is reflected in the ranking and values in the Young Child Outcomes Index below the national average of eight states of Assam, Meghalaya, Rajasthan, Chhattisgarh, Madhya Pradesh, Jharkhand, Uttar Pradesh and Bihar. They are poor performers in the Environment Index as well and need special focus.
- While the disadvantaged child remains relegated to the margins and is impacted by socio-cultural beliefs and gender relations, neglect and young child abuse has emerged as a serious concern that is not confined to any specific social group.

- The multiple problems of families, including poverty and lack of access to resources, necessitate for the State to step in as the primary duty bearer in enabling families to provide childcare. But its budgetary commitment is inadequate and the implementation of its policies and programmes has been weak. In addition, civil society and the corporate sector also have a vital role to play.

Notes

1 EU-UNICEF Child Rights Toolkit Integrating Child Rights in Development Cooperation, n.d.
2 National Census, 2011.
3 NFHS 4 (2015-16).
4 Data from NFHS 4 (2015–16). Cited in Ramachandran, 2018.
5 Ibid.
6 NCERT, 2006.
7 Ibid.
8 All boxes, figures and tables have been compiled by the research team and the contributors of the technical background papers unless stated otherwise.
9 UNICEF, 2001, p. 14.
10 Seuss, 1982.
11 UNICEF Innocenti, n.d.
12 Know Violence in Childhood, National Commission for Protection of Child Rights and ChildFund India, 2017.
13 UNDP, Human Development Report, 2018.
14 National Census, 2001, 2011.
15 Law Commission of India, 2015.
16 National Policy for Children, 1974, p. 1.
17 Talati et al., 2016. Also see Down to Earth, 2015.
18 Engel et al., 2007.
19 Quoted in the National Policy for Children, 2013, MWCD, GoI.
20 National Early Childhood Care and Education (ECCE) Policy, 2013.
21 NPA, 2016, p. 140.
22 MHRD, 1986.
23 Draft NEP, 2019, p. 46.
24 12th Plan Working Group Report, 2011.
25 The Protection of Children from Sexual Offences (POCSO) Act, 2012.
26 MWCD, WGREP Nutrition, 2011, p. 33. The Working Group on Child Rights Made Similar Observations (2011).
27 NITI Aayog, 2017. The VNR process was led 2017 by NITI Aayog.

Bibliography

Bajaj, M., 2018. *Childcare and the Childcare Worker*. Technical Background Paper for the Report 2020. Mobile Creches, New Delhi.

Bhatia, J., Z.A. Bhutta and S.C. Kalhan (Eds.), 2013. *Maternal and Child Nutrition: The First 1,000 Days* (Vol. 74). Karger Medical and Scientific Publishers.

Chopra, G., 2015. *Child Rights in India: Challenges and Social Action.* Springer.

Down to Earth, 2015. *ICDS Gets Packaged Food for the Malnourished.* Retrieved from www.downtoearth.org.in/news/icds-gets-packaged-food-for-the-malnourished-4301; date of access: 14 July 2019.

Engel, P. et al., 2007. Child Development in Developing Countries 3, Strategies to Avoid the Loss of Developmental Potential in More than 200 Million Children in the Developing World. *Lancet.* Vol 369, pp. 229–242. Retrieved from www.who.int/maternal_child_adolescent/documents/pdfs/lancet_child_dev_series_paper3.pdf; date of access: 22 May 2019.

EU-UNICEF Child Rights Toolkit Integrating Child Rights in Development Cooperation, n.d. Retrieved from www.childrightstoolkit.com/wp-content/uploads/toolkit/English/Child-Rights-Toolkit-Web-Links.pdf; date of access: 4 June 2019.

HAQ: Centre for Child Rights, 2018a. *Fact Sheet 1: The Profile of the Child Victims. Children's Access to Justice and Restorative Care.* Retrieved from http://haqcrc.org/wp-content/uploads/2018/04/childrens-access-to-justice-and-restorative-care.pdf-1.pdf; date of access: 4 July 2018.

HAQ: Centre for Child Rights, 2018b. *Union Budget 2018–19. Budget for Children in #New India.* HAQ Centre for Child Rights, New Delhi. Retrieved from http://haqcrc.org/wp-content/uploads/2018/02/haq-budget-for-children-2018-19.pdf; date of access: 4 July 2019.

Kaul, V. and D. Sankar, 2009. *Early Childhood Care and Education in India.* NUEPA.

Law Commission of India, 2015. *Early Childhood Development and Legal Entitlements.* Report No. 259. Retrieved from http://lawcommissionofindia.nic.in/reports/Report259.pdf; date of access: 15 December 2018.

Ministry of Health and Family Welfare, Government of India, 2017. *NFHS 4: State Fact Sheets.* New Delhi.

Ministry of Human Resource Development (MHRD), Government of India, 1986. *National Policy on Education, 1986.* New Delhi.

Ministry of Human Resource Development, Government of India, 2019. *Draft National Education Policy 2019.* Retrieved from https://mhrd.gov.in/sites/upload_files/mhrd/files/Draft_NEP_2019_EN_Revised.pdf; date of access: 14 January 2020.

Ministry of Statistics and Programme Implementation, Registrar General of India, GoI. Census of India 2001. New Delhi.

Ministry of Statistics and Programme Implementation, Registrar General of India, GoI. Census of India 2011. New Delhi.

Ministry of Women and Child Development (MWCD), Government of India, 2011. *Report of the Working Group on Child Rights for the 12th Five Year Plan (2012–17).* New Delhi.

Ministry of Women and Child Development, Government of India, 2013. *National Policy Children-2013.* Retrieved from http://india.gov.in/national -policy-children 2013; date of access: 12 September 2019.

Ministry of Women and Child Development, Government of India, 2016. *National Plan of Action for Children, 2016: Safe Children – Happy Childhood.* Retrieved from https://wcd.nic.in/sites/default/files/National%20Plan%20of%20Action%202016.pdf; date of access: 13 January 2020.

Mody, A. and S. Aiyar, 2011. *The Demographic Dividend: Evidence from the Indian States.* IMF Working Paper. Retrieved from www.imf.org/en/Publications/

WP/Issues/2016/12/31/The-Demographic-Dividend-Evidence-from-the-Indian-States-24660; date of access: 2 March 2019.

Murthy, R.K., 2018. *Parental Care and the Young Child*. Technical Background Paper for the Report 2020. Mobile Creches, New Delhi.

National Commission for Protection of Child Rights, 2017. *Know Violence in Childhood*. Retrieved from http://ncpcr.gov.in/showfile.php?lang=1&level=2&&sublinkid=1679&lid=1682; date of access: 22 July 2019.

National Commission for Protection of Child Rights and ChildFund India, 2017. *Handbook for Ending Violence Against Children—Situational Analysis of India*. Retrieved from http://ncpcr.gov.in/showfile.php?lang=1&level=2&&sublinkid=1679&lid=1682; date of access: 22 July 2019.

National Crime Records Bureau, Ministry of Home Affairs, Government of India, 2017. *Crime in India-2016*. NCRB, New Delhi.

National Early Childhood Care and Education (ECCE) Policy, 2013. Retrieved from https://wcd.nic.in/sites/default/files/National%20Early%20Childhood%20Care%20and%20Education-Resolution.pdf; date of access: 11 November 2019.

National Policy for Children, 1974. Retrieved from www.haqcrc.org/pdf/national-policy-for-children-1974/; date of access: 2 September 2019.

NCERT, 2006. *National Focus Group on Early Childhood Education*. Position Paper, September 2006. Retrieved from www.ncert.nic.in/new_ncert/ncert/rightside/links/pdf/focus_group/early_childhood_education.pdf; date of access: 2 July 2019.

NITI Aayog, 2015. *A Quick Evaluation Study of Anganwadis Under ICDS*. Niti Aayog, Programme Evaluation Organisation, June 2015.

NITI Aayog, 2017. *Voluntary National Review Report on Implementation of Sustainable Development Goals*. United Nations High Level Political Forum, India.

The Protection of Children from Sexual Offences (POCSO) Act, 2012. Press release. 19 December 2014. Retrieved from http://pib.nic.in/newsite/PrintRelease.aspx?relid=113750; date of access: 14 December 2018.

Ramachandran, V., 2018. *From the Womb to Primary School: Challenges, Policies and Prospects for the Young Child in India*. Technical Background Paper for the Report 2020, Version 3, 20 August 2018. Mobile Creches, New Delhi.

Ramani, V., 2018. *Physical Wellbeing of the Young Child in India: Challenges, Prospects and Way Forward*. Technical Background Paper for the Report 2020. Mobile Creches, New Delhi.

Save the Children, HAQ: Centre for Child Rights, Plan International, CRY: Child Rights and You and Terres des Hommes (Germany). *The South Asian Report on Child-Friendliness of Governments*. Retrieved from http://haqcrc.org/publication/south-asian-report-child-friendliness-governments/; date of access: 11 November 2019.

Seuss, 1982. *Horton Hears a Who!* Random House Books for Young Readers.

Talati, K.N. et al., 2016. Take Home Ration in ICDS Programmes: Opportunities for Integration with Health System for Improved Utilization Via Mamta Card and E-Mamta. *BMJ Global Health*. Vol 1, pp. A7–A8. Retrieved from https://gh.bmj.com/content/1/Suppl_1/A7; date of access: 14 July 2019.

UN Committee on the Rights of the Child (CRC) General Comment No. 7, 2005. *Implementing Child Rights in Early Childhood*, CRC/C/GC/7/Rev.1, 20 September 2006. Retrieved from www.refworld.org/docid/460bc5a62.html; date of access: 2 March 2019.

UNDESA, 2016 & 2017. *Synthesis of Voluntary National Reviews for 2016 and 2017.*

UNICEF, 2001. *State of the World's Children.* UNICEF, New York.

UNICEF, 2006. *A Guide to General Comment 7: 'Implementing Child Rights in Early Childhood'.* Bernard van Leer Foundation, The Hague.

UNICEF Innocenti, n.d. *The Convention on the Rights of the Child.* Retrieved from www.unicef-irc.org/portfolios/general_comments/GC7.Rev.1_en.doc.html; date of access: 30 December 2018.

United Nations Development Programme, 2018. *Human Development Indices and Indicators: 2018 Statistical Update.* UNDP, New York.

2 Advancing physical well-being

Physical well-being of children has been one of the most distressing issues for India for seven decades since independence. Persistent neglect or recurrent illnesses aggravate the vulnerability of the young child, resulting in development deficits and, in worst case scenarios, death. Infant and child mortality, malnutrition, stunting and wasting to chronic illnesses are preventable but remain pervasive. They are related to a wide range of factors beyond the utilisation of healthcare and emergency medical care, including the overall well-being and nutrition of women, infant and young child feeding practices, safe drinking water, sanitation, hygiene and a socio-cultural, natural and physical environment.

This chapter draws upon the available data to analyse the situation of the young child in India in terms of survival and physical development as well as the issues of nutrition, healthcare, safe water, sanitation, hygiene and socio-economic determinants that impact physical well-being. It takes cognisance of India's achievements in creating the conditions for the young child's physical well-being, the impediments that need to be addressed with a sense of urgency and concludes with recommendations and action points for improving the outcomes for the young child.

2.1 Young child mortality

2.1.1 Mortality rates decline but the number of child deaths is unacceptably high

India has witnessed significant decline in the IMR in the last two decades, yet it contributes the highest number of neonatal, infant and under 5 deaths in the world. The Sample Registration System (SRS) data, which the government often uses for estimating IMR, shows a decline from 44 per 1,000 live births in 2011 to 33 in 2017.[1]

The findings of successive NFHS further corroborate the steady decline in IMR – from 57 per 1,000 live births in 2005–2006 to 41 in 2015–2016.[2] Figure 2.1 highlights the trends in child mortality over the years.

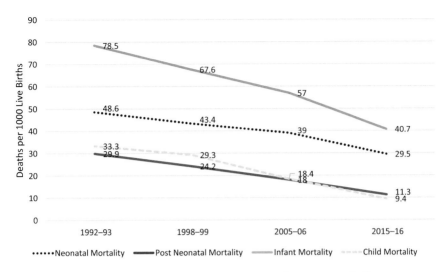

Figure 2.1 Child mortality rates from 1992 to 2016 show a steep decline
Source: NFHS 1–4

The under-5 mortality rate (U5MR) which indicates the prospects of new-born survival till their fifth birthday, also showed a marked decline from 55 per 1,000 live births in 2011 to 39 in 2016.[3] The NFHS-4 estimated a decline from 74 per 1,000 live births in 2005–2006 to 50 in 2015–2016.

Almost all studies conclude that the mortality rate among neonates, infants and children has declined but a child born in a remote rural area or an urban slum does not have the same chance of survival as a child born in a well-off household. The picture varies across different states in India, across rural and urban areas, across economic groups and social groups.

Indeed, the averages conceal significant inter and intra-state differentials in reduction in IMR and U5MR. Uttar Pradesh was at one end of spectrum with the highest IMR (73) and U5MR (96) in India and Kerala was at the other end with the lowest IMR (15) and U5MR (16) in 2005–06 (NFHS-3). The decline in U5MR has been uneven across states with 78 deaths per 1,000 live births in Uttar Pradesh as compared with 7 deaths per 1,000 live births in Kerala in 2015–2016 (NFHS 4). This is also reflected in the Young Child Outcomes Index (Table 1.1). It brings forth these inter-state differentials with Kerala scoring as high as 0.858 and Bihar as low as 0.452 in the 2015–2016 Index that takes IMR into account in addition to stunt-ing and net attendance at the primary level. The other states in the bottom five include Uttar Pradesh (0.460), Jharkhand (0.371), Madhya Pradesh (0.526), Chhattisgarh (0.55) all of which have an Index score lower than the all-India Index of 0.585. Goa (0.817), Tripura (0.761), Tamil Nadu (0.731) and Mizoram (0.719) are among the top five.

Chhattisgarh and Madhya Pradesh in the central region, Assam and Arunachal Pradesh in the north-east, Jharkhand, Orissa and Bihar in the east, and Rajasthan in the north have reported high levels of IMR and U5MR. In contrast, all states in south and west India fared much better. Indeed, the southern states, viz., Kerala, Tamil Nadu, Karnataka, Andhra Pradesh and Telangana with neonatal mortality rate (NMR) and IMR equivalent to developed countries have almost completed 'epidemiological transition,' which is characterised by a marked reduction in communicable, maternal, neonatal and nutritional diseases that have a major impact on child health.[4]

Higher than national average child mortality rates in the states like Bihar, Chhattisgarh, Jharkhand, Madhya Pradesh, Odisha, Rajasthan, Uttar Pradesh, Uttarakhand, Assam and Meghalaya, which are bigger in size and population than most countries of the world and lag behind in child mortality reduction, translate into a large number of infant and child deaths.

Lower child mortality rate in urban areas is not surprising in view of better developmental infrastructure, availability of health facilities and accessibility of basic services. The strategies seeking to improve child survival should specifically focus on the ways and means of reducing the IMR in rural areas, which have lagged behind urban areas. The rural IMR was 80 in 1994, 64 in 2004 and 44 in 2013 compared with 52, 40 and 27 in urban areas in the corresponding periods.[5] In 2015–2016, the U5MR was 56 deaths per 1,000 live births in rural areas and 34 in urban India (NFHS-4).[6]

It is worth reflecting on the main causes of child mortality for a better understanding of why some children are more likely to die early. WHO identified pre-term birth complications, acute respiratory infections, intrapartum-related complications, congenital anomalies and diarrhoea as the leading causes of death.[7] However, all these causes can be addressed through preventive measures involving immediate and exclusive breastfeeding, access to skilled health professionals for antenatal, birth, and postnatal care, access to nutrition and micronutrients, access to water, sanitation and hygiene, immunisation and knowledge of the danger signs that enable the caregivers and family members to seek immediate medical or emergency intervention.[8]

Still births and newborn deaths are usually related to maternal health, nutrition and timely access to ANC, skilled birth attendance and postnatal care (PNC), and if need be emergency obstetric care. On the other hand, later deaths among young children are more likely to be related to neglect, malnutrition and lower immunity to illnesses and environmental factors.

The inter and intra-state differentials in IMR and U5MR are pointers to the inability of the State to reduce vulnerabilities due to gender, caste and economic status, create high quality development infrastructure, ensure good quality health services and food security for all through social policies, financial investment and capacity development. While the inability to utilise good quality health services contributes to life threatening situations for the young child, discrimination in access to basic rights and entitlements has been a major factor in child mortality.

2.1.2 Reduction in perinatal and neonatal mortality is key to improving child survival

Globally, nearly 85 percent of child deaths occur in the first five years of life.[9] Following the global pattern, India has done relatively well in reducing mortality among children under 5 years of age. The loss of momentum in the decline in IMR and U5MR is partly due to a slower decrease in the neonatal mortality rate (NMR) or infant deaths from birth till the age of one month. The NMR in India declined from 33 per 1,000 live births in 2010 to 24 in 2016.[10]

About 30 percent deaths within the neonatal period are attributed to pre-term birth, which is intricately linked with maternal health and nutritional status, followed by respiratory distress syndromes. About 23 percent women in India have lesser than the lowest range of normal Body Mass Index and 53 percent women of reproductive age group are anaemic, which explains preterm and low birth babies.

The proportion of babies born with low birth weight is likely to be higher in India than the global average of 16 percent because of socio-economic factors. Globally, 20 million infants are born every year with low birth weight, out of which an estimated 7.5 million births occur in India,[11] and just less than half are prone to infection and premature death within first month of their lives. Around 600,000 children die within 28 days of their births in India.[12]

The success of southern states of the country – Kerala, Tamil Nadu, Karnataka, Andhra Pradesh and Telangana in reducing IMR and NMR is due to their ability to achieve marked reduction in communicable, maternal, neonatal and nutritional diseases that affect children the most. The states like Bihar, Chhattisgarh, Jharkhand, Madhya Pradesh, Odisha, Rajasthan, Uttar Pradesh, Uttarakhand, Assam and Meghalaya are still struggling to move in that direction.[13]

2.1.3 Social marginalisation and exclusion influence child mortality

Differentials in the intra-household distribution of food and other resources, delayed access to healthcare and other basic services, and possibly malnutrition are manifested in the consistently higher U5MR for girls. Social norms, which have contributed to abject or relative female neglect, have also led to the misuse of modern diagnostic technologies, resulting in skewed gender balance in the population. While research indicates widespread neglect of the girl child, there is anecdotal evidence of maltreatment.

Poorest households are unable to access, afford and utilise many of the basic entitlements and their coping strategies are often based on discriminatory social norms. In absolute numbers, 52.5 million Indians were impoverished due to health costs in 2011, almost half of the world's impoverished population.[14] Financial assistance under the *Janani Suraksha Yojana* (JSY) received for institutional delivery covered only 36.4 percent of all mothers, with out-of-pocket expenditure per delivery in a public health facility amounting to almost INR 3,200.[15]

Socio-economic status has an important role in child survival as it determines the quality of life and access to basic services that impact child health, as listed in Box 2.1. U5MR was 56 per 1,000 live births for Scheduled Castes (SCs) and 57 per 1,000 live births for Scheduled Tribes (STs). Similarly, it shows a decline with increasing household wealth – from 72 per 1,000 live births for the lowest wealth quintile to 23 deaths per 1,000 for the highest quintile.[16] Although STs have a lower IMR (62) than the SCs (66), U5MR was found to be higher among STs (96) than among SCs (88). Other Backward Classes (OBCs) have lower mortality (51) than SCs or STs but still higher than others who are not SC, ST or OBC (39).[17] Overall, U5MR is 23 percent higher among OBCs than among the population in the general category.[18]

Among religious groups, Hindus have the highest IMR (59), followed by Buddhists (53), Muslims (52), Sikhs (46) and Christians (42).[19] Christians and Sikhs have relatively low mortality rates at all ages under 5 years.

The Sachar Committee report in 2006 had noted that Muslim children exhibit lower child mortality than Hindu children, in spite of the fact that, on average, their mothers are poorer and less educated – characteristics typically associated with higher child mortality. Studies have not been able to come up with conclusive explanations for this paradox. Besides relatively higher urbanisation of the community, the additional time spent by Muslim women at home which translates into better childcare practices and lower child mortality could also be a contributing factor.[20]

Box 2.1   Various determinants impact child health

Essentially four key factors make a huge difference to child health.

1   *Access for women to nutritious food, timely healthcare and education up to or beyond secondary school.* This has been an

accepted social norm in several Indian states, which has resulted from a number of local historical factors.

2   *Access to safe drinking water, proper sanitation and related social/community hygiene.* Societal awareness that this reduces children's exposure to communicable diseases varies across states and communities.

3   *Levels of abject poverty.* Lack of access to government food security schemes and programme often compounds inequality in wealth. In many of the poor performing states, the functioning of the PDS system or the ICDS centre or any other pro-poor programmes aggravates distress among the very poor and marginalised.

4   *Gender relations and gender issues.* There have been inter-state and intra-state differentials in gender relations and for different social groups, castes or religions. The preference for sons and aversion to or neglect of daughters has been prevalent among the landed communities and the rich. But the preference for sons seems to be increasing even in areas and communities that were known for greater gender equality.

2.1.4 The first signs of disabilities tend to appear during the early years

India is the second most populous country with a large number of infants born annually with congenital birth defects or structural, functional and metabolic disorders, which contribute to infant mortality or disability. Due to plethora of risk factors, e.g., universality of marriage, high fertility, large number of unplanned pregnancies, poor ANC coverage, poor maternal nutrition, high consanguineous marriages and high carrier rate for haemo-globinopathies,[21] the prevalence of birth defects in India is in 61–70 per 1,000 live births range.[22] The application of various cost-effective community genetic services can prevent about 70 percent of these defects.[23]

Iodisation, double fortification of salt, flour fortification with multivitamins, folic acid supplementation, peri-conceptional care, carrier screening and prenatal screening are some of the proven strategies for control of birth defects. Consumption of iodised salt has been promoted since a long time but its consumption in India remains low.

Timely identification of impairments as well as secondary prevention can reduce the impact on the functional level of the individual and prevent it from becoming a disabling condition. Parents and family members at home and caregivers and service providers in the AWCs, schools and primary health sub-centres or at health camps should be able to identify early signs of impairments and risk of developmental delay. Specialists need to step in soon thereafter for clinical assessments and planning of necessary interventions.[24]

2.2 Sex selection and gender discrimination have major implications for the young child

2.2.1 *Adverse sex ratio at birth shows that girls are less likely to survive*

Adverse child sex ratio (CSR) and sex ratio at birth (SRB) in India, increasingly evident from surveys in the last few decades, reflect confluence of deep-rooted gender bias against females in social norms, and availability of modern technology that facilitates sex determination. It has been viewed as an outcome of technology facilitated gender-based violence. The findings of three successive national censuses in 1991, 2001 and 2011 rang alarm bells of a demographic crisis, which has led to concerns regarding the gross violation of the girl child's right to survival and its serious implications for the social fabric and economy.

Gender-based discrimination due to deep-rooted patriarchal social norms has for long been recognised as a social development and human rights issue, which poses a major challenge to realisation of sustainable development. It has been manifested in inequitable distribution of household resources and discrimination against women and girls in access to food and healthcare, restricted mobility and fewer educational and developmental opportunities. Complex issues related to lineage, labour and inheritance, interpreted to disadvantage females, contributed to pernicious practices such as female infanticide.

Experts have not reached a consensus on the positive or negative impact of higher levels of education and wealth on son preference. Most of them are inconclusive on the national trend in view of the rapidly changing situation on the ground and huge diversity across regions, communities and economic wealth quartiles.[25]

The economically better-off and better-educated classes in rural and urban areas have been using technology to identify the sex of the foetus and aborting the female foetus. Adverse sex ratios demonstrate clearly that improved education levels and economic standards have not overridden gender discriminatory social norms. The knowledge of these technologies and the ability to afford them have clearly been detrimental for the survival of the girl child.

2.2.2 *Exposure to violence, especially gendered violence, has adverse effects across childhood*

Exposure of the young child to violence has not received due attention in India. A global study in 2017, 'Know Violence in Childhood,' estimated that 1.3 billion children around the world experience harsh discipline at the hands of caregivers and that corporal punishment is the most commonly experienced form of violence against children, which could begin as early as age one. The report noted that children under the age of four are exposed to direct abuse by primary caregivers and other family members. Furthermore, children whose mothers are abused are at higher risk of being abused by the perpetrator of the violence or by their mothers due to marital stress.[26] Witnessing or experiencing violence at an early age has long-term effects on children.[27]

Although boys and girls are both vulnerable to violence, the former may experience somewhat greater levels of physical violence and the latter are likely to experience higher levels of sexual violence. These are patterns commonly visible in most countries, but they can vary according to social context. For example, societies where girls and women are restricted from appearing in public may see higher levels of sexual violence against girls.[28] Much of sexual violence against young girls is invisible and under-reported and typically comes to light through media reports.

Even though sustained efforts by many governmental and non-governmental agencies have challenged the culture of silence around the issue of violence against children, there is still limited public awareness of its nature, incidence and implications. Implicit in the data on sex ratio and gender imbalance is violence against the young child. Although there are anecdotal accounts, child neglect, shaken baby syndrome and physical and sexual abuse of the young child, have not been captured in empirical studies. A nuanced perspective is yet to emerge, which would enable a systemic response that integrates violence prevention strategies in spaces that young children inhabit.

2.2.3 Child health is closely linked with women's well-being and empowerment

Health and nutrition status of the mother has major implications for the health and nutrition status of the young child. NFHS-4 data on women in the 15–49 age group reveals that 11.1 percent were less than 145 centimetres in height and 22.9 percent had a Body Mass Index (BMI) below 18.5. Slightly over half (50.3 percent) of pregnant women in the 15–49 age group were anaemic. Both these conditions heighten the probability of preterm babies.

Mother's education levels contribute to lowering of infant and child mortality rates but is most effective in reducing mortality of older children. Available data shows that the decline in IMR was higher among children whose mothers had some schooling than among those with no schooling. In NFHS-3, the IMR was 26 for children whose mothers had twelve or more years of schooling, 50 for children whose mothers had five to seven years of schooling, and 70 for children whose mothers lacked schooling. An analysis of NFHS 4 in *IndiaSpend* (2018) notes that U5MR for children whose mothers had no schooling was 67.5 deaths per 1,000 live births compared to 26.5 for children whose mothers had twelve or more years of schooling.[29]

In several states in India women's access to nutritious food, timely health-care and education up to or beyond secondary school has been an accepted social norm. Some states and regions do better than others in terms of access to safe drinking water, sanitation and hygiene within households, surrounding spaces and communities, which reduces children's exposure to communicable diseases. The YCEI (Table 1.2), which includes an assessment of female literacy rate, sex ratio, immunisation coverage, poverty rate and safe water supply access – to rank states with regard to the overall environment in which children grow – notes the index score to be highest in Kerala (0.855) followed by Goa (0.846) and Sikkim (0.819). The low-ranking states include Arunachal Pradesh (0.533), Manipur (0.537) and Jharkhand (0.578), which along with Nagaland, Madhya Pradesh, Assam, Uttar Pradesh, Bihar, Rajasthan, Chhattisgarh and Gujarat score lower than the all-India index (0.672).

The Asian Enigma has ascribed the major reason for the exceptionally high rates of child malnutrition in South Asia as being "rooted deep in the soil of inequality between men and women." Women's disempowerment in Indian social ethos has undermined the nutrition status of children. Early marriage and childbearing, inadequate spacing between children and the poor nutrition status of women in the childbearing age group adversely affected the quality of infant and childcare. Social attitudes still militate against greater opportunities for women. Neighbouring Bangladesh has shown significant progress in child survival and development indicators through its focus on women's empowerment and maternal and child health programmes.

2.3 Ill health among young children

2.3.1 *Most causes of child mortality and ill health are preventable*

India has a long way to go before it can ensure that all children are able to go through early childhood without any major illness or trauma. Infants and small children are particularly vulnerable to respiratory infections, diarrhoeal diseases, measles, meningitis and other viral diseases. Poor sanitation, poor nutrition, non-availability of safe drinking water and overall environmental hygiene all exacerbate the situation.

As per NFHS-4, 18 percent of infants had low birth weight, which is an estimated 4.8 million children of the 26.9 million born every year, which is linked with maternal health and nutrition and contributes to infections and ill health. Safe practices during childbirth, proper nutrition and care, immunisation, safe water, sanitation and hygiene can prevent many childhood ailments, as Box 2.2 highlights. Continued prevalence of neonatal tetanus, diphtheria, whooping cough and measles among children raises questions about the effectiveness of maternal and child health initiatives and campaigns implemented over several decades.

Communicable diseases continue to affect children living in diverse poverty situation in almost all states of India. Malaria, alongside other mosquito-borne diseases like dengue, chikungunya and encephalitis, is a major public health challenge. Four states of India, viz. Uttar Pradesh, Bihar, West Bengal and Assam, share the maximum burden of encephalitis. The prevalence of cholera in 2014 was recorded in Gujarat, Karnataka, Madhya Pradesh, Maharashtra, Punjab, Rajasthan, Uttar Pradesh and West Bengal.[30]

Box 2.2   Various public health interventions prevent child mortality

1 Full immunisation among children under three years of age, and pregnant women
2 Full antenatal, natal and postnatal care
3 Skilled birth attendance with a facility for meeting need for emergency obstetric care
4 Iron and Folic acid supplementation for children, adolescent girls and pregnant women
5 Regular treatment of intestinal worms, especially in children and reproductive age women
6 Universal use of iodine and iron fortified salt
7 Vitamin A supplementation for children aged 9–59 months
8 Preventive and promotive health educational services, including information on hygiene, hand-washing and dental hygiene, use of potable drinking water, high calorie diet and obesity, need for regular physical exercise, advice on initiation of breastfeeding within one hour of birth and exclusively up to six months of age, and complementary feeding thereafter, adolescent sexual health, need for screening for NCDs and common cancers for those at risk
9 Home based newborn care, and encouragement for exclusive breastfeeding till the age of six months
10 Community based care for sick children, with referral of cases requiring higher levels of care
11 HIV testing and counselling during antenatal care
12 Free drugs to pregnant HIV positive mothers to prevent mother to child transmission of HIV
13 Malaria prophylaxis, using Long Lasting Insecticide Treated Nets (LLIN), diagnosis using Rapid Diagnostic Kits (RDK) and appropriate treatment

14 School check-up of health and wellness, followed by advice, and treatment if necessary

15 Management of diarrhoea, especially in children, using Oral Rehydration Solution (ORS)

16 Diagnosis and treatment of tuberculosis, leprosy including drug and multi-drug resistant cases

17 Vaccines for hepatitis B and C for high risk groups

18 Patient transport systems including emergency response ambulance services of the 'dial 108' model

(Planning Commission, 2013)[31]

2.3.2 Maternal and child health services are inadequately utilised

Utilisation of antenatal care may have improved but is below par. The NFHS-4 found that only 51.2 percent mothers had four ANC visits and full ANC coverage[32] was at an abysmal 21 percent, although the percentage of institutional delivery now touches almost 80 percent.

There are large inter-state variations in the coverage, utilisation and quality. While some states, notably southern states like Tamil Nadu and Kerala, provide fairly efficient ANC services, home-based neonatal care is relatively low even in these states. Kerala is now seeking to address this deficiency in services by screening all children immediately after birth. Even where ANC coverage rates are high, the issue of systematic follow-up by medical staff, leading to satisfactory outcomes for the health of the mother and the newborn persists. Weight gain in mothers during pregnancy is not satisfactory, leading to a high percentage of LBW babies. The NFHS-4 figure for India of children receiving a health check within two days of birth is a paltry 24.3 percent.

India has made considerable progress in management of diseases like diarrhoea or life-threatening illnesses. However, prevention, continuous care and support remain major concerns. Vast strides in female literacy in the 1960s, 1970s and 1980s helped to raise awareness of good practices for child health and nutrition and higher education levels in the general population sensitised families to women and children's health.

2.3.3 Full immunisation is still distant

Immunisation, so necessary for prevention against childhood illnesses, stands at an abysmal 62 percent (NFHS-4). Full immunisation of children in the 12–23 months age group has improved at a sluggish pace – from 35.4 percent in 1992–93 to 42 percent in 1998–1999 and 43.5 percent in

2005–2006 but accelerated to 62 percent in 2015–16. Figure 2.2 highlights the trends in immunisation by vaccine.

The pace of increase is even slower when compared with achievements in institutional births that improved from a similarly low level of 39 percent in 2005–2006 to 79 percent in 2015–2016. This raises questions about the effectiveness of publicly financed universal immunisation programmes[33] and ability of ICDS to deliver immunisation services.

Immunisation coverage ranges from 21 percent in Nagaland to 81 percent in Tamil Nadu.[34] It tends to be lower in states with high poverty, poor child health and human development indicators. The percentage of fully vaccinated children in Uttar Pradesh (23 percent), Rajasthan (27 percent), Assam (31 percent), Bihar (33 percent), Jharkhand (34 percent) and Madhya Pradesh (40 percent) is lower than the national average of 44 percent. In addition to Tamil Nadu, about three-fourths or more of children in Goa, Kerala and Himachal Pradesh are fully immunised. As the YCEI (Table 1.2) shows, states with a low ranking in Health Index that measures immunisation (including Arunachal Pradesh, Nagaland and Uttar Pradesh) rank low in the overall YCEI as well.

Between 2005–2006 and 2015–2016, immunisation coverage in India increased by 18 percent points (from 44 percent to 62 percent). Interestingly, much of the progress came from rural areas (from 39 percent to 61 percent) whereas urban areas show slower improvement (from 58 percent to 64 percent). Not too stark urban-rural differences in immunisation coverage in NFHS-4 – and the fact that most children received immunisation in

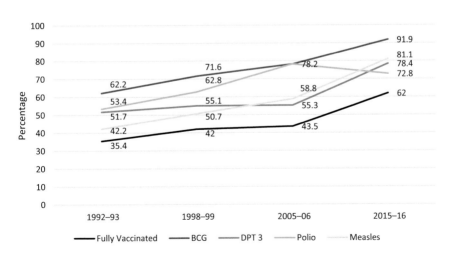

Figure 2.2 Trends in immunisation by vaccine, 1992–2016

Source: NFHS 1–4

public-health facilities, 82.1 percent in urban areas and 94.2 percent in rural areas – indicates the ability of public health facilities to provide the necessary services if there is political and administrative resolve.

Full immunisation is determined by supply side factors such as the availability of health facility and promoters and demand-side issues such as public awareness of the importance of timely immunisation and the number, types and sequence of prescribed vaccines. The improvements in coverage have been better among households in the lowest wealth quintiles compared to those from higher wealth quintiles.[35] Children belonging to mothers with secondary or higher education have high coverage (67 percent) than those without formal education (52 percent).[36]

The stagnation in coverage indicated by slower pace of improvement in full immunisation coverage in urban areas and just about 70 percent among households in the highest wealth quintile is worrying. Notwithstanding the progress dynamics, it is discernible that the rural-urban hierarchies as well as the socio-economic gradients in terms of wealth and social group affiliations are fully intact.[37] India does seem to deliver better results through vertical programmes administered in mission mode.

2.3.4 *Natural calamities and clear signs of climate change threaten child health*

India has always been prone to recurring natural disasters such as floods, droughts, cyclones, earthquakes and landslides. Out of 602 districts in the country, as noted in a 2011 study, 125 districts have been identified as most hazard prone areas in India.[38] **In the event of any natural calamities, children are more likely to be injured, more vulnerable to infections and malnutrition and are also exposed to greater danger through separation from their families or caregivers.**[39] Moreover, infants and young children may not be able to communicate necessary information if they become separated from their caregivers and remain at high risk of trafficking.

The WHO estimated that environment related causes and conditions contributed to 26 percent of the annual 6.6 million deaths of children under 5 in 2012.[40] More recently (WHO, 2017b), it attributed more than one in four deaths of the world's children under the age of 5 to unhealthy environments.

Climate change is a fast-emerging challenge for public health and sustainable development. Globally, over half a billion children are living in areas with extremely high levels of floods and nearly 160 million children live in areas of high or extremely high droughts (United Nations Children's Fund UNICEF, 2015).

Globally, environmental risks – such as air pollution, secondhand smoke, tainted water, lack of sanitation and inadequate hygiene – take the lives of 1.7 million children during their first five years every year.[41] Young children with developing organs and immune systems, smaller bodies and airways, are particularly at risk of ill health due to a polluted environment. Diarrhoea, malaria and pneumonia are the most common causes of death aged one month to 5 years.

Environmental issues are global in nature but India ranks very low on air and water pollution level compared to rest of the world.[42] Air pollution, which has become a perennial feature in India, increases the risk of respiratory infection, adverse neonatal condition and congenital anomalies and is the cause of about 600,000 deaths in children below the age of 15, and one in ten deaths in children under 5.[43] Respiratory infections, such as pneumonia, are usually due to indoor and outdoor pollution and second hand smoke. Diarrhoea is a result of poor access to clean water, sanitation and hygiene while malaria is caused by unrestrained breeding of mosquitoes at open water storage. Unintentional injuries due to environmental causes (such as poisoning, falls and drowning) are also preventable through childcare.

2.4 Several factors determine child nutrition

Experts and community workers argue that the first 1,000 days – the 270 days in the mother's womb and 730 days after birth are critical for overall child development (Box 1.1). Focussed attention to nutrition and overall well-being of the mother during pregnancy and focussed and targeted strategies to ensure proper feeding (from breastfeeding to complementary feeding), stimulation, timely immunisation and early childhood care and education can have significant impact on the child. A child's brain develops at a rapid pace till the age of three and poor nutrition at this stage can harm long-term cognitive abilities.

Malnutrition, as measured by the proportion of under-5 underweight children, acts as one of the single most causes for the child mortality arising from poverty, misconceptions pertaining to childcare practices, neglect and poor breastfeeding. Insufficient food intake or absorption makes children susceptible to infections and hampers their growth.

Estimates of child mortality ascribe up to 56 percent of child deaths to malnutrition, with even mild and moderate malnutrition contributing significantly to the death rate. A child who is left unattended, or in the care of a sibling is much more likely to be undernourished and prone to illness and developmental deprivation. Box 2.3 details the various factors that determine child malnutrition.

The findings of the Comprehensive National Nutrition Survey (CNNS) (2016–18), a third-party survey,[44] and the SRS (2018) indicate considerable progress made by India in malnutrition reduction in recent years. The CNNS recorded a decline since NFHS-4 in stunting from 38.4 percent to 34.7 percent, wasting from 21 percent to 17.3 percent and underweight from 35.7 percent to 33.4 percent.

Box 2.3   Several factors determine child malnutrition

The conceptual framework on the causes of child malnutrition was developed in 1990 as part of the UNICEF Nutrition Strategy and refined by other researchers. Individual related *immediate determinants* depend on the dietary intake (of proteins, calories, fat and micronutrients) and health status. Inadequate dietary intake lowers immunity to disease, and in turn, depresses appetite and reduces energy. They are influenced by the following three household related *underlying determinants*, which are further aggravated by poverty:

1   **Access to food** is contingent on access to means of production, income-earning livelihood and/or transfers in cash or kind (as in provision of social security or humanitarian relief).
2   **Nurture and care** refers to the time, attention and support given to meet the physical, mental and social needs of the child and other members of the family, especially the mother.
3   A **healthy environment** mainly comprises of safe water, sanitation, healthcare and environmental safety, including shelter.

(UNICEF, 1990)

The *State of the World's Children* (UNICEF, 2019) notes that poor families usually tend to buy low-quality food which costs them lesser, subsequently resulting in the most disadvantaged children facing the "greatest risk of all forms of malnutrition." As growth and development occurs at a rapid pace during childhood, chronic malnutrition essentially affects the child for a lifetime.

A World Bank document (*Snakes and Ladders*, 2004), argues that families and communities that have lived in abject poverty for over two or three generations, migrant communities have gradually lost their traditional knowledge related to child nutrition and child health. As a result, most of them are not in a position to draw upon traditional knowledge to improve the health and well-being of their children. For example, nutritious traditional food is substituted by ready to eat biscuits and salty snacks. This problem is far more severe among SC communities than ST.

2.4.1 India faces multiple burdens of child malnutrition

Wasting, a major threat to public health, contributes to sharply raising child mortality rates in combination with stunting in India. With 58.7 million stunted children, South Asia tops the list of five regions of the world which register stunting rates of over 30 percent. Even more distressing (and even alarming) are the high wasting rates in South Asia, far higher than elsewhere in the world. As the biggest country in this region, India shoulders the largest burden of stunted and wasted children. India with a wasting rate of 21 percent, is very close to the bottom of the international ladder, along with Sri Lanka, Djibouti and South Sudan.[45]

India has about 26 million wasted children of which nearly 9 million are severely wasted children. Pakistan has a higher stunting rate than India while Bangladesh and Indonesia have broadly comparable percentages. Nepal also performs slightly better in comparison, as noted in Box 2.4. However, where wasting rates are concerned, nearly all the countries are better placed than India, the surprising exception being Sri Lanka which has a wasting rate higher than India. Placed 113th (based on NFHS-4 figures) in 132 countries in stunting prevalence and 127th out of 130 countries in wasting prevalence, India has a fair way to go to reach the WHO 2025 goals.

Box 2.4   Nepal and Bangladesh perform marginally better than India

Neighbouring Nepal and Bangladesh still keep company with India in stunting percentages, but their performance is marginally better (Global Nutrition Report, 2018). Noticeable improvement in these countries over the past fifteen years is significant – Nepal from 57.1 percent in 2001 to 35.8 percent in 2016 and Bangladesh from 50.8 percent in 2000 to 36.8 percent in 2014. In addition to improvements in income and wealth, it has been driven by increased access of women to education and, in the case of Bangladesh, employment opportunities.

Women's access to health services, particularly during pregnancy, has increased significantly in both countries. The coverage and use of toilets has also increased in both countries, which has contributed to reduced stunting among children below the age of five. However, as in India, nutrition-specific interventions and programmes, especially in relation to IYCF practices, need a major boost to address the nutritional deficits of U5 children effectively.

There has been a decline in stunting but increase in wasting in India in the decade between NFHS-3 and 4. Wasting rate increased from 19.8 percent to 21 percent in the same decade. NFHS-4 data shows that all states and UTs have registered appreciable reductions in stunting rates, including the eight Empowered Action Group (EAG) states. The variations between states in the different nutrition indicators, viz., stunting, underweight and wasting, are noticeable. Stunting percentages range from a high of 48.3 percent in Bihar to a low of 19.7 percent in Kerala, underweight percentages from 47.8 percent (Jharkhand) to 16.1 percent (Kerala) and wasting rates from 27.6 percent (Dadra and Nagar Haveli) to 6.1 percent (Mizoram). In line with these indicators, Kerala is the top performer while Bihar is at the bottom of the Young Child Outcomes Index (Table 1.1). Interventions in nutrition have enabled Odisha to show marked improvement in the health status of children, as mentioned in Box 2.5.

Box 2.5 Odisha has shown noteworthy progress in child nutrition

Odisha's performance in improving nutrition and health status of children below the age of five in the last decade has been encouraging. Between 2005 and 2015, the IMR and U5MR declined from 65 and 91 to 40 and 49 respectively, institutional births increased from 36 percent to 85 percent, the proportion of women receiving at least four ANC visits increased from 37 percent to 62 percent, full immunisation of children increased from 52 percent to almost 79 percent and stunting among children reduced from 45 percent to 34.

High-level political and bureaucratic support for policies and programmes and a stable political environment facilitated a vision-led approach, capacity development for planning and implementation, and adequate allocation of funds. Improved road connectivity, availability of safe drinking water and increased thrust on gender equity and equality contributed to the state-wide scale up of the *Mamata* conditional cash transfer programme for pregnant and lactating women, promotion of education of girls, especially from the STs, and women's rights to property.

Nutrition-specific and nutrition-sensitive interventions, such as *Ami Bhi Paribu* (We too can), promoted positive deviance, the screening and referral of severely malnourished children for special health and nutrition support, and engagement of women's self-help groups for supplementary nutrition. The improvements in service delivery and infrastructure have contributed to behavioural change and increased public confidence in the state capacities and demand for services.

(Venkatesan, 2018)

Full immunisation of children in the 12–23-month age group has gone up from 43.5 percent in NFHS-3 to 62 percent in NFHS-4, still a far cry from the goal of universal immunisation. Early and exclusive breastfeeding rates are at 41.6 percent and 54.9 percent and only 9.6 percent of children between 6 and 23 months receive an adequate diet. What the figures clearly reveal is the need to stress interventions in the critical 'first thousand days' of life, from conception till the child reaches two years of age.

A comparison of states with different rates of stunting and wasting presents an interesting paradox. **The states with high stunting rates often display lower wasting rates but states faring well in stunting rates show very high wasting rates, including fairly high severe wasting rates.** While Madhya Pradesh, Jharkhand and Chhattisgarh could be expected to have high wasting rates, states like Karnataka, Gujarat and Maharashtra figure in the list of high wasting states. There are no specific studies as yet which analyse this phenomenon but one possible reason could be that since wasting is based on weight in relation to height, the states/districts which registered slower declines in stunting rates relative to underweight rates in the NFHS-4 (as compared to NFHS-3) would show lesser wasting rates as compared to states where stunting rates have fallen significantly in relation to underweight rates.

A comparison of some of these states is instructive in this regard. States like Bihar, Madhya Pradesh, Himachal Pradesh and Tripura showed significant decline in wasting rates over the decade because of a sharp decline in underweight rates relative to the decline in stunting rates. However, Maharashtra and Karnataka registered major increases in wasting rates in the same period even though their U5MR are far lower than Bihar and Madhya Pradesh. This seems to indicate that while the reach and quality of health services may be far better in Maharashtra and Karnataka, there is need to look into the causes for the very slow decline in underweight rates in these states.

Child nutrition and health indicators also vary across three other strata – gender, social background and rural-urban residence. While there is some difference in U5MR as between males and females, 51.5 versus 47.8 deaths per 1,000 live births, it is significant that U5MR in rural areas at 55.8 far outstrips the urban rate of 34.4, a pointer to the lower standards of healthcare in rural India. Again, the incidence of child mortality is far higher for socially disadvantaged groups like the SCs and STs as compared to the general population.

Variations in nutrition indicators are equally pronounced when one looks at variations between districts of a particular state and even between urban and rural differentials in a state. Although Odisha has a stunting rate of 34.1 percent, the districts of Cuttack and Puri have stunting rates of 15.3 percent and 16.1 percent respectively. In Karnataka, Mandya district has a stunting rate of 18.6 percent as compared to Koppal district with a stunting percentage of 55.8 percent. Barddhaman district in West Bengal shows a stunting prevalence in urban areas of 19.3 percent as opposed to 42.7 percent in rural areas.

There are also variations between ICDS projects within a district, which have significant implications for the directions that public policy needs to take, focussing on a much smaller sub-district area (lesser than even a block) as opposed to a district-level approach. While NFHS-4 data at the sub-district level is not available, the ICDS Monthly Progress Reports (MPR) of two states, Maharashtra and Karnataka, reveal huge differences in underweight rates of under-5 children within a district.

- Nashik district in Maharashtra has ICDS projects in Harsul and Tryambakeshwar in the western tribal hilly regions with underweight rates of 25.08 percent and 21.02 percent respectively. In contrast, Sinnar and Niphad ICDS projects in the prosperous irrigated eastern regions have underweight percentages of 4.31 percent and 4.92 percent respectively.[46]
- Gulbarga (Rural) and Chincholi ICDS projects in Gulbarga district of Karnataka have underweight rates of 9.90 percent and 11.47 percent respectively while two other ICDS projects in the district, Chitapur and Sedam, have underweight rates of 46.66 percent and 47.53 percent respectively.[47]

India is home to one-third of the world's stunted population. UNICEF (2014) reports that one among three children who are malnourished globally belong to India. Global Hunger Index (2018) ranked India at 103 out of 119 assessed countries with a score of 31.1. India fell under the category of 'serious' level of hunger with 14.8 percent undernutrition, 21 percent wasting and 38.4 percent stunting among children under 5 years of age.[48] Even poorer countries in the region like Bangladesh have better child survival and development indicators, which have been largely attributed to their focus on women's empowerment, increasing attention to children's health and childhood programmes.

Children in India fare poorly on several anthropometric indices that are used to estimate the prevalence of under-nutrition. Height-for-age, weight-for-age and weight-for-height capture the cumulative effect of under-nutrition during the life of the child. It has also been established that the risk of mortality is inversely related to children's height-for-age and weight-for-height.

About 21 percent children below age 5 in India are malnourished and only 9.6 percent of children between 6–23 months in the country receive an adequate diet (NFHS 4, 2015–16). Furthermore, 38 percent (1 in 3) of children under 5 years of age are stunted, 21 percent (1 in 5) of the children suffer from wasting, 36 percent of children under 5 years of age are underweight, 58 percent of children between 6 months–5 years are anaemic in the country and the total immunisation coverage in the country stood at 62 percent in 2015–2016.[49] Table 2.1 categorises states as per stunting levels.

Table 2.1 States by stunting (%), (NFHS 4)

Category A >38 (%)		Category B < 38 (%), >30 (%)		Category C < 30 (%)	
Bihar	48.3	Chhattisgarh	37.6	Sikkim	29.6
Uttar Pradesh	46.3	Assam	36.4	Arunachal Pradesh	29.4
Jharkhand	45.3	Karnataka	36.2	Manipur	28.9
Meghalaya	43.8	Maharashtra	34.4	Telangana	28.9
Madhya Pradesh	42.0	Odisha	34.1	Nagaland	28.6
Rajasthan	39.1	Haryana	34.0	Mizoram	28.0
Gujarat	38.5	Uttarakhand	33.5	Jammu and Kashmir	27.4
		West Bengal	32.5	Tamil Nadu	27.1
		Delhi NCR	32.3	Himachal Pradesh	26.3
		Andhra Pradesh	31.5	Punjab	25.7
				Tripura	24.3
				Puducherry	21.1
				Goa	20.1
				Kerala	19.7

Source: Ramani, 2019

Micro-nutrient deficiencies among children are major impediments to their development. Anaemia prevalence among children aged 6–59 months is more than 70 percent in Bihar, Madhya Pradesh, Uttar Pradesh, Haryana, Chhattisgarh, Andhra Pradesh, Karnataka and Jharkhand. Anaemia prevalence among children (6–59 months) is less than 50 percent in Goa, Manipur, Mizoram and Kerala. For the remaining states, the anaemia prevalence is in the range of 50 to 70 percent.

Anaemia prevalence among male and female children (6–59 months) was reported as 69 percent and 69.9 percent respectively; severe anaemia was reported for 3.2 percent male children and 2.7 percent female children. About 76.4 percent of children (6–59 months) in the lowest wealth index are suffering from anaemia, whereas 56.2 percent children of the highest wealth index are suffering from anaemia.[50]

With over 48 million children malnourished and high levels of stunting and micronutrient deficiencies, maternal nutrition and infant and young child feeding practices deserve particular attention. Infant and Young Child Feeding is determined by various factors, highlighted in Box 2.6. The national guidelines do refer to the crucial importance of initiating timely and appropriate complementary feeding as soon as the child is six months of age. The NFHS-4 reported that merely 9.6 percent children aged 6–23 months receive an adequate diet, including 14.3 percent of non-breastfeeding children and 8.7 percent of breastfeeding children, with urban indicators better in most cases by a few percentage points. It also shows a decline in timely complementary feeding rates from 52.6 percent to 42.7 percent (2015–2016) in the backdrop of increase in exclusive breastfeeding from 46.4 percent to 54.9 percent since NFHS-3.

Box 2.6   Various factors determine infant and young child feeding

Early initiation, delay or inadequacy (consistency, number of feeds and quantity), practice of the popular notion of 'feeding on demand', autonomy of decision-making, poor control over time spent on care and feeding, knowledge gap of mother/caregiver on complementary feeding, and the need to resume work by mother – are factors that determine quality infant and young child feeding.

Mothers' engagement in household chores, livelihood and respon-sibility of children leave them with little time and choice to cook and prepare age-appropriate complementary foods.[51] Women engaged in wage employment in the informal sector face considerable difficulty in feeding their infants and young children while caregivers (siblings, elders or neighbors) are unable to serve as an adequate alternative for care. They often lack childcare facilities at workplace or an alternative for childcare, which could allow them to practice exclusive breastfeed-ing or timely complementary feeding.

(Dasgupta et al., 2018)

Early initiation of complementary feeding is reported among low birth-weight and preterm infants.[52] Children are thus often initiated complemen-tary feeding before 6 months of age, and with food that is low in nutrition and diversity but high in calories (packaged/convenience foods). Children are primarily looked after by the caregivers who feed children "whenever the child is hungry" or "whenever the child asks for food."[53]

The states with high levels of chronic poverty and repeated cycles of male migration have poor Infant and Young Child Feeding (IYCF) indicators.[54] Children in households with multiple migration cycles, and who are left behind, face the consequences of early initiation – inadequacy as well as low quality of complementary feeding.[55] Feminisation of agriculture and wage labour with the increase in migration cycles and male migrants has implications on childcare and feeding (especially when elder siblings step in to take care). Over-burdened women get little time for food-gathering (green vegetables, fruits or tubers from commons) or cooking food separately for children, who end up eating diets meant for adults (with little diversity).[56]

The *Anganwadi* Workers (AWWs) and Accredited Social Health Activists (ASHAs) are trained to promote IYCF and counsel caregivers of children but the emphasis during training and the knowledge and focus of the work-ers is disproportionately on breastfeeding than age-appropriate complemen-tary feeding.[57] It is also important to note that children who received extra nutrition through government-run programmes from the time they were in their mothers' wombs until age three were 11 percent more likely to acquire a graduate degree than those who received them between ages 3 and 6.[58]

India is possibly in the throes of double burden of malnutrition (also known as malnutrition paradox), which is the coexistence of undernutrition along with overweight and obesity. This phenomenon is largely due to poor quality of food and dietary practices. According to a recent study, India had the second highest numbers of obese children in the world.[59] The findings of NFHS-4 that the number of obese people in India has doubled since NFHS-3 lends credence to this finding. Most of the states have experienced sharp rise in the number of obese people. Andhra Pradesh, Andaman and Nicobar, Puducherry and Sikkim have more than 30 percent of their populations falling under the 'obese' category. More than 10 percent of the population in Bihar, Madhya Pradesh, Meghalaya, Tripura and West Bengal is obese; doubling since NFHS-3. As Box 2.7 notes, malnutrition has severe economic consequences.

Box 2.7   Malnutrition results in economic loss

Calculations for adult productivity from Administrative Staff College (1998) and AERC (1998) studies show that stunting accounts for 1.4 percent, iodine deficiency for 0.3 percent and iron deficiency for 1.25 percent of loss in GDP in India, making a total of almost 3 percent GDP lost. The losses including childhood cognitive impairment associated with iron deficiency account for almost 1 percent of GDP in India, when cognitive and manual work are both factored in. At an estimated GDP of INR 13 million crores for 2017–18, this loss would translate to about INR 4 lakh crores annually.[60]

2.5 Safe water deficit, open defecation and poor hygiene undermine child health

Open defecation has been a perennial problem in India. **The high prevalence of several preventable communicable ailments has been attributed to the large number of households without access to toilets.** A National Sample Survey Office (NSSO) survey covering Rajasthan, Bihar, Madhya Pradesh and Uttar Pradesh, where two-fifths of India's rural population resides, reported over 68 percent open defecation in 2016. Although in 2015, the World Bank noted that 40 percent of the Indian population resorts to open defecation, a paper authored by its researchers in December 2018 stated, "A staggering 48 percent of Indians continue to defecate in the open despite large scale efforts from the government to raise awareness about the harmful aspects of open defecation and subsidize latrine construction, and growing latrine ownership."

There has been significant political commitment and policy thrust on construction of toilets in the last five years. According to the National Annual Rural Sanitation Survey 2018–2019, 93.3 percent of rural households had access to toilets, 96.7 percent of the people who had access to toilets used them and 90 percent of verified open defecation free villages were confirmed as Open-Defecation Free (ODF).

Many critics have expressed their scepticism regarding the strategy, data on toilet construction and household usage of the newly constructed toilets. In 2018, a study found that more rural Indians owned a latrine, but 44 percent still defecated in the open. Almost a quarter (23 percent) were latrine owners who defecated in the open largely due to deeply entrenched beliefs about caste 'impurity' associated with emptying latrine pits.[61] It found that most of the new structures were based on the single pit design that require undecomposed sludge to be emptied manually or through expensive suction machines whereas the government recommended twin-pits that allow decomposition of faecal sludge and are easy to empty, without disrupting the use of toilets.[62]

According to critics, *Swachh Bharat* has focussed on latrine construction without addressing adequately the attitudes to latrine pits, which are rooted in notions of purity and pollution. Further, open defecation among toilet owners has not declined significantly due to poor quality and maintenance issues. According to the 2017 national sample report,[63] no more than 56.4 percent of urban households, where 377 million people live, in India are connected to sewer lines (36.7 percent of rural areas, where 833 million people live, have drainage). Further, India has the capacity to treat only 37 percent of the sewage generated in urban areas.[64]

Initiatives for behavioural change comprise of IEC (Information Education and Communication), films like *Toilet, Halkaa* or *Gutrun Gutargun*, and a cadre of *swachhagrahis* who undertake inter-personal communication for achieving sustainable sanitation outcomes.[65] *Swachhagrahis* are being enrolled as motivators for bringing about behavioural change with respect to key sanitation practices in rural areas.

2.6 Key issues

2.6.1 Multi-pronged approach to public health has eluded policymaking

Complex problems like public health require complex solutions, which require strategic responses at different levels in multiple sectors and arenas. Experience across the world has shown that a holistic approach to development – which includes education, overall living environment, clean drinking water, proper sanitation and a reliable primary healthcare service – is critical for making a difference.

The rapid progress made by China on a range of child development indicators could be attributed to a multi-pronged approach. Similarly, Bangladesh has also adopted a more holistic strategy not only towards child development but also health and well-being of women. Similarly, the impressive improvement in the overall child health indicators in Malaysia, Bhutan, Lao PDR, Vietnam and several countries in South East Asia show that what works is a multi-pronged approach. In India, various state initiatives are noteworthy (refer to Box 2.8 and 2.9 for Maharashtra, and 2.10 for Kerala)

Box 2.8   Maharashtra's Rajmata Jijau Mother-Child Health and Nutrition Mission is noteworthy

The Mission was the offshoot of a successful effort from 2002 onwards in eight districts of Aurangabad division of Maharashtra (the 'Marathwada initiative') to reduce child malnutrition. The first of its kind State Nutrition Mission was set up with technical and financial support from UNICEF following media reports of child deaths due to malnutrition in the tribal areas. It began functioning in April 2005 from the city of Aurangabad and extended its scope in three phases, starting with the five tribal districts with highest child malnutrition in the first year, ten other districts with significant tribal populations in the second year and the entire state in the third year.

The attempt was to universalise the ICDS by registering every child with the AWC, monitor overall growth (instead of the weight till 2009) to identify and provide medical attention and appropriate nutrition to severely underweight children and those with faltering growth. The training of AWWs in IYCF regimens and capacity development of the supervisory and field staff of the ICDS and health departments was accorded priority and efforts were made to raise the staff morale by attending to various operational impediments, such as the vacancies, minor infrastructural requirements of the AWCs, and recognising their performance. They were encouraged to interact with the community regularly and hold growth monitoring meetings with caregivers.

The Mission promoted close convergence between the ICDS and the health department for a state-wide six-monthly campaign for Vitamin A supplementation and deworming of children 2007 onwards, which has shown promising increase in the percentage of children who received Vitamin A supplementation. This convergence was evident when the Child Development Centres, the Maharashtra version of the Nutritional Rehabilitation Centres, began in 2008 to tackle severe malnutrition. The Mission trained the ICDS and health staff in the WHO Growth Standards after the Central government adopted by them in August 2008.

Public policy and cooperation of the government departments and agencies at different levels of governance, convergence of the health and the ICDS machineries, especially from the block to the village levels, are crucial for improving outcomes for children at scale.

2.6.2 *Weak convergence and collaboration have hampered partnerships with civil society*

The merits of public-civil society partnership in reducing child malnutrition reduction have been recognised but the dialogue and engagement between governments and opinion makers and researchers on jointly evolving strategies to combat child malnutrition and promoting behavioural change in families and communities has been limited.

Active and enthusiastic State intervention can galvanise the CSOs.

Box 2.9 Bhavishya Alliance Initiative in Maharashtra: connecting government, corporates and NGOs

A multi-sectoral partnership, the Bhavishya Alliance Initiative was implemented from 2006 to 2011 in 10 blocks in five tribal districts and an urban ward in Mumbai in Maharashtra where child malnutrition was most prevalent. It developed pilot initiatives for rural and urban areas through a Change Lab process involving various organisations and sectors. The focus was on: (1) community empowerment and ownership; (2) strengthening ICDS and Health management systems; (3) capacity building and education; (4) management information systems; and (5) information, education and communication. Bhavishya Alliance led the coordination, project planning and monitoring of the outcomes while different government agencies, corporate bodies and NGOs were responsible for implementation.

A major lesson was that strong local administrative support and continued government funding is crucial for the success, upscaling and sustaining of such programmes. Most of the initiatives were promising but did not continue beyond the pilot stage due to bureaucratic apathy and delays. The State Nutrition and Health Mission provided a contact point but there was still a need to interact with different departments of the state government to enlist their support and cooperation in deployment of personnel and financial resources for implementing pilot projects. Staff turnover further undermined planning, implementation and upscaling efforts. The investment in the Change Lab process was never fully realised since many team members, both from the corporate and government sectors, were reassigned to new responsibilities within a year or two.

Community involvement was noticeable where those with major stake in successful outcomes, like adolescent girls and young women, were involved. However, funding constraints, lack of capable local NGOs and CBOs to assist in implementation, and inadequate or no support from the field-level government machinery prevented the implementation of pilot projects to all the 10 tribal blocks and an urban ward that were originally envisaged. As an integrated plan for implementation of various initiatives in different areas was lacking, a holistic strategy for reducing child malnutrition in an area like an ICDS block and a plan for upscaling successful pilot initiatives could not be developed. Funds from different sources were inadequate for creating a corpus that could meet overhead expenditures and fund some pilot initiatives. Absence of mechanisms to facilitate interactions among partners, limited high-level engagement with the government and the media, and distrust of the corporate sector in certain quarters weakened public policy advocacy.

A review of the Bhavishya Alliance advocated a multi-sectoral corporate, CSO and government partnership. It proposed corporate involvement through core business practices, public-private partnerships, philanthropy and social investment, and public policy dialogue, an important role of NGOs and CBOs in community mobilisation, monitoring project implementation and outcomes, and possibly fund raising. As it recognised that the CSOs have been wary of the role of corporates in such programmes, it expected trust building measures.

Four areas were identified for strategic thrust, viz.,

1   Binding agreements with the concerned government regarding the funding and upscaling of pilot initiatives, oversight and progress of projects;
2   Scaling up of successful pilot initiatives, including *anganwadi*-cum-day-care centres within and outside Maharashtra;
3   Engagement with corporates to advocate inclusion of child malnutrition reduction in their core business practices and their involvement in public-private partnerships and public policy advocacy; and
4   Association with organisations engaged in research and publication on education, health and nutrition for public education campaigns.

(Ramani, 2011)

The engagement with corporates, as was visualised in the Bhavishya Alliance Initiative, was also done at the level of utilisation of technology in Kerala to counter the high rates of infant and child mortality in the Attapady block in the Palakkad district. The initiative is notable for the government's commitment which allocated adequate financial and human resources for specific objectives and achieved them. It has been extended to three more blocks in tribal areas of other districts. A change in the political regime in Kerala in 2016 did not diminish the commitment to the reduction of child malnutrition and mortality.

Box 2.10   Kerala: determination to change matters

Attappady block has a tribal population of nearly 50 percent residing in the hilly areas of the Western Ghats. Socio-economic factors like alienation of tribals from their land, reduced access to forest produce and lack of gainful employment explain high maternal and child malnutrition rates in the area. Teams of experts visited the area following media reports of exceptionally high infant mortality in mid-2013. A team from the National Institute of Nutrition reported that the IMR in Attappady was sixty-six as compared to fourteen deaths per 1,000 live births in Kerala and observed very high rates of stunting, underweight and wasting in children attending the health camps at the Tribal Specialty Hospital in Kottathara in Palakkad. Another team from UNICEF identified weaknesses in the local healthcare systems in delivering proper ANC and PNC to women and attending to neonates and infants as a major cause of high rates of infant and child mortality.

The Kerala government swung into action almost immediately after public attention was drawn to the media reports. A Special Task Force under senior IAS officers devised measures for dealing with the problem. It commissioned Riddhi Management Services, a Kolkata based GIS solutions provider with extensive experience in the social sector, to customise the Jatak software for tracking the nutrition status of children to Attappady. The training of AWWs in the use of software enabled communication of the weight of each child in the AWC through voice data to the server every month. The health staff accessed the data on severe underweight children and measured their height at the nearest health facility to identify severely and moderately acute malnourished children. The Medical Officer examined these children and admitted those who had medical complications to the NRC in the block for six weeks. Other severely acute malnourished children were attended to at the community level employing CMAM protocols.

The health and ICDS workers conducted community outreach and organised 'Village Health Sanitation and Nutrition Days' to educate mothers on childcare and improving the nutrition and health status of their children. Supervisors use 'Nireeksha' *Anganwadi* Centre Monitoring System to provide information on the state of infrastructure and delivery of services through mobile telephony and web-based systems. The programme for treatment of severely acute malnourished children, employing the Jatak software, has been extended to three blocks of Wayanad, Kannur and Idukki districts.

Informed and intelligent use of real-time data forms the fulcrum for informed policymaking and implementation. The voluminous data generated monthly by the ICDS and health sectors has not been used to plan budgets, devise policies and deploy manpower. While the Mother and Child Tracking System (MCTS) was launched in 2011 by the Ministry of Health and Family Welfare (MoHFW), the government has never used the information to empower field health workers to deliver services more effectively to women and children. The ICDS MPRs are sent monthly by states to the MWCD, but not only is this data not in the public domain; no state uses this data (or improves on its accuracy) to reach children in need of interventions.

2.6.3 Legislation alone cannot change social norms and behaviours

The Central government has tried to control sex-selection through prenatal diagnostic techniques and female infanticide through legislation and socio-economic programmes. In the 1980s, the government and civil society recognised that prenatal diagnostic technologies were being misused for sex-selection due to deep-rooted socio-cultural preference for sons in India.

The Government of India enacted the Prenatal Diagnostic Techniques Act (PNDT) in 1994 and amended it further through the Pre-Conception and Prenatal Diagnostic Techniques (Regulation and Prevention of Misuse) (PCPNDT) Act in 2004 to foster positive change legally. The 2004 Act holds the service providers accountable for disclosing the sex of foetus but not the parents who demand and avail such services. In view of the persisting social norms that place a premium on a male child, its implementation has been weak. A study by civil society organisations found that only 600 cases had been booked under this law in fifteen years[66] with roughly twenty convictions.

The *Beti Bachao Beti Padhao* scheme seeks to address the declining child sex ratio through empowerment of girls. It was initiated in 2014–2015 in

100 selected districts low in CSR, covering all states and UTs, with three-fold objectives, viz., (1) prevention of gender biased sex selective elimination, (2) ensuring survival and protection of girl children and (3) ensuring education and participation of girl children. In 2015–2016, the scheme was introduced in sixty-one more districts.[67]

Three ministries, viz., MWCD, MoHFW and Ministry of Human Resource Development (MHRD), implement the scheme through the District Collector. The states are expected to operationalise multi-sectoral district action plans, and provide training to district level officials and frontline workers, who then make efforts to engage with children through interesting activities, including street plays, signature campaigns, *Guddi Gudda* (girls-boys) Boards[68] and live your dream for one day initiative (e.g., be a police woman).

The effectiveness and efficiency of the scheme is difficult to ascertain. According to an MWCD report in April 2016, forty-nine of the 100 districts covered under the *Beti Bachao Beti Padhao* programme witnessed a positive SRB but not the others.[69] Deep-rooted gender discriminatory social norms are difficult to change. There are concerns that the gender discriminatory norms may resurface once the scheme ends. Under-utilisation of the funds allocated for the scheme, indicative of sub-par implementation, has also been reported.

The growing popularity of surrogate parenthood has increased the risks for the care and upkeep of the child. There are guidelines but no law to regulate this phenomenon and to protect the rights of children born through surrogacy. The efforts to bring in a legislation have been going on for years. More recently, the Assisted Reproductive Technology (Bill), 2017, proposes a ban on the use of ART for sex selection and transfers the rights over the child after the birth from biological parents to the commissioning parents.[70] The bill has been criticised on the grounds that it could lead to weak health of poor surrogate mothers and their children, and that it violates the right of a child, albeit born through surrogacy, to know his or her biological parentage. Article 7 of the CRC upholds the child's right to know his or her origin and identity.[71]

Signalling political consensus on the urgent need to reduce child malnutrition, the government has begun setting priorities, specific quantitative targets and the areas where action is required, identifying the implementing agencies, and guiding efforts at the state and local levels. The National Nutrition Policy in 1993 prioritised children below six years as a high-risk group, but it took the National Nutrition Strategy (NNS) in 2017 to provide a roadmap for child malnutrition reduction in India. This strategy focuses on interventions in the states, districts and specific pockets, identified by the NITI Aayog and the MWCD using a new Nutrition Monitoring System (NMS), as lagging behind others in improving child nutrition status.

The MWCD and the NITI Aayog have set up the National Nutrition Mission (NNM) or the *Poshan Abhiyaan* with specific goals for time-bound improvements in the nutrition status of under-6 children and pregnant women/lactating mothers. These targets, listed in Table 2.2, are undoubtedly ambitious as they are expected to be achieved over a three-year period beginning 2017–18.

Poshan Abhiyaan has been allocated a three-year budget of INR 904.6 million commencing from 2017–18. All the states and districts will be covered in a phased manner, i.e., 315 districts in 2017–2018, 235 districts in 2018–2019 and the remaining districts in 2019–2020. More than 100 million people are expected to benefit from this programme.

The NNM is a comprehensive approach towards raising nutrition levels in India. It is expected to map and galvanise the existing schemes, put in place a robust convergence mechanism, undertake Information and Communications Technology (ICT) based real-time monitoring, and provide incentives to states and Union Territories for achieving targets. At the community level, it is expected to introduce measurement of height of children, nutrition resource centres, and social audits at AWCs, provide IT based tools to AWWs while rationalising reporting requirements and mobilise communities on nutrition through *Jan Andolan*.

The inauguration of *Swachh Bharat Mission* (SBM) on 2 October 2014, heralded the high priority of sanitation on the government's agenda. In addition to the creation of quality infrastructure and delivery of services, a greater thrust on behavioural change for improved sanitation is required especially as attitudes and practices related to sanitation are rooted in notions of purity and pollution.

To address the environmental issues, the Indian government has about 200 laws dealing with environmental protection, and environmental regulations

Table 2.2 Poshan Abhiyaan: programme targets

S. No.	Objective	Target
1	Prevent and reduce stunting in children (0–6 years)	By 6% (@ 2% p.a.)
2	Prevent and reduce undernutrition (underweight prevalence) in children (0–6 years)	By 6% (@ 2% p.a.)
3	Reduce the prevalence of anaemia among young children (6–59 months)	By 9% (@ 3% p.a.)
4	Reduce the prevalence of anaemia among women and adolescent girls in the age group of 15–49 years	By 9% (@ 3% p.a.)
5	Reduce Low Birth Weight (LBW)	By 6% (@ 2% p.a.)

Source: MWCD, GoI. National Nutrition Mission: Administrative Guidelines

dating back to the 1970s. As various types of calamities occur in different regions due to variations in geographical, topographical and geological features, many states (e.g., Odisha) have formulated their own State Climate Change Action Plan.

But none of the laws and policies related to environment have considered the implications for children, especially their protection before, during and after a disaster. The inclusion of child-focussed disaster risk management and reduction in the disaster mitigation policy with sound investments in developing safe infrastructures, particularly well-located schools and health facilities with good road access is being discussed in several government and CSO fora.

2.6.4 *The availability, utilisation and quality of services faces multiple issues*

The performance of AWCs under the ICDS is by and large uneven with some states being active and others being passive or dormant in implementing various programmes. A longitudinal study of 200 AWCs in six states,[72] viz., Tamil Nadu, Himachal Pradesh, Maharashtra, Chhattisgarh, Rajasthan and Uttar Pradesh, showed considerable improvement in the services between 2006 and 2016.[73] The proportion of mothers who reported having an AWC in their neighbourhood increased from 72 to 85 percent. The availability of nutrition for children under 6 years of age, and weight monitoring services at the AWC also improved. However, 59 percent of mothers reported that they distributed THR among family members, thereby reducing the share of children.[74]

The proportion of centres open for more than four hours was higher in Tamil Nadu, Himachal Pradesh and Maharashtra (termed as 'active states') while Chhattisgarh, Rajasthan and Uttar Pradesh were termed as 'dormant states' due to their weaker performance. Home visits were a low 46 percent in the active states, and even lower at 30 percent in dormant states. Among these, the active states score better than the all-India average on the overall Environment Index, as the YCEI (Table 1.2) focussing on policy and environment enablers shows, while the three dormant states are poor performers, scoring lower than the all-India average Index. States like Karnataka (Box 2.11) and Odisha (Box 2.12) have initiated noteworthy interventions in terms of *anganwadis* and AWW salaries and community participation respectively.

Nutritional health education meetings with mothers showed a decline between 2004 and 2014. The exception was Maharashtra where they increased ostensibly due to the NRHM, which celebrates village health and nutrition days at the AWCs. The meeting under ICDS and Village Health and Nutrition Day (VHND) engaged mainly with mothers. As mothers and grandparents come to the centre more, low rates of home visits points to the possibility of low engagement with fathers on parenting.

Box 2.11   Karnataka: Mathrupoorna – when good economics and politics go hand in hand

Significant regional economic and social disparities are manifested clearly in the inter-district variations in child nutrition status in Karnataka. Nine districts, all located in the northern parts of the state, are part of the NNM, and three of them, Koppal, Yadgir and Gulbarga, having child stunting rates of over 50 percent. Even overall, Karnataka is characterised by stunting and underweight percentages in the mid-30s and very high rates of wasting and severe wasting (26.1 percent and 10.5 percent respectively).

In view of the role of maternal health in child malnutrition, the Government of Karnataka initiated the comprehensive maternal nutrition, *Mathrupoorna* programme in February 2017 on a pilot basis in four backward talukas in different geographical regions. Drawing on the lessons from the pilots the government rolled it out across the state on 2 October 2017. The programme provides a full cooked midday meal to pregnant and lactating women to bridge the gap between what they eat and what they should eat. They receive milk and eggs in addition to calcium and iron supplements.

Whereas the SNP provides only INR 9.50 per mother per day, the Karnataka government spends INR 21. With over eight lakh women already enrolled in this programme in 65,911 AWCs, the state government will incur an annual expenditure of INR 60 million, including its share of the official SNP component.

Karnataka has also taken a number of proactive measures to improve ICDS outreach and improve the quality of nutrition to under-6 children. All children in AWCs receive two eggs twice a week, with a five days a week egg supply to severely underweight children throughout the state and to moderate underweight children in five northern districts of the state. The *Ksheera Bhagya* milk supply scheme provides whole milk to over 10 million children aged 6–59 months five days a week.

The monthly payment of INR 8,000 to the AWWs and INR 4,000 to the AWHs is among the highest in the country, which is aimed at motivating them to deliver the highest quality of services to mothers and children. They are also eligible for medical reimbursement, paid leave and a contributory pension scheme. All AWCs in the state have been geotagged to enable monitoring from higher levels to improve service delivery. Efforts on a pilot scale have been initiated to track the nutrition status of every under-5 child through the use of online software to enable health and nutrition services to reach the child in time.

The supplementary nutrition component of the ICDS has often been criticised for corruption, pilferage and delays. A centralised system supplies food for cooking to AWCs across the country resulting in recurring complaints of poor quality of grains and limited storage space. While one of the responsibilities of the AWWs is to plan the menu based on local food availability for supplementary nutrition, they do not have any control over the quantity and quality of the supplies.

Several independent enquiries have found that neither THR nor hot-cooked meals are being provided to U6 children in some states,[75] and leakages often impede spending of the allocated funds for THR/hot cooked meals for the intended beneficiaries. Instances of discrimination against children on grounds of their caste and disabilities have also been reported. Furthermore, the NNM neglects the non-food component of these measures. For the Take Home Ration (THR), for example, the design with regard to under-3 children is flawed, and there are serious logistic issues in it as the mother is expected to collect the THR, which may not be possible always.

Severe Acute Malnutrition (SAM) programmes in different states also do not follow any systematic pattern. The decision to entrust the recording of height of children to the AWW has not produced the desired results. The experience with getting AWWs in some states to record lengths/heights has not been encouraging.

The Supreme Court issued orders in 2001 and 2004 and followed up with a landmark judgment in 2006 to ensure a time-bound 'universalisation with quality' of the ICDS. It prescribed the guarantee of a minimum nutrition provision and supported decentralisation of procurement by eliminating contractors and engagement of local Self-Help Groups (SHGs) and *Mahila Mandals* in supply and distribution to improve the system and services.

Box 2.12　Reorganisation of the delivery system in Odisha has led to greater community participation

Following the Supreme Court order, the State Government of Odisha took steps in April 2011 to decentralise, streamline and strengthen the supplementary nutrition component of the ICDS with greater participation from local communities. Contractors have been replaced by Women's Self-Help Groups (SHGs) for providing the beneficiaries with ration according to a standard weekly menu, which meets the prescribed protein and calorie norms and is within the allocated cost. About 71 percent of the respondents in a social audit reported that the menu chart was being followed. The AWWs procure all materials locally, except rice and wheat, to curb pilferage during transportation.[76]

2.6.5 *Financial resource allocation is inadequate*

The Government of India provides 50 percent financial support to the ICDS Supplementary Nutrition Programme (SNP). The norms for SNP have been reviewed in November 2017, but it needs to be assessed whether the existing norms need to be revised upwards to provide each child a healthy nutritious nutrition supplement. Budgets for SNP are based on coverage. This would mean that states with poor coverage have lower allocation. There is need to align budgets to the child population and ensure universal participation. There is also a need to provide additional allocations to states that have poor child indicators.

Other components such as honorarium to AWWs, capacity development and provision for ECCE materials also need to be enhanced. All childcare workers, including *Anganwadi* Workers and helpers, ASHA workers and crèche workers need to be recognised as professional workers and remuneration fixed based on their role as full time workers.

Even the funds allocated are not properly utilised. Independent reports suggest that there are states where neither the THR nor hot cooked meals are being provided to U6 children. There is also the issue of leakages, i.e., whether the amount shown as spent on THR/hot cooked meals actually reaches the intended beneficiaries.

The issue of accountability is often referred to in the public and policy discussions, but mechanisms that would permit comprehensive oversight at all levels are not in place. Media have been reporting cases of misappropriation of social sector funds (e.g., SNP) of the Centre and the states, and some CSOs and networks often hold social audits or *jan sunvayees* to verify the claims of various government departments through feedback from local communities. But a more systematic arrangement needs to be considered.

The budgetary allocations and the gaps are detailed in Chapter 6

2.6.6 *Capacities and competencies are severely limited*

The delivery of services that are essential for arresting child mortality and ensuring child and maternal health and nutrition is dependent on the ASHAs, ANMs and AWWs. **Common concerns of these frontline workers relate to inadequate remuneration, weak supervision, insufficient pre-service and in-service training, weak supervision and lack of coaching and mentoring.** A system for ongoing capacity building of AWWs under the ICDS has not evolved. Centralisation of administrative and financial powers at the level of the ICDS Directorate or Commissionerate has led to major inefficiencies in programme performance. While the position of staff in place is good in the AWCs, the vacancies are significantly high at supervisory levels, namely Child Development Project Officers (CDPOs) (both urban and rural/tribal) and supervisors or *Mukhya Sevikas*, which negatively impacts their ability to perform their roles.

There is an overall shortage of health personnel in remote tribal areas in particular, and the shortage of Statistical Assistants in CDPO and district offices creates difficulties for data management.

2.6.7 Women's empowerment efforts and maternal entitlements fall short

Given the critical role of the mother's health and physical condition in foetal growth and nutritional status of the child, attempts at maternity support have been made since 1987, starting with the Dr Muthulakshmi Reddy Childbirth Assistance Scheme in Tamil Nadu. A few other states introduced similar schemes in the following years and the Central Government stepped in with the National Maternity Benefit Scheme (NMBS) in 1995–1996, which offered a one-time payment of INR 500 between eight to twelve weeks before childbirth. The NMBS was subsumed into the *Janani Suraksha Yojana* in 2005, which made payment to the mother conditional on institutional delivery.[77]

The Scheme introduced by the Tamil Nadu Government could be said to be the inspiration for the provision of maternity benefit of not less than INR 6,000 to the pregnant woman and lactating mother in the National Food Security Act (NFSA), 2013. The law entitles the pregnant woman/lactating mother to free meals during pregnancy and for six months after childbirth through the local AWC.

However, the *Pradhan Mantri Matru Vandana Yojana* implemented since 1 January 2017, has diluted the provisions of the NFSA and provides only INR 5,000 to the mother, and that too for only one living child. Tamil Nadu, Andhra Pradesh and Telangana have been providing hot cooked meals to pregnant women and lactating mothers. Karnataka has now joined them with the launching of the *Mathru Poorna* maternal nutrition scheme on 2 October 2017.

2.7 Recommendations and action points

2.7.1 Focus on reducing perinatal and neonatal mortality

The Central and state governments should accelerate their efforts to curb child mortality and malnutrition, especially in the disadvantaged geographical pockets that are lagging behind.

Priority interventions in problem regions: The state governments should employ strategies for the reduction of perinatal mortality rates and the NMR (e.g., home-based neonatal care), promote registration of every pregnancy with the ICDS and public health services, and seek the expansion of the coverage of maternal nutrition, ANC and PNC for major favourable spin offs for child health and well-being.

Preventive health interventions through the Primary Health Centres (PHCs): The PHCs need to maintain lists of high-risk mothers, viz., those with a history of anaemia, previous obstetric complications and high blood pressure, and ensure skilled birth attendance.

Where the IMR is below the national average, the state governments need to bolster their investment in management of various causes of infant mortality. But where the national goal of IMR reduction has been achieved, they should consider integrating community genetic services in the PHCs for the control of birth defects.

Parental entitlements: Universal maternity entitlements, discussed in Chapter 5, could enable the mother and child to stay in close proximity and facilitate breastfeeding and emotional bonding.

Parental and family counselling: ICDS and health services in nearly all states need to intensify the counselling of mothers, caregivers and families in responsive childcare, especially in the period of infancy, covering the areas of early and exclusive breastfeeding, full immunisation and introduction of timely complementary feeding.

2.7.2 Direct attention to states and regions with high levels of child malnutrition

MWCD and NITI Aayog could bring some urgency to malnutrition reduction by coordinating implementation of measures through the *Poshan Abhiyaan*. Such a platform also enables sharing of good practices and experiences among states. The *Poshan Abhiyaan* should serve as a clearing house for keeping implementation machinery at the state and local levels informed of the latest developments in international nutrition practices.

The *Poshan Abhiyaan* targets are ambitious but with political and administrative commitment they offer an opportunity for galvanising national efforts to reduce child malnutrition and achieve the SDG targets.

Identifying problem regions for priority interventions can be a viable strategy.

Priority interventions in problem states and districts: The focus should be on the states with poor child development indices and districts which are the worst-off in terms of stunting, wasting and underweight indices. The NNM identified 315 districts for coverage in the first year, 235 for the second year and the balance of all states and UTs for 2019–2020. Utilisation of technology could help identify the areas with the worst child nutrition indicators where the efforts to reduce malnutrition could be intensified to optimise outcomes for young children.

2.7.3 Harness multi-sectoral expertise for capacity development

Involvement of reputed persons with expertise in areas which have an impact on child malnutrition, such as agriculture, education, health, nutrition, livelihoods and women's empowerment, would help contribute to changes in public systems and governance and in shaping public policy in these areas. Universities, nonprofits and think tanks should be engaged to analyse the extent and nature of child undernutrition, especially in those districts and blocks identified as particularly vulnerable. Their research inputs should be used to tailor policies and programmes to align with what mothers and children really need. Wherever possible, the assistance of active NGOs should be used to supplement the activities of field-level functionaries, provide crucial technical inputs to them and monitor the health and nutrition status of U6 children. Print and electronic media can be used to report on how well programmes are really working on the ground and the responses of communities and families to programmes aimed at their welfare.

Private sector as a partner in malnutrition reduction: The corporate sector has been recognised as an important stakeholder in the collective efforts to provide basic services with quality and arrest malnutrition. The government needs to secure a regulatory regime which could ensure the withdrawal of products injurious to the future health and nutrition of the mother and child along with transparency and accountability. Alongside, it needs to foster a collaborative environment to facilitate partnerships for health and nutrition-specific initiatives.

2.7.4 Ensure smart allocation and efficient utilisation of financial resources

General budgets of state governments should incorporate a specific 'child budget' which focuses on U6 children. The budgets of the Departments of Health (DoH) and Departments of Women and Child Development (DWCD) in particular should list schemes or programmes that directly or indirectly impact on the health and nutrition status of the U6 child. The budgets should be disaggregated to the ICDS project level to facilitate monitoring of the allocations to (and expenditures in) the areas with the highest incidences of child malnutrition and child (and infant) mortality. Chapter 6 refers to this in greater detail.

As referred to earlier, the Central and state government should seriously consider augmenting its share of the monthly honorarium paid to AWWs/ AWHs, ASHA and crèche workers in order to motivate these critical field functionaries. Simultaneously, they should work out financial allocations with a view to reaching the package of services offered by the programme to the entire mother and child population and revise the cost norms (e.g., for SNP) periodically to provide realistic financial support to mothers and children.

Timely allocation of funds from the Centre to states and further on to PRIs and urban bodies could enhance performance, encourage innovations to deal with barriers and bottlenecks in implementation at the field level and promote accountability for outcomes. The Government of India could consider drawing up a scheme for rewarding better performing states with higher fund allocation even while tackling the inefficiencies in service delivery in the states with relatively poor performance.

An independent mechanism for verifying the efficiency of SNP service delivery needs to be devised to ensure that limited social sector funds (of the Centre and states) are used efficiently and the leakages are plugged.

PRIs and urban local government bodies must provide for schemes aimed at improving the nutrition and health status of women and U6 children in their annual budgets. Maharashtra has a provision where a percentage of the revenue received from government is earmarked by rural local bodies for schemes designed to improve the welfare of women and children. Many of these schemes are uncoordinated, often duplicating programmes of other departments. Specific funding for maternal and child health and nutrition would help augment receipts from the Government of India and state governments. This would also enthuse elected local government officials to play a more active role in promoting schemes that further the objective of enhancing maternal and child health and nutrition.

Since financial resources are always a problem, the thrust of action could be areas that are worst off in terms of stunting, wasting and being underweight. For instance, the worst affected blocks in the worst affected districts drawn from NITI Aayog's list of aspirational districts.[78] Technology could be employed to identify specific blocks with the worst child nutrition indicators. Intensive efforts to reduce malnutrition in these blocks could provide valuable lessons for subsequent upscaling and facilitate interventions that respond to local conditions. For instance, the THR could comprise of locally available nutritious foods.

Focus on child malnutrition in urban areas. India's urban areas, especially its sprawling urban agglomerations, with their slum areas and areas where the socially disadvantaged are concentrated, need special focus. With moderate and severe malnutrition levels as significant in some urban ICDS projects as some of the more severely affected rural ICDS projects, greater municipal government involvement is essential if urban child malnutrition is to be successfully tackled. Municipal corporations and larger municipal councils need to take on the responsibility in their areas, while smaller municipal council areas could continue to be looked after by *Zilla Parishads*.

2.7.5 Decentralise and recalibrate the ICDS

The ICDS should be overhauled to facilitate an integrated set of services, including improved health and nutrition services for the holistic development of children under-6 age group. The NFHS-4 has provided evidence that nutrition and health interventions influence both height and weight-related growth patterns in the first five years of life. The role of caregiver/family counselling by ICDS/health frontline workers will be particularly crucial in initiating nutrient supplementation and improved hygiene to tackle stunting or chronic malnutrition.

In a phased manner, *anganwadis* should also make provision for crèche services. This is critical to ensure enhanced participation of the under threes as well as ensure adequate care of the young child as most poor households with working women are unable to take care of their young ones. The need for crèches has been spelt out in great detail in Chapter 5.

Decentralisation of management: The ICDS management and supervision of AWCs should be decentralised to the district level to facilitate adaptation of inputs to ground level realities and local needs. The state governments should allocate discretionary funds to the districts for innovations and responses to local issues.

Innovations for human resource development: Innovative policies are required to address human resource deficit, either through contractual appointments and/or making postings in such locations, along with meeting desired service standards, mandatory for future career advancement. Speeding up recruitment processes, including at the Public Service Commission levels, is crucial to achieve the ambitious goals set by the NNM.

Two-pronged approach to tackle acute and chronic malnutrition: Community-based Management of Acute Malnutrition (CMAM) and Nutritional Rehabilitation Centres (NRC) should be set up in the vicinity of AWCs with a higher preponderance of SAM children. The follow-up of such SAM children for a year after their discharge from the treatment should be mandatory to prevent relapse and continued chronic malnutrition since frequent episodes of weight loss tend to impact linear growth.

The AWW could continue with the practice of recording the weight of the child, and the health staff should step in to examine all children whose heights fall in the < -3SD category and treat them for SAM through NRCs/CMAM. This practice needs to be followed in every state so that systematic identification and treatment of SAM children is possible.

Multiple and decentralised modes of food delivery: The Central government should encourage various channels of food delivery to make available local and culturally appropriate food practices and facilitate monitoring. The state governments should provide options of childcare, including child feeding support for children who are left unsupervised due to lack of adult/family care. In addition, they should consider expanding the scope of midday meals schemes to public and private pre-schools. Additional provisions of breakfast to freshly cooked lunches, served in hygienic environments, could benefit young children immensely.

Comprehensive SAM programme: The ICDS should link the AWCs with high preponderance of SAM children with NRCs or CMAM centres. These children should be monitored for at least a year after their discharge from treatment to prevent relapse and the chances of continued chronic malnutrition due to the impact of frequent episodes of weight loss on linear growth.

2.7.6 *Invest in capacity development and motivation of frontline workers*

The AWWs and AWHs should receive due appreciation and recognition through better remuneration and working conditions. Increased remuneration, together with funds to carry out localised activities, including minor purchases and repairs and timely payments could motivate them to give their best. Capacity enhancement, supportive supervision and the resolution of their problems at the supervisory level could motivate them and create enabling conditions for performance and accountability.

Improved remuneration for the frontline workers: Central and state governments need to revisit the issue of remuneration and professionalisation of all childcare workers, including AWWs, AWHs, ASHA and crèche workers. The Central government should consider raising its share in the payment to AWWs from the existing national level average remuneration of INR 4,500 to INR 10,000, benchmarked to the wholesale price index (WPI) and increased on a pro-rata basis for each rise in the WPI. The monthly honorarium of INR 4,500 in addition to the incentives for ASHA should be increased to INR 8,000 plus performance incentives, with pro rata revision of the remuneration with increases in WPI. For the AWH and crèche worker, the payment should be 10,000 and 8,000 INR respectively, the additional budgetary requirement for which is detailed in Chapter 6.

Workforce for nutrition education and counselling: Although nutrition education and counselling is a component of the *Poshan Abhiyaan*, a workforce to carry it out has to be provided for. In case the ASHA worker is to be vested with the task for health and nutrition counselling, allocation for their capacity development needs to be increased substantially.

Supportive supervision: The government should take immediate steps to fulfil supervisory level vacancies in order to improve supervision and monitoring of the functioning of AWCs and roll out a comprehensive capacity development programme to enable the supervisors to provide technical support to the frontline workers, including coaching and mentoring, in addition to monitoring of processes and outcomes.

Accountability for performance and outcomes: The government should establish a system of accountability for improving the health and nutrition status of children from the top of bureaucracy, viz., the Secretaries in the DoH and DWCDs (and the departmental heads under them, like the Director of Health Services, the Mission Director, NHM and the ICDS Commissioner/Director), to the middle level functionaries, the CDPOs and supervisors, to the frontline workers.

2.7.7 *Reinvigorate national campaigns and parental education programmes*

Two national flagship programmes, *Swachh Bharat* and *Poshan Abhiyaan*, provide windows of opportunities for sustained nationwide campaigns and parental education programmes.

National nutrition education campaign: The government should mount an overarching nationwide door-to-door nutrition education campaign, similar to the Pulse Polio Immunisation campaign, to reach every household. While raising public awareness about the cumulative burden of poor nutrition and frequent childhood illnesses on the overall health and development, its design should have scope for addressing local specificities. The key messages should highlight the importance of locally available food sources, improved food intake of mothers and regular feeding of babies from the time they are weaned.

Expansion of family counselling: The Central and state governments need to assume greater responsibility for family counselling on good nutrition practices. ICDS and health services in nearly all states need to intensify the counselling of mothers, caregivers, and families in proper childcare, especially in the period of infancy, covering the areas of early and exclusive breastfeeding, complete immunisation and introduction of timely complementary feeding.

Renewed focus on water handling, hygiene and use of improved toilets: Hygiene and improved practices for handling and storing water should be integrated in the *Swachh Bharat*, the national sanitation programme, for influencing routine practices of communities and households to curb the spread of infectious diseases.

School-based health and nutrition programmes: Comprehensive programme(s) need to be designed, tested and rolled out to enable regular check-ups of young children, to initiate them to healthy food habits, regular intake of water, proper handwashing and hygienic practices, and to enrol those who have been identified as malnourished or have other health issues for special interventions.

2.7.8 *Technological solutions can improve systems, services and outreach*

Improvement in data generation systems: Central and state governments need to invest in improving the quality of data generation systems and harnessing the potential of technology for identifying geographical areas as well as specific disadvantaged groups that require concerted action.

Dissemination of quality data: The data related to young child development, especially the utilisation of health, nutrition, water and sanitation services and social behaviour in terms of hygienic practices should be placed in the public domain without delay to enable other stakeholders the opportunity to develop support strategies and plans.

Key Messages

- A holistic approach to development, including public awareness and parental education, improved living environment with access to clean drinking water, proper sanitation and a reliable primary healthcare service is critical for making a difference to the health and nutritional standards among children.
- India continues to contribute the highest number of neonatal, infant and under-5 deaths in the world notwithstanding the significant decline in IMR in the last two decades.
- An estimated 4.8 million children of the 26.9 million born every year in India have low birth weight. Many are born with congenital defects and disabilities, and many are vulnerable to infections. Poor nutrition, inadequate immunisation, low access to safe drinking water and well-maintained sanitation facilities and overall environmental hygiene exacerbate the situation.
- Persistently adverse child sex ratio indicates deep-rooted gender bias and neglect of the girl child. The health and nutrition status of mother is intricately linked to pre-term birth and impacts the health and nutrition status of infants and young children.
- Economic status of the households influences the availability, accessibility and utilisation of basic health, nutrition and social development services. Sub-optimal functioning of government systems, flagship programmes and schemes in many states subject the very poor and marginalised to greater distress and further compounds inequality in wealth.
- Child nutrition cannot be ensured through the supply of food or meals alone. The presence of an adult caregiver who can feed the child, maintain hygiene and provide adequate care is equally important.

Notes

1 SRS, 2019.
2 NFHS-3 and NFHS-4. Retrieved from http://rchiips.org/nfhs/pdf/NFHS4/India. pdf; date of access: 29 October 2019.
3 Ministry of Statistics and Programme Implementation, 2018.
4 ICMR, 2016.
5 Central Bureau of Health Intelligence et al., 2015.
6 India's Infant Mortality Down 42% in 11 Years Yet Higher than Global Average.
7 WHO, 2017a.
8 Ibid.
9 UNICEF et al., 2018.
10 Data: Children in India 2018: A Statistical Appraisal, 2018.
11 Balarajan et al., 2013.

12 Ending Preventable Maternal, Newborn and Child Deaths, n.d.
13 ICMR, 2016.
14 World Bank, 2017.
15 Gupta et al., 2012.
16 NFHS 3
17 NFHS 4, India Report, p. 187.
18 NFHS 3 National Report, Vol. 2, p. 183.
19 Salve, 2018.
20 Guillot and Allendorf, 2009.
21 It is a medical term used to refer to the group of blood diseases and disorders affecting the red blood cells.
22 Sharma, 2013.
23 Ibid.
24 Identification and Assessment, n.d.
25 Gaudin, 2009.
26 National Commission for Protection of Child Rights and ChildFund India, 2017.
27 Ibid.
28 Ibid.
29 See, www.indiaspend.com/mothers-education-household-wealth-decide-survival-of-infants-in-india-51235/; date of access: 2 December 2019.
30 Mukherjee, 2017 (NHP 2015, Table 3.1.6, p. 103).
31 Planning Commission, Government of India, 2013. The list also included interventions aimed at parents and guardians, such as a basket of contraceptives and safe abortion services, awareness regarding RTI/STI and the importance of helmets on two-wheelers and seat-belts in four wheelers and advice against tobacco and alcohol consumption, which also impact children.
32 Full ANC coverage includes at least four ANC visits, at least one tetanus toxoid injection and iron folic acid tablets or syrup taken for 100 or more days.
33 Rudra, 2017.
34 NFHS 3.
35 Ramachandran, 2018.
36 Rudra, 2017.
37 Ibid.
38 Vranda and Sekar, 2011.
39 Kousky, 2016.
40 Pross et al., 2016.
41 The Cost of a Polluted Environment: 1.7 Million Child Deaths a Year, n.d.
42 Chandra, 2015.
43 WHO, 2017a.
44 CNNS (2016–18) assessed the nutritional status of children from birth to 19 years. The survey collected data of more than 112,000 children and provided state-level estimates. India Preliminary Fact Sheet. Retrieved from https://nhm.gov.in/index1.php?lang=1&level=2&sublinkid=1332&lid=713; date of access: 22 November 2019.
45 NFHS-4 figures for India, Global Nutrition Report 2016 for the other countries.
46 Maharashtra ICDS MPR March 2017.
47 Karnataka ICDS MPR October 2016.
48 Global Hunger Index India, n.d.
49 NFHS 4.
50 MOSPI, 2017, p. 11.
51 Nair et al., 2014.
52 Chaturvedi et al., 2016.

53 Ibid.
54 Ibid.
55 Horo, 2017.
56 Dasgupta et al., 2018.
57 Breastfeeding Promotion Network of India (BPNI).
58 Nandi et al., 2018.
59 Murray et al., 2017.
60 Cited in Horton, 1999.
61 Research Institute for Compassionate Economics and Accountability Initiative, 2018.
62 Ibid.
63 Swachhta Status Report 2016, n.d.
64 NSSO, 2017.
65 July 2018 circular on revised guidelines for swachhagrahis. Swacch Bharat Mission, n.d.
66 Public Health Foundation of India et al., 2010.
67 MWCD, 2016. Beti Bachao Beti Padhao Scheme Expanded in Additional 61 Districts, n.d.
68 Ministry of Women and Child Development, n.d.
69 Cited in Save the Children, 2018.
70 Department of Health Research, 2017.
71 European Institute for Law and Justice, 2012.
72 Dreze et al., 2006.
73 Kapoor et al., 2016.
74 Ibid.
75 Media reports have noted, for example, that THR or hot-cooked meals were not provided in Uttar Pradesh. See https://scroll.in/pulse/829945/uttar-pradesh-starved-an-old-nutrition-scheme-to-fund-a-new-one-neither-is-working; date of access: 15 November 2019. The report highlighted that hot-cooked meals had not been provided for a year. Likewise, in Maharashtra, it was decided in 2017 to replace hot cooked meals with ready to cook food mixes in *anganwadis*. See www.business-standard.com/article/economy-policy/children-to-lose-their-hot-cooked-meals-in-maharashtra-117082600036_1.html; date of access: 15 November 2019.
76 UNDP, 2017.
77 Venkatesan, 2018.
78 In January 2018, the Government of India launched the *Transformation of Aspirational Districts* programme, which has identified districts across the country with relatively low levels of progress for more focussed policy intervention to ensure inclusivity and sustainability with growth.

Bibliography

Balarajan, Y., S.V. Subramanian and W.W. Fawzi, 2013. Maternal Iron and Folic Acid Supplementation Is Associated with Lower Risk of Low Birth Weight in India. *The Journal of Nutrition*. Vol 143. No 8, pp. 1309–1315.

Barker, D.J.P., 1998. *Mothers, Babies and Health in Later Life* (2nd Ed.). Churchill Livingstone, Edinburgh, London, New York, Philadelphia, San Francisco, Sydney and Toronto.

Beti Bachao Beti Padhao Scheme Expanded in Additional 61 Districts, n.d. Retrieved from https://pib.gov.in/newsite/PrintRelease.aspx?relid=136289; date of access: 29 October 2019.

Breastfeeding Promotion Network of India (BPNI). *Report on Capacity Building Training Course on Infant and Young Child Feeding Counselling for Development of Middle Level Trainers in 2 Districts of Punjab (NRHM)*. Retrieved from www.bpni.org/Training/Report-capacity-building-IYCF-MLTs-Punjab.pdf; date of access: 4 November 2019.

Central Bureau of Health Intelligence, Directorate General of Health Services Ministry of Health and Family Welfare (MoHFW) and Government of India, 2015. *National Health Profile 2015*. Table 1.2.7. New Delhi. Retrieved from www.indiaenviron mentportal.org.in/files/file/NHP-2015.pdf; date of access: 23 November 2019.

Chandra, M., 2015. Environmental Concerns in India: Problems and Solutions. *Journal of International Business and Law*. Vol 15. No 1, Article 1. Retrieved from https://scholarlycommons.law.hofstra.edu/cgi/viewcontent.cgi?article=1278& context=jibl; date of access: 12 November 2019.

Chaturvedi, S., S. Ramji, N.K. Arora, S. Rewal, R. Dasgupta and V. Deshmukh, 2016. Time-Constrained Mother and Expanding Market: Emerging Model of Under-Nutrition in India. *BMC Public Health*. Vol 16, p. 632. Retrieved from www.indianpediatrics.net/apr2018/284.pdf; date of access: 1 November 2019.

The Cost of a Polluted Environment: 1.7 Million Child Deaths a Year, n.d. Retrieved from www.who.int/news-room/detail/06-03-2017-the-cost-of-a-polluted-environment-1-7-million-child-deaths-a-year-says-who; date of access: 11 November 2019.

Dasgupta, R., I. Chaand and K.R. Barla, 2018. The Slippery Slope of Child Feeding Practices in India. *Indian Pediatrics*. Vol 55. No 4, pp. 284–286. Retrieved from www. indianpediatrics.net/apr2018/apr-284-286.htm; date of access: 22 November 2019.

Department of Health Research, 2017. *The Assisted Reproductive Technology (Regulation) Bill, 2017*. Retrieved from www.prsindia.org/uploads/media/draft/ Draft%20Assisted%20Reproductive%20Technology%20(Regulation)%20 Bill,%202014.pdf; date of access: 18 August 2018.

Development Initiatives, 2018. *Global Nutrition Report: Shining a Light to Spur Action on Nutrition*. Development Initiatives, Bristol.

Dreze, J. et al. (Eds.), 2006. *Focus on Children Under Six*. Edition: Abridged Report. Citizens' Initiative for the Rights of Children Under Six, New Delhi.

Dube, R., V. Nandan and S. Dua, 2014. Waste Incineration for Urban India: Valuable Contribution to Sustainable MSWM or Inappropriate High-tech Solution Affecting Livelihoods and Public Health? *International Journal of Environmental Technology & Management*. Vol 17. No 2–4, pp. 199–214.

Echavvari, R. and R. Ezcurra, 2010. Education and Gender Bias in the Sex Ratio at Birth: Evidence from India. *Demography*. Vol 47. No 1, pp. 249–268.

Ending Preventable Maternal, Newborn and Child Deaths, n.d. Retrieved from https://unicef.in/Uploads/Publications/Resources/pub_doc30180.pdf; date of access: 20 November 2019.

European Institute for Law and Justice, 2012. *Surrogate Motherhood: A Violation of Human Rights*. Report Presented at the Council of Europe, Strasbourg. Retrieved from www.ieb-eib.org/en/pdf/surrogacy-motherhood-icjl.pdf; date of access: 12 November 2019.

Gaudin, S., 2009. *Son Preference in Indian Families: Absolute Versus Relative Wealth Effects*. Retrieved from http://www2.oberlin.edu/faculty/sgaudin/research/India-Gender_Demography_AcceptedVersion.pdf; date of access: 11 November 2019.

Global Hunger Index India, n.d. Retrieved from www.globalhungerindex.org/india. html; date of access: 20 November 2019.

Guillot, M. and K. Allendorf, 2009. *Hindu-Muslim Differentials in Child Mortality in India*. Paper Prepared for the XVI IUSSP International Population Conference,

Session "Mortality Differentials in Multi-Ethnic Societies," 2 October 2009, Marrakech, Morocco. Retrieved from https://iussp2009.princeton.edu/papers/92861; date of access: 8 November 2019.

Gupta, S.K. et al., 2012. Impact of *Janani Suraksha Yojana* on Institutional Delivery Rate and Maternal Morbidity and Mortality: An Observational Study in India. *Journal of Health Population and Nutrition*. 30(4): 464–71.

Horo, M., 2017. *Health Problems of Left Behinds: An Exploratory Study of Chronically Poor Blocks of Ranchi District* (unpublished thesis). Jawaharlal Nehru University. Retrieved from www.indianpediatrics.net/apr2018/284.pdf; date of access: 1 November 2019.

Horton, S., 1999. Opportunities for Investments in Nutrition in Low-Income Asia. *Asian Development Review*. Vol 17. No 1,2, pp. 246–273. Retrieved from https://pdfs.semanticscholar.org/2a1a/b227f0fe442d440a774e4546fda3673c8c24.pdf; date of access: 3 December 2019.

Identification and Assessment. *Guidelines for Parents of Children with Disabilities. Parents of Children with disabilities – Planning Commission*, 2002. Retrieved from www.planningcommission.nic.in/reports/sereport/ser/stdy_ied.pdf; date of access: 10 November 2019.

India Preliminary Fact Sheet. Retrieved from https://nhm.gov.in/index1.php?lang=1&level=2&sublinkid=1332&lid=713; date of access: 22 November 2019.

Indian Council for Medical Research, 2016. *India Health of Nation's States: The Indian State Level Disease Burden Initiative*. Indian Council for Medical Research, New Delhi.

India's Infant Mortality Down 42% in 11 Years Yet Higher than Global Average. Retrieved from www.indiaspend.com/indias-infant-mortality-down-42-in-11-years-yet-higher-than-global-average/; date of access: 1 November 2019.

International Institute for Population Sciences (IIPS) and Macro International, 2007. *National Family Health Survey (NFHS-3), 2005–06: India: Volume II.* IIPS, Mumbai. Retrieved from http://rchiips.org/nfhs/NFHS-3%20Data/VOL-2/Front%20Matter.pdf; date of access: 19 November 2019.

Kamath, S.S., 2015. Child Protection During Disasters. *Indian Pediatrics*. Vol 52, pp. 467–468.

Kapoor, A., D. Sinha and G. Meera, 2016. *Progress of Children Under ICDS: Revisiting the Focus Districts*. Centre for Equity Studies, New Delhi

Kaur, R., S.S. Bhalla, M.K. Agarwal and P. Ramakrishnan, 2016. *Sex Ratio at Birth: The Role of Gender, Class and Education*. UNFPA, New Delhi.

Kousky, C., 2016. Impacts of Natural Disasters on Children. *The Future of Children*, pp. 73–92.

Kulkarni, P., 2012. Comments, India's Child Sex Ratio: Worsening Imbalance. *Indian Journal of Medical Ethics*. Vol 9. No 2.

Ministry of Health and Family Welfare, Government of India, 2017. *NFHS 4: State Fact Sheets*. New Delhi.

Ministry of Statistics and Programme Implementation, 2018. *Children in India 2018: A Statistical Appraisal*. Retrieved from www.mospi.gov.in/sites/default/files/publication_reports/Children%20in%20India%202018%20%E2%80%93%0A%20Statistical%20Appraisal_26oct18.pdf; date of access: 12 November 2019.

Ministry of Statistics and Programme Implementation, NSSO, Government of India, 2017. *Swachhta Status Report 2016*. Retrieved from https://factchecker.in/modis-report-card-evaluating-ndas-flagship-programmes-in-the-run-up-to-2019-elections/; date of access: 19 November 2019.

Ministry of Women and Child Development, 2016. *Beti Bachao Beti Padhao.* Retrieved from http://wcd.nic.in/bbbp-schemes; date of access: 12 August 2018.

Ministry of Women and Child Development, n.d. *2019 Beti Bachao Beti Padhao Scheme Implementation Guidelines.* Retrieved from https://wcd.nic.in/sites/default/files/Guideline.pdf; date of access: 16 November 2019.

Mother's Education, Household Wealth Decide Survival Of Infants In India. Retrieved from https://www.indiaspend.com/mothers-education-household-wealth-decide-survival-of-infants-in-india-51235/; date of access: 15 January 2020.

Mukherjee, S., 2017. Emerging Infectious Diseases: Epidemiological Perspective. *Indian Journal of Dermatology.* Vol 62. No 5, pp. 459–467.

Murray, J.L., J.E. Shaw, J.-C. Tardif, M.V. Perez, A. Eskander and Institute for Health Metrics, 2017. *Health Effects of Overweight and Obesity in 195 Countries Over 25 Years: NEJM,* 6 July 2017. Retrieved from www.nejm.org/doi/full/10.1056/NEJMoa1614362; date of access: 6 November 2019.

Nair, M., P. Ariana and P. Webster, 2014. Impact of Mothers' Employment on Infant Feeding and Care: A Qualitative Study of the Experiences of Mothers Employed Through the Mahatma Gandhi National Rural Employment Guarantee Act. *BMJ Open.* Vol 4, p. e004434. Retrieved from www.indianpediatrics.net/apr2018/284.pdf; date of access: 1 November 2019.

Nandi, A., J.R. Behrman, S. Kinra and R. Laxminarayan, 2018. *Early-Life Nutrition Is Associated Positively with Schooling and Labor Market Outcomes and Negatively with Marriage Rates at Age 20–25 Years: Evidence from the Andhra Pradesh Children and Parents Study (APCAPS) in India,* 25 January 2018. Retrieved from https://academic.oup.com/jn/article/148/1/140/4823713; date of access: 6 November 2019.

The National Annual Rural Sanitation Survey 2017–18. Retrieved from http://pib.nic.in/newsite/PrintRelease.aspx?relid=178030

National Commission for Protection of Child Rights and ChildFund India, 2017. *Handbook for Ending Violence Against Children—Situational Analysis of India.* Retrieved from http://ncpcr.gov.in/showfile.php?lang=1&level=2&&sublinkid=1679&lid=1682; date of access: 22 July 2019.

National Sample Survey Organisation, 2012. *Employment & Unemployment and Migration Survey: NSS 64th Round: July 2007–June 2008.* NSSO, Ministry of Statistics and Programme Implementation, Delhi.

NFHS-3 and NFHS-4. Retrieved from http://rchiips.org/nfhs/pdf/NFHS4/India.pdf; date of access: 29 October 2019.

Olofin, I., C.M. McDonald, M. Ezzati, S. Flaxman, R.E. Black, W.W. Fawzi, L.E. Caulfield, G. Danaei and Nutrition Impact Model Study, 2013. Associations of Suboptimal Growth with All-cause and Cause-specific Mortality in Children Under Five Years: A Pooled Analysis of Ten Prospective Studies. *PLoS One.* Vol 8. No 5, p. e64636.

OneIndia News, 26 September 2017. *How Beti Bachao Campaign Failed to Live Up to Its Claim in Modi's Home Turf Varanasi.* Retrieved from www.oneindia.com/india/how-beti-bachao-campaign-failed-to-live-up-to-its-claim-in-modis-home-turf-varanasi-2551080.html; date of access: 12 August 2018.

Parks, N., 2009. UN Update: Climate Change Hitting Sooner and Stronger. *Environmental Science & Technology.* Vol 43. No 22, pp. 8475–8476.

Planning Commission, Government of India, 2013. *Twelfth Five Year Plan (2012–2017). Social Sectors,* p. 14. Retrieved from http://planningcommission.gov.in/plans/planrel/12thplan/pdf/12fyp_vol3.pdf; date of access: 21 November 2019.

Pross, O.A., J. Wolf, C. Corvalan, R. Bros, M. Niera, 2016. *Preventing Disease Through Healthy Environments: A Global Assessment of Burden of Disease from Environmental Risk*. World Health Organisation, Geneva.

Public Health Foundation of India, Centre for Youth Development and Activities, Prayatn, ADITHI and Vimochana, 2010. *Implementation of the PCPNDT Act in India: Perspectives and Challenges*. Public Health Foundation of India, New Delhi.

Rajan, S.I., S. Srinivasan and A.S. Bedi, 2017. Update on Trends in Sex Ratio at Birth in India. *Economic and Political Weekly*. Vol 52. No 11, 18 March 2017, pp. 14–16.

Ramachandran, V., 2018. *From the Womb to Primary School: Challenges, Policies and Prospects for the Young Child in India*. Technical Background Paper. Mobile Creches, New Delhi.

Raman, S., 2018. Gujarat Declared Free of Open Defecation a Year Ago. But in 4 Districts, Toilets Without Walls, Water and Unconvinced Locals. *Factchecker.in*, 24 November 2018. Retrieved from https://factchecker.in/gujarat-declared-free-of-open-defecation-a-year-ago-but-in-4-districts-toilets-without-walls-water-and-unconvinced-locals/; date of access: 21 November 2019.

Ramani, V., 2011. *Bhavishya Alliance: Lessons from Its Efforts to Tackle Child Malnutrition in Maharashtra (2006–2011)*. Retrieved from https://vramani.files.wordpress.com/2018/08/bhavishya-alliance-analysis-and-learnings.pdf; date of access: 22 November 2019.

Ramani, V., 2018. *Physical wellbeing of the Young Child in India: Challenges, Prospects and Way Forward*. Technical background paper for the Report 2020. Mobile Creches, New Delhi.

Ramani, V., 2019. Fixing Child Malnutrition in India: Views from a Public Policy Practitioner. *The Hindu Centre for Politics and Public Policy*. Policy Watch No. 8. Retrieved from https://www.thehinducentre.com/the-arena/article26397464.ece; date of access: 16 January 2020.

Research Institute for Compassionate Economics and Accountability Initiative, 2018. *Changes in Open Defecation in Rural North India: 2014–2018*. A Working Paper. Retrieved from https://riceinstitute.org/research/changes-in-open-defecation-in-rural-north-india-2014-2018-2/; date of access: 7 January 2019.

Rudra, S., 2017. *Immunisation Coverage: India Far Away from Meeting Targets*. Observer Research Foundation. Retrieved from www.orfonline.org/expert-speak/immunisation-coverage-india-far-away-from-meeting-targets/; date of access: 22 November 2019.

Salve, P., 2018. *Muslims Have Highest Fertility Rate, Lack Access to Healthcare*, 27 April 2018. Retrieved from www.indiaspend.com/muslims-have-highest-fertility-rate-lack-access-to-healthcare-36353/; date of access: 21 November 2019.

Save the Children, 2018. *Understanding the Benefits of Beti Bachao Beti Padhao Scheme, Save the Children*, New Delhi.

Sharma, R., 2013. Birth Defects in India: Hidden Truth, Need for Urgent Attention. *Indian Journal of Human Genetics*. Vol 19. No 2, pp. 125–129. doi:10.4103/0971-6866.116101. Retrieved from www.ncbi.nlm.nih.gov/pmc/articles/PMC3758715/; date of access: 2 November 2019.

Smith Lisa, C. and L. Haddad, 2000. *Explaining Child Malnutrition in Developing Countries: A Cross-Country Analysis*. International Food Policy Research Institute, Washington, DC.

SRS, 2019. Retrieved from www.censusindia.gov.in/vital_statistics/SRS_Bulletins/SRS_Bulletin-Rate-2017-_May_2019.pdf; date of access: 23 November 2019.

Swacch Bharat Mission, n.d. *SBM(G) guidelines—Swacch Bharat Mission*. Retrieved from http://swachhbharatmission.gov.in/sbmcms/writereaddata/images/pdf/Guidelines/Complete-set-guidelines.pdf; date of access: 7 November 2019.

UNDP, 2017. *Decentralisation of ICDS Supplementary Nutrition Programme: Ensuring Timely and Quality Nutrition to All Beneficiaries in Odisha*. Retrieved from https://niti.gov.in/writereaddata/files/bestpractices/Decentralisation%20of%20ICDS%20Supplementary%20Nutrition%20Programme%20Ensuring%20timely%20and%20quality%20nutrition%20to%20all%20beneficiaries%20in%20Odisha.pdf; date of access: 24 November 2019.

UNICEF, 1990. *Strategy for improved nutrition of children and women in developing countries*. Retrieved from http://www.ceecis.org/iodine/01_global/01_pl/01_01_other_1992_unicef.pdf; date of access: 16 January 2020.

UNICEF, 2014. *The State of the World's Children*. UNICEF, New York.

UNICEF, 2019. *The State of the World's Children*. UNICEF, New York.

UNICEF, WHO, the World Bank and United Nations, 2018. *Levels and Trends in Child Mortality. Report 2018. Estimates Developed by the UN Inter-Agency Group for Child Mortality Estimation*. Retrieved from https://childmortality.org/wp-content/uploads/2018/12/UN-IGME-Child-Mortality-Report-2018.pdf; date of access: 4 November 2019.

United Nations Children's Fund (UNICEF), 2015. *The Impact of Climate Change on Children*. Retrieved from https://www.unicef.org/publications/files/Unless_we_act_now_The_impact_of_climate_change_on_children.pdf; date of access: 16 January 2020.

Vranda, M.N. and K. Sekar, 2011. (A298) Assessment of Psychosocial Impact of Flood on Children—Indian Experience. *Prehospital and Disaster Medicine*. Vol 26. No S1, pp. S83–S84. Cambridge University Press.

Welt Hunger Hilfe, 2018. *Global Hunger Index*. Retrieved from https://www.globalhungerindex.org/pdf/en/2018.pdf; date of access: 16 January 2020.

World Bank, 2017. *Universal Health Coverage Global Monitoring Report*. Retrieved from http://datatopics.worldbank.org/universal-health-coverage/; date of access: 12 November 2019.

World Health Organisation, 2016. *Health Situation and Trend Assessment: Sex Ratio*. Retrieved from www.searo.who.int/entity/health_situation_trends/data/chi/sex-ratio/en/; date of access: 15 November 2019.

World Health Organisation, 2017a. *Causes of Child Mortality. Global Health Observatory Data*. Retrieved from www.who.int/gho/child_health/mortality/causes/en/; date of access: 1 December 2018.

World Health Organisation, 2017b. *Don't Pollute My Future—The Impact of Environment on Children's Health*. World Health Organisation, Geneva.

3 Promoting early childhood learning

A good start to life, aided and abetted by optimal utilisation of opportunities offered by the 1,000 days window, lays the foundation for cognitive, intellectual and skills development. Persistent equation of early learning with pre-school education, which essentially serves the older early childhood age group (viz., 3–6 years) has resulted in the neglect of infants and toddlers. The process of learning begins at birth, initially through stimulation, play, interactions, non-verbal and verbal communication and gradually through observation and cues from the immediate environment and increasingly structured activities.

Guided by the ambition of SDG 4.2 which calls for all efforts to ensure that all girls and boys have access to quality early childhood development, care and pre-primary education so that they are ready for primary education, this chapter explores the state of early childhood learning in India – within homes, in crèches, day-care facilities and pre-schools, the nature and scope of public and private services and the key impediments in the expansion of ECCE with quality. It culminates with recommendations and action points based on an analysis of the key impediments in the expansion of ECCE with quality.

3.1 Early learning matters

3.1.1 Early years are the foundation for life-long learning and development

Learning begins at birth as the infant begins to respond to external stimuli and signals from the parents, caregivers and immediate environment. Gradually the interactions with others help the young child acquire the abilities to communicate through expressions and verbal cues, and gradually through language. The exposure to 'print rich' environment initiates the child into the world of illustrations, stories and games, and boosts her imagination, logical reasoning and self-expression. With the development of emotional bonds and relationships, improved fluency in verbal and non-verbal expression, the young child increasingly makes sense of the surroundings and, in due course, begins to imbibe values and social norms.

3.1.2 Home-based early learning is crucial for infants and toddlers

Newborns are dependent for their survival on their parents and other caregivers within the household who feed, care, comfort and protect them. This dependence evolves into opportunities for emotional attachments, and the foundation of social relationships, language, cultural and cognitive learning. Regardless of where children are located and the differences in childcare practices, social norms have favoured warm, responsive, linguistically rich and protective relationships during critical periods of their development. Children have typically been raised in the company of other children, even cared for by other children, siblings or cousins.[1]

Parents and other caregivers promote early learning when they engage with the young child through early stimulation – be it in the form of cuddles, tickling or making soothing sounds – and gradually progressing to conversations and games. Several age-appropriate games, which do not require any aids or use local materials, help infants and young children to develop locomotor skills and social engagement progressively. Interactions, including conversations, play, lullabies and songs with vivid imagery in local languages, or more specifically the mother tongue, help to develop proficiency in language, especially the mother tongue. Storytelling initiates them into understanding the complexities of life and familiarising them with good conduct and values.

Globalisation, urbanisation, migration and changing family structures and dynamics could be pushing the rich tradition of early childhood practices towards extinction. Empirical research is limited but anecdotal accounts of the growing use of mobile phones and cartoon networks on the television, of course depending on the socio-economic status of the family, are hard to miss.

Ubiquitous mobile phones may keep young children occupied while the parents and caregivers are busy with other chores while the television may be an effective incentive for finishing meals or behaving well but together they signal the devaluation of human contact. Technological advances can be enabling in many ways, but not as a substitute for the touch and feel in human interactions. The contribution of physical and mental stimulation and emotional bonding is most significant when brain development is at its peak and children are naturally inclined to exploration.

Parents and other caregivers facilitate such learning in early childhood through stimulation, physical care and play, along with health, nutrition and clean environment. Although there cannot be a substitute for parental inputs to early learning birth onwards, well-designed ECCE programmes can address any deficit or enhance young child's early cognitive, physical, social and emotional development.

Ultimately, it is the social environment, socio-economic conditions and exceptional situations being experienced by the household that influence young children.

3.1.3 Child play is an important learning opportunity in early childhood

Stimulation and play are age-appropriate facilitators of child development and learning. Box 3.1 highlights the importance of play in ECD. Theories in child development promote the idea that play is children's work and that particularly in the early years, children learn through playful encounters with their environment. Play invokes autonomy and provides space and scope for guided self-learning, especially at the early childhood stage, albeit it is not a substitute for collaborative learning. Both solitary and cooperative play contributes to children's well-rounded engagement with the world.[2]

Box 3.1   Play is important to facilitate early childhood development

The significance of play is in the practice with symbolic action or learning to represent objects in the world around them with symbols, which comes naturally to children. Other than an area of exploration and some materials, this playful engagement with the environment does not require intervention from adults. Some theories promote specific strategies and materials for play whereas others support a more natural engagement and unstructured play. These experiences undeniably hold a great significance for children. The significance of folk interpretations of play and traditional games need not be underestimated.

These early learning opportunities have helped in transmitting social and cultural norms and practices. Many of the games, songs and stories are repositories of culture and identity as they are passed on from one generation to the next. Notwithstanding their value in providing socio-cultural continuity, many of the early learning traditions and opportunities as well as songs and games may also reflect social and gender discriminatory norms.

Young children in many rural and tribal communities, with a large repertoire of traditional games and activities, do not perceive play and work separately. Community living conceives childhood and adulthood in continuity and opens most spaces to children as well as adults. It has an important impact on the way children play, what they play and who they play with. By and large adults perceive play as children's engagement and do not feel the need to actively interact with children while they are playing.

Cultural diversity in play activities demonstrates that work and play need not be mutually exclusive. Indeed, the boundaries between these two sets of activities do not exist in some cultures and even young children participate in work around the household and play. Implicit in the expectation from a young child in a rural Indian household assigned with the responsibility for the care for a younger sibling and some household chores is that there would be play opportunities.

Well-trained educators at crèches and day-care centres, and later at pre-schools, are able to provide favourable and desirable experiences for all children, irrespective of their background, while adapting them to specific individual developmental needs. They introduce the young child to increasingly structured and organised instruction outside of the family context and help to develop socio-emotional skills necessary for participation in school and society as well as readiness for primary education.

3.1.4 Acquisition of linguistic skills occurs through early interactions

Young children acquire proficiency in language at a rapid pace. Their brains are wired for making sense of the sounds in their environment, and adults assist them with linguistic skill development. According to child development experts, newborns are capable of categorical speech perception and are sensitive to a wider range of speech categories than exists in their own language.

At about two months of age, they begin cooing. Around six months, they begin babbling and continue to expand the repertoire of such sounds over the first year.[3] Between 6 and 8 months, they begin organising speech into phonemic categories of their mother tongue. The sound and intonation patterns start to resemble those of the mother tongue, as they get ready to talk. At 10 to 11 months, their skills at establishing joint attention improves, and generally by their birthday they engage in turn-taking games, directing attention to an object, action or entity, pointing to or a whole hand or swiping motion towards the desired object, often with a whine or grunt to communicate and influence others' behaviour.[4]

The quality of interaction between the young child and adults largely determines language development, which is critical for subsequent learning and development. Adults ease language learning for infants through infant directed speech.[5] Conversations in mother tongue are crucial for the comprehension and comfort of pre-school age children, as is noted in Box 3.2. Learning is compromised when the language spoken at home is treated as informal and crude, and the child is compelled to disregard familiar tongues and adopt new languages. The consequences are detrimental for the young child who should be getting ready for basic concepts in school instead of struggling to make sense of a new language.[6]

Box 3.2   Multilingualism cannot undermine the criticality of the mother tongue

India's children speak one of the nearly 780 languages Devy identified through the People's Linguistic Survey of India, with the possibility of at least another 100 that they had been unable to reach. This was at least about 500 languages more than what the languages survey during the 2011 Census had counted. This uncovers the extensively multilingual nature of the country, a problem that has proved to be a challenge in the planning for school languages. For Devy, the survey and its findings relates not only to the preservation of languages, but also the particular past that is contained in them (Devy, 2014). Mohanty argues that for a child to have a firm foothold in school, the foundation must be built through the mother tongue, with a phased introduction of other languages.

In an attempt to resolve the tension between language of knowledge and home language that continues to haunt the country, Devy (2018) extends a proposal wherein the two (or more) need not be separated through the establishment of regional Special Language Resource Centres (SLRCs) that provide support to school going students and others to support the construction of bridges between the several languages in India. This also needs the support and action of citizens themselves, which is now clearly directed towards the ambition to study the English language that is seen as a path to success. The participation of government organisations, NGOs, and schools is essential for the success of such an experiment. In fact everyone has to work concertedly towards ensuring that children's home languages are preserved and respected.

One in every six of school-going children in the world is waiting for the bridge between the word "future" in her home language and the same word in the language of "power" and "knowledge". This done, the "logocide" let loose upon young minds can be arrested at least partially. India can find its honourable place in the world's knowledge community not by becoming monolingual and culturally uprooted but by remaining multilingual and culturally productive.

(Devy, 2018)

Various approaches to early childhood education in multiple languages, especially mother tongue, are being tried and tested in different states in India. The distance between the languages spoken at home, in the local community and in the school often aggravates the discrimination experienced by children belonging to ethnic minority.[7]

3.1.5 *Young children imbibe values through early education*

Moral development is a process of internalisation of societal standards, which begins in early childhood and gradually proceeds into adolescence and adulthood. Morality has been attributed to various factors, including pre-wired emotional reactions, exposure to and internalisation of societal standards or through active reflection on situations in which social conflicts arise.

Young children may internalise pro-social norms by exposure to warm, responsive, competent and powerful words and deeds, which are consistently reiterated and reinforced. Conversely, frequent harsh punishment can weaken moral internalisation and hinder adjustment. Young children, who frequently witness domestic violence or receive harsh and inconsistent discipline, are exposed to negative models. They may develop social-cognitive deficits and distortions that contribute to long-term maintenance of aggression. Poverty, insecurity and inadequate schooling may advance their propensity to anti-social acts.

Young children can view moral rules in terms of realism or flexible, socially agreed upon principles. Pre-school and early school age children consider intentions when making moral judgements although they interpret intentions rigidly. They may have differentiated notions about the legitimacy of authority figures. They also understand gender in a specific way as they grow up, as Box 3.3 highlights.

Box 3.3   How children understand gender

Kohlberg's theory of gender identity development describes how young children learn to understand their gender and what being that gender means in their everyday life. Kohlberg theorised that there are three stages to this process.

1   During the early pre-school years (ages 3–4), young children engage in gender labelling. They can tell the difference between boys and girls, and label people accordingly. But they still believe that gender can change and have trouble understanding that males and females have different body shapes but share characteristics.

2   They obtain a better understanding of gender identity as they mature. They understand that gender is stable over time but often think that changing physical appearance or activities can change them into the other sex.

3   By the early school years (ages 6–7), most children understand gender consistency, the idea that they are one gender and will remain that gender for life. A few of them, however, struggle with their gender identity and continue to struggle with their true identity through adulthood.[8]

Gender-based socialisation also impacts the choices households make regarding care and education of young girls. A larger proportion of boys than girls attend private institutions. Similar trends are visible in the case of pre-school aged children as well, confirming that gender discrimination begins very early in a child's life. As characteristics like mother's education and family income are important positive triggers, it is the poor families and those where the mother is not literate or barely literate that seems to be disadvantaged.

3.1.6 Home-based early learning has several shortcomings

The Indian family system has been characterised by family bonds and multiple caregivers, but this homogenised perception overlooks the factors that undermine its ability to create conducive conditions for the young child due to a variety of factors. For instance, poverty and livelihood insecurity, chronic ill health, domestic violence and other stresses and strains within the household undermine early learning experiences. According to an estimate, "more than 200 million children under 5 years fail to reach their potential in cognitive development because of poverty, poor health and nutrition, and deficient care."[9]

Many parents, however, neither have the resources nor an understanding of their role and responsibility in ECCE. Most of them want the best for their child but have a blinkered view of early learning. They often see pre-schools as a medium for children to learn reading, writing and arithmetic – basically as a downward extension of primary school while untrained or poorly trained teachers use formal learning techniques and primary school curriculum. Due to popular demand, private pre-schools have mushroomed and have a formal and distant approach to teaching and learning. Primary education continues to overshadow pre-school education in the current literature on the private-public learning gap in India,[10] which is perhaps a reflection of the collective failure to appreciate and encourage early learning that responds to the unique needs of infants, toddlers and pre-school going age group.

The interaction between ECCE workers, including pre-school teachers, and parents is central to ECCE, but parents are neither encouraged nor motivated enough to engage with childcare centres and pre-schools. The formality associated with any kind of teaching and learning creates a chasm between the teachers and the parents. Many parents remain unfamiliar with the scientific underpinnings of ECD and do not appreciate their own role and the importance of engaging with ECCE workers. Many parents, economically stressed but seeking social mobility, accept the exposure of their young children to repetition of alphabets and numbers as long as they can learn to write and count in preparation for the entry to a private primary school of their choice.

Mass media and social media have also flooded the public domain with advice on bringing up children. Living in an aspirational social environment, parents have a fear of missing out as they struggle to make choices based on their own normative framework and experiences as well as such information and debates about schooling. For those who do not have this access, prevailing public opinion guides their beliefs and actions.

Several children and families need support and the argument is not about whether they need special services to support early development, the concern is how this care and education is presented, by whom and for what purpose. The success of service delivery is dependent on how the children and families are approached and the nature of interface between people. Although problems exist, it has to be understood that the dynamics of the problems and workable solutions are rooted in local contexts.

Opportunities for acquiring learning experiences are crucial for children, especially when they are living in difficult and unsafe conditions. Moreover, the vision of ECCE centres has to expand beyond one where food is being provided, and secondly, the unnecessary comparison and competition with private schools leads to a preference for fee-paying centres.

3.2 Early childhood education services are crucial for cognitive development

3.2.1 ECCE services are currently inadequate to complement home-based early learning

Drawing upon empirical research, the current discourse on child development calls for collective and complementing ECCE involving both parents, other family members, caregivers in crèches, day-care, pre-schools and other spaces situated by infants and young children for their optimal cognitive development. Notwithstanding the sparse research on popular perceptions of ECCE in India, experts have noted several lacunae in social norms and behaviours that impede convergence of early learning interventions within and outside the home for optimal outcomes for the young child.

ECCE programmes propose standard procedures but flexibility in implementation has not been built in to address the local concerns of the young child and to sustain different models that may be located within divergent frameworks (e.g., those related to improved schooling, women's work and employment, democratic principles, poverty alleviation).

The limited data on pre-school education enrolment indicates that a large number of children do not have access to pre-primary education provided by the government. In 2015–2016, U-DISE data showed a 10.72 percent enrolment in pre-primary classes to total enrolment in primary classes while UNESCO Institute of Statistics in 2017 noted 13.8 percent pre-primary Gross Enrolment Ratio (14.3 percent for boys and 13.1 percent for girls).[11]

One in four schools (24.1 percent) had the pre-primary section attached to the primary section and there were wide regional and state-wise differences. Nagaland was on top with 96.5 percent of primary schools having the pre-primary section. It was followed by West Bengal (93.6 percent), Meghalaya (82.3 percent), Sikkim (81.1 percent), Assam (74.7 percent), Kerala (69 percent), Jammu and Kashmir (60.1 percent), Haryana (51.2 percent) and Delhi (50.5 percent).[12] Government pre-school sections in many of these states are characterised by low enrolments and fewer teachers relative to private schools.

3.2.2 All children do not have access to ECCE services

There is no consolidated data available to enable an accurate assessment of the extent of provisions for ECCE across India. Various data sources indicate that the largest provider of pre-school education in India is the ICDS followed by the private schools, and centres run by NGOs, experimental schools run by academic institutions, day-care programmes and crèches, as well as international agencies.

In the 2011 Census, around 76.5 million children or 48 percent of 158.7 million children under 6 years reportedly accessed the ICDS, which includes ECCE in its package of services. The remaining 30 to 40 million children – in all probability belonging to the most disadvantaged and the very poor – did not access these services.

A rapid survey commissioned by the MWCD in 2015 revealed rural-urban differences, social category and wealth index differences in participation in the AWCs and private pre-schools and education centres, as shown in Table 3.1. A significant percentage of children from the lowest wealth index attended AWCs whereas children from the highest wealth index attended private pre-school centres. The AWCs catered to 37 million children. Just over 3 million children attended a formal pre-school centre or a pre-primary section in primary schools in 2014–2015. Close to 27 percent of children aged 3–6 years did not attend any pre-school facility, and just about 58 percent of those enrolled attended regularly.

Table 3.1 Participation in pre-school education varies by extent of disadvantage (2013–2014)

	Residence			Gender		Social category				Wealth index	
	Total	Rural	Urban	Male	Female	SC	ST	OBC	Other	Lowest	Highest
3–6 year olds attending PSE (%)											
- AWC	37.9	45.1	21.6	36.6	39.3	41.6	50.9	34.8	33.9	51.4	15.4
- Privately run institution	30.7	22.0	50.3	31.7	29.6	25.0	17.3	32.1	32.1	8.6	61.5
- Not attending	26.9	28.0	24.5	27.3	26.6	29.1	27.3	28.3	22.9	34.7	19.9
3–6 year olds attending PSE in AWC for 16+ days in the month prior to the survey (%)	58.1	58.6	55.5	57.2	58.9	57.2	58.0	58.4	58.9	56.6	56.6

Source: MWCD, 2015 (RSOC), p. 4

A policy brief based on an assessment sponsored by UNICEF[13] found that four out of every seven children attended pre-school centres. Despite that, children's participation does not follow a linear trajectory as prescribed by policy. Attendance in pre-school centres often extends to 7 years of age, and attendance in school stabilises only after 8. At age 5, preparedness for school is low, and pre-school quality is poor and inappropriate, and as children grow older there is a rising distance between expectations from children and their performance.

3.2.3 ICDS has consistently faced a relative neglect of early education

The neglect of pre-school education is a persistent criticism of the ICDS since the 1980s. A study by Centre for Early Childhood Education and Development (CECED), Annual Status of Education Report (ASER) and UNICEF in 2017 noted that with few exceptions, AWCs generally act as a place where children come primarily to collect their mid-day meal and spend some time while their parents are away at work. It is quite common for families to send their children to the AWC for supplementary feeding, and then onto a private school for classes, even at a young age.

The AWCs are not known for delivering good quality ECCE. Most *anganwadi* workers (AWWs) lack the basic qualifications required for pre-school teachers training, and the in-service training system is weak. Furthermore, when one AWW with a helper is expected to manage supplementary nutrition, immunisation, health check-up, referral services, the care of pregnant women and interventions for adolescent girls, ECCE is likely to be put on the backburner.

There is generally no planned activity, and children can be found playing among themselves while the AWW is busy with administrative work. Activities, if any, are invariably recitation of poems or rhymes or learning of letters or numbers. Play materials are not available in appropriate numbers and AWWs rarely take them out for children fearing they will get damaged.

The study also expressed concerns about the location of the centres, cleanliness and safety. It found that most AWCs in the three states had limited infrastructure. Typically, they were running from rented accommodation while others operated from primary school campuses or in a separate room allocated on the outskirts of the village. Almost 50 percent of these centres did not have enough space for children and the AWW to move around freely, let alone conduct group activities. In about 54 percent of AWCs in the absence of proper seating facilities children had to sit on torn mats or on a bare floor. Basic amenities such as toilets were rarely available, and in most cases, children used open spaces to urinate and defecate.

A study of the ICDS services in south India highlighted the poor standard of records although community relationships were maintained well (Tripathy et al., 2014). Despite irregular supply of stock, health and nutrition services were effective. Almost half the centres had inadequate space, and almost 40 percent workers ran the centres in their own homes. Although drinking water facilities were available in around 87 percent centres, sanitation was poor in around half the centres visited.[14]

Several studies have shown that the support of local communities, local NGOs and the administration is not always available to the AWCs. As and when the community engagement is strong, there is a visible difference in the services available to children. In 2000, the M S Swaminathan Research Foundation argued in favour quality improvement over the mere establishment of childcare or AWCs under the ICDS. Expansion of the existing programmes such as the ICDS and the National Crèche Scheme without addressing the fundamental weaknesses in the design and implementation of the programme cannot be expected to improve health, learning and other macro human development indicators. It is also important to design pre-school activities in the home language of the child, to the extent possible. A recent report noted that the ICDS has failed to achieve desired outcomes like improving the quality of pre-school education (IndiaSpend, 2018).[15]

3.2.4 *The quality of pre-school education in government and private schools is uneven*

A position paper on ECCE by National Council of Educational Research and Training (NCERT) (2015) found that the age of entry into pre-school significantly impacts performance. If children join before 4 years of age, their long-term indicators are better, making a strong case for early entry into pre-school. It also associated positive indicators with income levels, social status and maternal and paternal educational levels.[16]

However, there is considerable scope for interventions geared towards bringing and retaining children aged 3–6 years in pre-school.

There are also a significant number of private players in the field of pre-school education, largely also English medium schools, and it is unwise to ignore this massive uprising of small and large players in the game. Research has identified that private schools are only a downward extension of primary school curriculums.[17]

Low-fee paying private schools have become an important phenomenon in the field of ECCE[18] and it is no longer possible to ignore their popularity. In the same report by NCERT (2015) it was discovered that children's performance is somewhat better when they emerge from private pre-schools as assessed through their performance on selected standardised tests despite the scepticism related to the downward extension of primary school activities. The authors report that the validity of these findings needs to be taken with due attention to the design and testing limitations. Another study found significantly better performance by children attending private pre-schools.[19] Furthermore, parents are more satisfied with private schools.[20]

Although school participation is an important objective of ECCE, research findings related to preparedness and participation for school have shown negative results. Pre-school centres, especially run by government, are ill-prepared for preparing young children for primary school. They are constrained by the non-availability of teachers and inadequate infrastructure. Nationally, there are 86,319 teachers in pre-primary sections in government schools. But more significantly, 65 percent of schools with pre-primary section did not have a teacher. In a study, it was found that both government and private pre-schools had the play component largely missing from their programmes, and activities were restricted to rote and repetitive learning (UNICEF, 2017).[21]

A large number of children make the transition to primary school with inadequate preparedness and tend to demonstrate low learning levels and high probability of dropping out in the early primary classes. A standard pattern of ECCE that follows national guidelines but is flexible enough to be contextualised and adapted by the implementers is still lacking. In the absence of guidelines and monitoring, private pre-schools cater to the popular demand for formalised teaching of children in pursuit of profits.

Various studies have highlighted the significance of the quality of programmes in determining children's scores on child development measures. If the ECCE programme is of good quality, they tend to score higher in comparison to children who do not experience such quality care and early education.

Due to the absence of data on pre-school attendance, studies of primary schooling in India cannot with certainty attribute the difference in test scores to pre-primary education. It is likely that any such gap is due to differences in pre-school attendance and that such divergences persist beyond pre-school years into primary school. A policy implication of a comprehensive exercise considering both pre-school and primary school attendance could be investment in pre-school education for remediation of gaps in future outcomes.

3.3 Innovations in ECCE have been notable, many with relevance for policy

3.3.1 Wide-ranging benefits of formal ECCE programmes have been identified

Families have conventionally assumed responsibility for children's early learning whereas formal institutions step in to impart skills and knowledge to children during and after middle childhood. The age of entry into pre-school significantly impacts children's performance. Studies have shown that the outcomes in long term are better if children join before 5 years of age.[22] Positive indicators were also associated with income levels, social status and maternal and paternal educational levels. Over the decades since its emergence, ECCE has become accepted as an eventuality and it is important to periodically revisit the original ideas behind its assumed relevance in global and local policy for young children.

Researchers broadly point to the four broad benefits of formal ECCE programmes, based on review of literature and practices. ECCE is a developmentally appropriate activity that responds to the developmental needs and learning patterns of young children, favourable for peer interactions and preparation for school, as Box 3.4 notes. Equity in ECCE means equal access to good quality programmes, in a level playing field (NCTE, 2016). Young children's participation in such ECCE services improves their chances for age-appropriate entry and participation in school. This further establishes ECCE as a solution to reducing poverty through better developmental outcomes of children, influencing their adult lives. ECCE also provides an immediate support in the form of care arrangements for children of working mothers.

Box 3.4   ECCE programmes have major benefits

Optimising children's cognitive abilities through developmentally appropriate activities: The ideas of theorists such as Montessori, Froebel, Piaget and Vygotsky about development have influenced educational institutions the world over. The term kindergarten is associated with the German educationist Froebel, whose attention to children's unique abilities and needs was path breaking in the early 1800s. Piaget and Vygotsky placed a great deal on children's experiences while differing on the role of language and significance of a teacher. They focussed on the importance of developmentally appropriate activities and children's capacities for learning. Maria Montessori emphasised the natural desire of children to learn with the caveat that as they begin to explore, adults tend to hinder that progress. She believed that adults misunderstand children because they view themselves 'as the child's creator' whereas the child is a separate being. Instead of teaching, education should guide a child's development.

Interrupting the cycle of poverty: It is widely assumed that the poor need assistance in bringing up children on account of inadequate resources and incapability attributed to their dispositions. ECCE, now recognised internationally through the policy and programmes, is best explained in the Care for Child Development package of UNICEF. The focus is on care and stimulation for under twos and learning through play for children between two and six years of age.

A more popular argument for the provision of quality childcare services is based on the perspective of women's empowerment instead of child entitlement. The women's rights groups have advocated for institutional care of children outside the home during the early years to enable their mothers to leave home for work without worries.

Preparing children for school: Arrangements for fulfilling societal roles for the care of young children between birth and six years have evolved over centuries and remain varied across cultures. Informal care and learning arrangements began being formalised in the 19th century with the establishment of kindergartens and nursery schools for educational purposes in Europe and North America.

Pre-schools, especially private, market the 'high quality' of their services. The argument forwarded is that in order for the child to 'become brilliant' parents should invest in their programme early. The prevalence and popularity of such teaching shops cannot be ignored.

3.3.2 *Varied NGO innovations have complemented the public education system*

Estimation of the number of young children accessing ECCE through programmes run by NGOs is nearly impossible. It is acknowledged generally, even by them, that they serve a tiny fraction of the young population. There is no way that they can provide services at a scale that could improve outcomes for children in a country like India. They envisage their role in innovation and creating replicable models for service delivery and capacity development and advocacy.

Various NGOs complement the public education system through their initiatives seeking to improve the effectiveness of ECCE provided by the government. The experimental approaches of the NGOs have successfully tackled many shortcomings in schooling and innovative models help in providing new solutions in ECCE. Many of them engage volunteer teachers and para-teachers where possible to reduce costs of a programme and established alternative schools with community support with limited infrastructure support and less qualified teachers.

Many of them offer ECCE services to children from poor families, children with disabilities, children of migrants and street children, who are either neglected or hard to reach by the services provided by the Government or the private sector. The role of NGOs is particularly significant in preparing the first generation learners and over-age children for primary school. Organisations like the MV Foundation, Pratham and BODH have demonstrated that even among the very poor, families are eager and willing to contribute towards school participation for their children. The services for children, as well as engagement with parents go a long way when sustaining their interest and preparing them for schools, are the main challenges.

A key factor of NGO involvement in ECCE is commitment to the community. Organisations like BODH, Mobile Creches, Pratham, *balwadis* sponsored by the Society for Elimination of Rural Poverty, Government of Andhra Pradesh and *Ka Shreni* centres attached to the government primary schools in Assam, have innovated and experimented with community engagement. For instance, mother teachers are the backbone of BODH's ECCE programme and many of them are former students. They have intimate knowledge of the community and act as a key link between BODH and centres. Box 3.5 provides more details about the various initiatives.

Box 3.5   Civil society initiatives have led to promising community-based ECCE programmes

Pratham began with a campaign to enrol all children in Mumbai into schools and set up a few *balwadis* in 1995 with active involvement of mothers to address the absence of pre-school facilities for the urban

---

poor. The *balwadis* have demonstrated that community-based ECCE programmes of good quality can be run with limited resources. The community contributes towards the space for the centre and the fees charged from the parents go towards the salary of the instructor. Locally recruited young pre-school teachers are trained, are provided with learning materials and teaching aids, and posted at the *balwadis*. Local youth, who have been the strongest allies of the programme, are being encouraged to facilitate the movement of children from local play schools to schools and coordinate between providers of various essential services.

The need to strengthen community based ECCE programme led to other areas of work like training, creating print rich media and developing innovative pedagogy. Community based training of women combined self-development approach with skill training on interactions with children. Although the payment of honorarium instead of a salary led to high turnover of *balwadi* workers, the demand for the training programme was high because they got new jobs easily.

BODH Shiksha Samiti has been guided by the imperative of ensuring quality education to children belonging to deprived communities. It is recognised as a pioneer in the field of education for the urban deprived as well as a resource agency for training on child centred pedagogy and community involvement in education. Its first school was set up in 1987 in partnership with a group of social activists with an urban community in Gokulpuri. It works intensively with selected hamlets of extremely backward communities in Rajasthan to spread public awareness on the importance of education in the early years and to set up community-based *Bodhshalas*. In addition to reaching out to more than 26,000 children in both urban and rural areas of Jaipur and Alwar through *Bodhshalas* and Government schools, it has expanded its area of operations to Ahmedabad in Gujarat and Leh in Ladakh.

Centre for Learning Resources (CLR) in Maharashtra, has built a repertoire of materials and people skills to improve the quality of ECCE and elementary education in the public sector. It undertook an action research project in Dharini, a tribal block in Amravati district, to strengthen the ECCE component in 215 AWCs in a bid to improve the school readiness of children. It developed 19 AWCs as model centres through training and mentoring of AWWs and upgraded the facilities and learning materials. For long-term sustainability of the initiative, CLR worked closely with the AW training centre so that there were adequate technical capacities, skill-sets and model centres to serve the entire block. In Chhattisgarh, CLR has tried to improve homebased holistic childcare through the training of caregivers under its Sajag project.

Among the UN organisations, a significant component of UNICEF's five-year Country Programme Action Plans (CPAP), which guides its work with the Government of India, is ECCE. The World Food Programme (WFP) provides technical assistance to the MWCD for the implementation of ICDS and other core activities. Among the bilateral donors, UK Department for International Development provides technical assistance to ICDS in Odisha, Madhya Pradesh and Bihar and also at the central level to support in ICDS (MWCD, 2017).

The Bernard Van Leer Foundation (BVLF) has provided research support for testing models of mother-tongue based ECCE in Odisha and worked with the state WCD to take the programme models to scale, training over 8,000 AWWs and supervisors engaged in working with children across the state. BVLF has been at the forefront in promoting ECD and brings out a range of publications on the subject, including the series titled 'Early Childhood Matters' and 'Early Childhood in Focus.'

3.4 Key issues

3.4.1 Indian laws encourage but do not guarantee ECCE

Educationists, CSOs, activists and planners have articulated the demand for inclusion of children below the age of six within the ambit of the fundamental right to education, for quite a while. The Right to Free and Compulsory Education (RTE) Act, 2009, essentially applies to the 6–14 age group even though its Section 11 recommends necessary arrangements by the state governments for pre-primary education to prepare children for elementary education. The exclusion of children under 6 years is viewed as dilution of the national commitment to universalisation of elementary education. The argument is that the framing of early childhood education as a fundamental right can expedite the planning and delivery of services across India, and that national and state level guidelines regarding ECCE cannot have the kind of impact that a legal entitlement can ensure.

The demand for including early education within the purview of RTE has been taken seriously. The MHRD appointed sub-committee of the Central Advisory Board of Education (CABE) to examine the feasibility of extending the RTE to children below 6 years.[23] The 12th Five Year Plan for Elementary Education established the target of at least a year of well-resourced pre-school education in primary schools to all children, particularly in educationally backward blocks.[24] In 2015, the Law Commission Report on Early Childhood Development recommended for free pre-school education for all children aged 3–6 years and pre-school centres in all government and aided schools in a phased manner,[25] and the 22nd Joint Review Mission (JRM) of the *Sarva Shiksha Abhiyan* (SSA) endorsed the suggestion that all states introduce pre-school sections in all primary schools to cater to 4–6 year-olds.[26]

Finally, the draft of the new National Education Policy released in 2019 (NEP, 2019) has laid emphasis on ECCE and supported the extension of RTE below 6 years and public investment in education.[27] A comprehensive set of recommendations related to ECCE in the draft policy has been put forth forcefully and convincingly. The recommendations include the need to focus on the 3–8 year age range as the foundational stage, strengthening ECCE in *anganwadis* run under the ICDS and integration of health and nutrition services at all pre-school centres.

3.4.2 The emerging ECCE policy agenda holds promise but faces implementation challenges

Regarding the nature, scope and content of early childhood education, the educationists and CSOs welcomed the clarity provided by the National ECCE Policy, 2013, and the accompanying National ECCE Curriculum Framework. The National ECCE Policy seeks to promote inclusive, equitable and contextualised opportunities for the optimal development of all children below the age of 6. It seeks to regulate and improve the quality of pre-school establishments across the country over a prescribed time period. It recommends the inclusion of play and activity, learning by doing in a child-friendly, manner to encourage self-expression, self-esteem and confidence among young children.

The National ECCE Curriculum Framework lays emphasis on strengthening capabilities of families, communities and service providers to ensure quality care and education for children in the early years. It seeks parental commitment to timely enrolment of children in ECCE programmes. Going beyond the National ECCE Policy, it proposes gender training of ECCE teachers, equal treatment of boys and girls, and the use of gender sensitive stories and play-way methods. It also encourages the regular communication of AWWs with parents on children's progress, the tapping of parents' and grandparents' knowledge of folk tales for learning in AWCs, early identification by ECCE teachers of disabilities and medical conditions and counselling of parents. The focus on inclusion of children with special needs and on reading, and the extra attention to the setting up of library facilities is another positive step.

The draft NEP 2019 has recognised several quality related deficiencies in the existing ECCE programmes, including the curriculum not geared to meet the developmental needs of children, lack of qualified and trained teachers and substandard pedagogy. It recommends a curricular framework for the 3–8 year age group that would be transacted as a learning continuum, by provisioning good quality ECCE at AWCs, at AWCs co-located in primary schools, at pre-primary sections of primary schools and at standalone pre-schools.

***Samagra Shiksha Abhiyan*, the latest scheme of the MHRD, can also mark the shift towards comprehensive and holistic education of the young child.** It proposes a consolidation of education services from pre-nursery to Class 12 under one umbrella, subsuming the three schemes: SSA, *Rashtriya Madhyamik Shiksha Abhiyan* (RMSA) and Teacher Education (TE), in order to streamline budgetary allocations and improve implementation. The scheme's objectives include reducing gaps based on gender, region, ethnicity and ability, ensuring the quality and relevance of education and strengthening local bodies like DIETs and SIEs (State Institutes of Education) and SCERTs towards realising RTE.

A centrally sponsored scheme, it has a distinct thrust on ECCE to be achieved by consolidating all Government funded pre-school programmes (viz., AWCs, *balwadis*, nursery, pre-school, preparatory, pre-primary, lower and upper kindergarten), locating pre-schools within the school campuses to the extent possible, special training initiatives for ECCE staff, involving institutions of higher education, strengthening existing linkages and building new ones and development of age appropriate programmes and materials. Albeit the scheme is an opportunity, its implementation by the Centre and states facilitated by effective monitoring processes, accountability and evaluation procedures shall determine its worth. There are concerns about effectively integrating the necessary health, nutrition, care and family support needs required by children in the three to six age group, accessing education in the pre-primary sections of the primary schools, at the co-located *anganwadis*. Distance for children to receive pre-school education at the primary school, whether in co-located *anganwadi* or at the school, is another concern.

The policy documents and curricular frameworks essentially provide structure to ECCE settings but the field-level ECCE service providers do not always translate them into action. Diversity and equity related issues of children and families in ECCE settings need to be assessed. The pivotal roles and relationships in the community and ECCE settings will influence the quality of transactions, as well as the child's learning and adaptability to vital aspects of the curriculum, thereby affecting the success of the programme. The teacher is looked upon as a key figure, more so in poverty settings, and parents look up to her in the quest for a bright future for their child. If the teacher is an untrained figure, their faith in the relevance of the ECCE programme will fade.

The implementation of several policies related to ECCE in India with progressive principles and promising approaches has been weak and plagued by capacity deficits. Additionally, there are some gaps and grey areas that need to be addressed through new or revised policies and guidelines, or enhancing capacities and accountability, and may even require further enquiry. The affirmation of the importance of ECCE for universalisation of elementary education took time and how the recommendations from the draft NEP 2019 will translate into plans, programmes and financial allocations is still a moot question.

Interventions seeking to strengthen early learning from birth till the age of six or eight need to be nuanced in their design and delivery by factoring in the socio-cultural milieu, economic conditions and marginalities of the young child and incorporating developmentally appropriate activities and support for newborns, toddlers and pre-school goers incrementally.[28] A holistic approach to ECCE facilitates child development, which occurs within the immediate and distant context of the child. It entails programmatic response to improve the overall environment within which the child is situated and to create a system that is equipped for attending to the unique development needs of each child. Furthermore, as child development is a continuous and cumulative process, and what precedes influences what follows, programmatic interventions need to plan for and address the entire childhood continuum, from prenatal to the end of the primary stage, as opposed to intervening during any one sub-stage exclusively.[29] The implications of this approach on systems strengthening, delivery of quality services and influencing social behaviours and norms are many.

Early learning has received a boost through policies and legislation, be it the National ECCE Policy and the draft NEP, 2019, but it needs to be taken a few notches higher in terms of public awareness and consciousness through political thrust. A comprehensive ECD framework, which situates a culturally relevant position on ECCE and views early learning in conjunction with childcare, is still elusive notwithstanding the abundance of policy statements. As the issues related to ECCE are located within various laws, sectoral policies and ICDS, sector-specific policymaking tends to obstruct the formulation of a holistic perspective and approach required for dealing with issues related to the young child.

3.4.3 Government and private ECCE and pre-school education fall short of expectations

ICDS may have the responsibility of delivering a comprehensive package of services for the young child, it is widely seen for its nutrition component and its ECCE component has been widely viewed as its weakest link. Accordingly, there has been a demand for restructuring the ICDS with a holistic approach to ECD and strengthening of the ECCE component.

The India Early Childhood Education Impact (IECEI) study, a collaborative, three-tier longitudinal study of ECCE service provision in rural areas in three states identified some of the key problems. It found that the AWCs had inadequate facilities like buildings and water supply. The location of AWCs was not always conducive for ECCE, and in some places they were located in the homes of the AWW. A significant 40 percent of workers lived outside the village in spite of the fact that a majority of them had been working for over five years (78 percent) and a significant 80 percent had received refresher training in the previous year.[30]

On the other hand, public and private sector pre-schools provide a different set of challenges with inconsistent quality and resource deficits. The government pre-schools have limited early learning resources, training for teachers and higher pupil teacher ratios. Private pre-schools, especially the low fee paying schools, employ untrained teachers, have poor space and infrastructure, and few early learning materials. Only the high-end pre-schools that cater to socio-economically better off group, are able to pay salaries to their pre-school teachers that are equivalent to primary grade teachers by charging high fees and payments for other expenses.

3.4.4 *Management challenges compromise performance*

Early learning programmes come under the ambit of two ministries, viz. the MWCD, which manages the ICDS, and the MHRD, which is responsible for school education, including pre-primary. The efforts to universalise ECCE programmes with quality need to factor in their overlapping roles, responsibilities and systems. Consistency with the National ECCE Policy, 2013, a common approach to ECCE and the basis for budgetary allocation, monitoring and evaluation would be imperative for efficiency and improved outcomes for young children.

In the ICDS, weak supervision has seriously undermined the monitoring of AWCs and performance of the frontline staff. While the field level staffing is good, the vacancies at supervisory levels are generally very high. The remuneration structures vary between the states and low pay impedes recruitment, especially of knowledgeable, skilled and motivated individuals. This results in infrequent visits by supervisors to AWCs, especially in rural, tribal and even in urban areas to monitor their performance. Even among the existing supervisory staff, the perception of their roles and responsibilities is limited. While holding the ICDS accountable for performance may be easier, the private ECCE centres are generally unlisted and unregulated.

While some states have gone ahead with including one to two years of pre-school, there are multiple curriculums available in the states, and there is lack of clarity and training on which curriculum to follow. Considerable work is needed on developing a single developmentally appropriate curriculum, which facilitates smooth transition from pre-schools to early grades with a curriculum that is in continuum and has flexibility for children to learn at their own pace. It needs to be applied in age-appropriate teaching learning processes in a language that contributes to cultural continuity in addition to facilitating expression and learning.

3.4.5 *The critical role of family in early learning needs to be upheld and strengthened*

The debates on the inclusion of the under 6 years age group in the RTE raise a valid concern regarding the role of the family. Will it diminish the importance of the family in the upbringing of the young child? **The importance of keeping the young child at home for the longest possible time during early childhood need not be undermined by the universalisation of ECCE.**

As early learning can happen simultaneously within and outside the home at crèches, day-care facilities and pre-schools, the challenge essentially is to ensure that both the family as well as the ECCE providers complement each other in order to optimise cognitive development of young children. Parents and other members in the family have a crucial role in early childhood learning, especially among the under three age group, through nurturing care of infants and young children.

Gender and socially transformative parenting visualises both parents playing an active role in parenting as well as avoiding inequalities and stereotypes relating to access to food and nutrition, early education, the nature of games and toys they introduce their children to. It has the potential to help break gender norms on emotional, physical and intellectual parenting.

There is greater emphasis on education of mothers on ECCE than fathers through home based and centre based stimulation for 'mother and child' to strengthen parental interventions. For instance, the pictures illustrating parental interactions with ECCE centres in the guidelines feature only mothers. It refers to the need for gender-neutral play way methods but does not address stereotypes based on factors such as caste, class, religion and ethnicity.[31]

Community participation in ECCE programmes can foster healthy relationships between teachers, families and local communities, community identities and promote a sense of belonging. It is not just important to acknowledge and accept cultural difference, to work towards removing discrimination and bias, social, ethnic and individual; it is also important to go further to implement knowledge, skills and products of the local culture to facilitate regard for the community, neither overly celebratory nor with contempt.

Social mobilisation processes may benefit from communication of appropriate messages that take cognisance of the aspirations of parents for good quality education for their children and encourage their engagement in the learning processes. Simultaneously, programme organisers need to maintain contact with educators, participate in programmes, provide regular opportunities for an interface between state and field level workers and mediate with the community on objectives and practices.

3.4.6 *There is a weak thrust on the young child in disadvantaged communities*

Research has shown that ECCE benefits the most vulnerable children significantly, and early intervention has immense benefits, especially under conditions of destitution, disability and conflict.[32] With a large percentage of children in vulnerable circumstances, questions are legitimately raised about India's preparedness to prepare its children for the new world, to provide the skills, attributes and knowledge required for contemporary career options. Although there have been several schemes for enhancing children's access to quality education – through the expansion of educational infrastructure, the inclusion of disadvantaged groups and weaker sections, and incentives to states for improving the systems, performance of schools and outcomes for children have been neglected.

There is still a lot that needs to be learnt about the early learning processes in disadvantaged communities, such as those experiencing poverty and deprivation, marginalisation due to socio-cultural distinction and living in remote habitats, as well as children with disabilities and transgender children. These lessons need to be integrated in ECCE programmes to make early learning a meaningful process for the young child, her family and community.

Schools promote independence and autonomy in learning and development but learning among communities, especially those in rural and tribal areas is cooperative and collaborative. One can use the expression 'distributed intelligence' to describe the knowledge that children have. Information is not expected to reside inside people, but among them. Siblings, neighbours and cousins teach each other and care for each other.

Gender transformative ECCE programmes engage parents, caregivers, community leaders and educators to change the way that children are taught so that unjust gendered norms and attitudes are challenged from an early age; ensure that girls and boys are provided with equal care and opportunities; promote men's support for care work and emotional engagement in the upbringing of children; and support women's rights to health, freedom from violence and empowerment.[33]

The demand for homework and the participation of parents in children's learning may be an unreasonable expectation, especially for first generation learners. Children are expected to care for bags, books and stationery and face a lot of negativity from schools for not being able to 'take care' of their materials.

It is in this context that the person facilitating pre-school education, whether a teacher or AWW, should have the aptitude, skills and knowledge to engage with young children and their families. It has been noted that wide cultural differences among children and their families can be a stumbling block, with pre-school teachers' attitudes towards children guided by social status and economic progress and in many instances, treatment of first generation learners with contempt. Proper selection, orientation, sensitisation, training and performance monitoring are therefore crucial.

In the absence of a cadre orientated, trained and dedicated to ECCE, professionalised ASHAs and AWWs may be mobilised to counsel parents on its basic principles and their role and responsibility in creating a supportive learning environment at home and holding the local service providers accountable.

3.4.7 *Resource deficits hinder the delivery of ECCE services*

Limitations of financial, human and technical resources have prevented the translation of progressive policy provisions into action, and thereby undermined the up-scaling and quality of ECCE services. Unless ECCE is injected with enhanced financial resources for improving the capacities, competencies and remuneration of personnel, securing adequate space, infrastructure and materials and developing age-appropriate curricula, and alternative approaches are taken to scale, then the government's commitment to ensure school readiness of all young children entering cannot be realised.

The funding for ECCE is currently subsumed within the inadequate budgetary allocations for the ICDS run by MWCD, and the *Samagra Shiksha Abhiyaan* managed by the MHRD. The bias of ICDS towards services such as supplementary nutrition and immunisation has relegated early learning to the margins. The Innovation Fund under the *Sarva Shiksha Abhiyaan* had allowed some initiatives for strengthening ECCE in ICDS, including the attempts at curriculum renewal. The state governments could utilise the amount of INR 1.5 million per district per year for a few options, which included the ECCE. Various states availed of the available funding, howsoever insubstantial, for pilot programmes to establish pre-primary education models that could be taken to scale. But this source dried up around 2012–2013 possibly due to lack of convergence between MHRD and MWCD, and concerns regarding duplication of resources.[34]

Once the framework for AWWs and government pre-schools is strengthened, there could be enhanced central provision for funding and the Innovation Fund could be revived with substantially enhanced funds for pre-school education to enable states to localise ECCE. India's diversity necessitates a flexible and contextual approach to ECCE.

The National ECCE Policy, 2013, and the National ECCE Curriculum Framework lack clarity on budgetary allocation for gender and social sensitisation of AWWs, helpers, CDPOs, parents and caregivers and material development and production. They also fall short in addressing the costs related to ECCE services for young street children, migrant workers' children, children of construction workers, children whose parents are in bonded labour, children of sex workers and child protection, including the identification and referral of cases of child sexual abuse to Child Protection Officers and parents (in case they are not involved).[35]

The working conditions, workload and remuneration of the AWWs and pre-school teachers need to be revisited in this context. According to several accounts, the AWWs are overwhelmed by the administrative functions, especially the maintenance of records. Most of the 60 AWWs in a study mentioned they were overworked and reimbursements for expenses were frequently delayed. They also felt they were being paid poorly for the amount of work they were expected to do.[36]

The issue of remuneration is important because a duly qualified teacher should provide education in the foundational stages.

The AWWs already carrying out multiple responsibilities is less likely to be equipped for ECCE through courses of short duration. They receive, at best, short trainings before and during their appointment. The promise of technical support, coaching and mentoring often remains unrealised as the Supervisors and the CDPO themselves may not have the orientation and training for ECCE. The status, motivation and accountability of AWWs also suffer when they are viewed as a 'volunteer' worker and paid an honorarium. For several decades now, experts have advocated for a two-year pre-primary teachers' education programme. It raises a set of issues about the system of training as well as the content for pre-school teachers, curriculum for *anganwadis* and pre-schools and the language in interactions.

Autonomous institutions like the National Institute for Public Cooperation and Child Development (NIPCCD) and some of the state branches in the ICDS have been conducting training for AWWs but they seem unable to provide training consistently to the large numbers of frontline staff across the country. The distribution of training institutions across states is uneven and most trainings are of short duration, which cannot instil the sensitivity, knowledge and skills for ECD, especially the early learning and childcare components, among them.

The dearth of recognised training facilities, which could provide specialisation in ECD and ECCE, is not surprising. Lack of a holistic perspective on ECD and consensus on professionalisation of core service providers has hampered the development of capacities for delivery of good quality services to young children. The fragmented components of ECD fail to coalesce when the roles and responsibilities of the service providers are fragmented.

The creation of a cadre of pre-school teachers' trainers also deserves particular attention. The training of trainers is exceptionally important for an endeavour that seeks to create a young child centred ECD system.

3.4.8 The collaboration with academia and CSOs is negligible

There is a significant knowledge deficit, which impedes the provision of affordable, scalable and culturally appropriate ECCE to the sizeable numbers of children who are disadvantaged and marginalised. Academic institutions like the Centre for Early Childhood Education and Development (CECED), Ambedkar University, New Delhi, and Azim Premji University, Bengaluru, have lately been active in the discussions on ECD policy and practice at the national level. But the involvement of institutions of higher learning with trainings, technical assistance, coaching and mentoring as part of scalable capacity development endeavours has been negligible.

The contribution of several NGOs has been significant in innovative programmes involving children of working mothers, children in difficult circumstances, children with disabilities, urban poor communities, remote villages and tribal areas. NGOs like BODH, PRATHAM, and Mobile Creches have pioneered high quality training programmes for educators.[37] Some of them with considerable experience of innovating and implementing promising ECCE models have cooperated with state governments and government agencies on pilot projects and piecemeal training processes. Although the NGOs appear keen to work with the government agencies to share and upscale their models, the collaboration has been fragmented. An institutional mechanism is required for GoI-NGO dialogue, which could lend credibility and independence to NGO action. Different models need flexibility to sustain, as discussed in Box 3.6.

Box 3.6   Different strategies for similar goals can be effective

India has a wide range of models in the field of ECCE including AWCs, private pre-schools, government/private schools having a pre-school section and AWCs located in government primary schools. Some of these models are nationwide whereas others are single centres or clusters of centres providing for local communities. Of late, there has been a focus-shift for making ICDS and other successful early childhood programmes to local programmes with strong early education component.

Although schemes propose standard procedures, flexibility in implementation is needed so that different models can sustain. An analysis of the findings from a nationwide qualitative study to document lessons from case studies of effective ECCE programmes by CECED in 2013 identified multiple pathways to successful programming. These organisations differed in terms of mandate, priorities and organisational structure. Inevitably, they had taken different routes to success with vastly different objectives, starting points, coverage and funding, but a commitment to children was the common theme. ECCE was not a goal but a means of achieving their goals, including promotion of democratic principles; poverty eradication; community mobilisation, participation and development; pre-school education,; and timely entry and retention for universalisation of elementary education.

3.5 Recommendations and action points

3.5.1 *Situate ECCE within a comprehensive ECD framework*

A shared understanding of ECD and its components needs to guide the commitment, policy shifts and expansion of programmes for achieving universalisation of ECCE services. Government agencies and CSOs should promote ECCE, which encapsulates the under 3 and 3–6 year age groups, continuing until 8 years, by advocating synergetic action by parents and family members, as well as service providers.

National ECD campaign: A nationwide campaign for ECD with strong ECCE component similar to the *Poshan Abhiyaan*, the national flagship nutrition campaign backed by the Prime Minister, must be followed up with persistence and consistency in utilisation of available options and opportunities, and ensuring accountability through tools such as *jan sunwaayi* (social audits). The overarching strategy should have enough flexibility for adaptation to local situations and social dynamics.

Common pre-school curriculum: The Central and state governments, through NCERT and State Councils of Educational Research and Training (SCERTs) should consider formulating a pre-school curriculum which is developmentally appropriate, inclusive and flexible enough for young children in different socio-cultural, economic and geographical contexts to learn at their own pace and transition to primary school smoothly. Such a curriculum must draw the curricular goals and pedagogy from the National Curricular Framework, ECCE 2014.[38] It would help in addressing the common misconception among parents and the general public as well as undertrained pre-school teachers, including AWWs, of pre-school education merely being a downward extension of primary school.

Thrust on equity and social inclusion: The ECD Framework needs to be bolstered by a strategy articulating equity and inclusion through capacity development of ECCE teachers, appropriate rules and regulations to ensure non-discrimination and inclusion of all young children, mechanisms to identify young children with disabilities, children from different social groups, children at risk of abuse and disadvantaged by multiple socio-cultural, geographic, political and economic barriers.

Promotion of gender and socially transformative parenting practices through ECCE: The School Management Committee (SMC), Village Education Committees, *Gram Sabhas* and other forums for sensitising teachers, parents and village leaders on gender/socially transformative parenting and the importance and holistic nature of ECCE should be integrated within the guidelines on *Samagra Shiksha Abhiyan*.

3.5.2 Seek extension of RTE to include early childhood age group

The Central Government needs to act upon the recommendations made in the draft NEP 2019, to extend the RTE Act 2009, to include all children under 6, within the ambit of a justiciable right to education. Further the state must expand its vision for education by addressing the holistic needs of children under three, through an institutional mechanism, namely the ICDS. The framework of the comprehensive RTE should give adequate thrust to early education while maintaining the primacy to health, nutrition, nurturing care and protection. A consultative process involving relevant government ministries, departments and agencies, academia and research institutions, CSOs and private service providers, and organisations with global experience and knowledge could add value to the drafting of the law to extend the RTE Act 2009 to cover children under 6 years.

The current policy framework also needs to be revisited in order to bring consistency in provisions for ECCE across all settings, private and public, and provide norms around the age of admission to pre-primary, teacher pupil ratio, curriculum, trained teachers, essential infrastructure and other inputs. The direction provided by the National ECCE Policy, 2013, and the draft NEP, 2019, needs to be pursued to move towards a continuous and integrated ECCE experience for children aged 3 to 6 in the pre-schools and pre-primary classrooms and their transition to primary school.

3.5.3 Strengthen trainers' capacities and competencies for early education

A clear vision towards teacher training for the ECCE sector needs to guide the Central and state governments. Given the large number of qualified early childhood education teachers required to universalise ECCE in India, capacity enhancement at multiple levels is imminent.

Revamp the existing training institutions: The Central and state governments should expand the network of training institutions that offer trainings as per National Council for Teacher Education (NCTE) norms to train pre-school teachers. The District Institutes of Education and Training (DIETs), SCERT and NIPCCD regional offices can support in the formulation and standardisation of training curriculum for ECCE workers.

Transition to higher education in ECCE: The Central and state governments should consider operationalising a four-year integrated B.Ed. programme focussing on the early years, in accordance with the recommendations of the Draft NEP 2019. A two-year pre-service diploma from a recognised institution after class 12 could address immediate human resource requirements till the four year B.Ed. becomes operational nationwide.

Interim short-term courses for ECCE providers: The government should consider granting a period of five years in order to encourage the AWW and other in-service pre-school teachers to upgrade their qualifications and become eligible for ECCE. They may be provided with NCTE approved courses of six months or more, which can be taught on campus and through distance, Massive Open Online Courses (MOOC) mediums to learn the theoretical and practical dimensions of ECCE, based on their current qualifications and experience. NIPCCD may collaborate with government, private and CSO institutions for training the AWWs for delivering quality ECCE at the AWCs.

Collaboration with academia and CSOs: The government should encourage and mobilise academic institutions and CSOs with experience and expertise to upgrade the capacities and competencies of AWWs and other caregivers till more training institutions with appropriate facilities are established.

3.5.4 *Professionalise ECCE workforce for universalised quality service provision*

Central and state governments need to work in tandem towards transforming the ICDS frontline workforce into formally recognised AWWs/ECCE workers who are caregivers for children under three years and educators imparting ECCE to children between 3–6 years at AWCs. It would entail investment in one additional worker at the AWC level, development of capacities and competencies of AWWs and ECCE teachers, as per requisite norms of NCTE for pre-school teachers.

Provision for a second AWW: In view of the multiple roles and responsibilities of the AWW under the ICDS, a provision for a second AWW, perhaps identified as the ECCE teacher, needs to be made, who provides early education at the AWC and supports families to create a learning environment at home as well. ECD with strong early education component requires quality time and interactions with young children, which the sole AWW clearly cannot provide while delivering the existing package of services, in addition to responding to demands for periodic work by local administrators during elections, public campaigns and festivals. In order to optimise the utility of available spaces, the timings of AWCs could be extended with two shifts of six hours each to accommodate children from six months to six years. Two trained workers – AWW and ECCE teacher and one helper – could work in two shifts at an AWC for effectively covering developmental needs of children under 3, and 3 to 6 years.

Remuneration commensurate with the role and responsibility: Essentially, two workers need to be employed, one trained to work with children under 3 years and the second AWW trained to work as an ECCE teacher for children in the 3–6 year age group, and remunerated as per their qualifications and roles. Recommendations for enhancing AWW and helper remuneration are made in Chapter 6.

Rationalisation of roles and responsibilities of ECD/ECCE service providers: The government should revisit the role, responsibilities and essential qualifications of all categories of frontline workers and supervisors while framing the profiles of AWWs and ECCE service providers. A certain degree of rationalisation of their roles and responsibilities would be required in view of the existing overlaps. ECCE teachers must be duly qualified and understand their roles to create opportunities and incentives for delivery of ECCE, within AWCs and across other ECCE services.

Supportive supervision and accountability: The government should make concerted efforts to promote supportive supervision processes of ICDS towards ensuring performance, accountability and outcomes. The appointment of mid-level staff through direct recruitment and internal promotion may help to address the human resource deficit at supervisory levels but a system for capacity development – including in-service training, coaching, mentoring, exposure visits and other learning opportunities on a regular basis – should be established. Ultimately, the system should integrate norms, practices and process and outcome indicators for performance accountability at different levels.

3.5.5 Increase budgetary allocation for quality ECCE

The Central government should seriously consider the amendment of the RTE Act to put the onus of free, quality and equitable pre-school education for all children fairly and squarely on the state governments and develop a formula for financing through the *Samagra Shiksha Abhiyan*, ICDS and other budget lines.

3.5.6 Activate ECD or ECCE councils at the national, state and district levels

As per the provisions in the National ECCE Policy, the national and state level ECCE councils need to be established or reactivated with a coherent agenda for action and to bring all actors to the discussion on convergence. These ECCE Councils can explore ways to strengthen governance, mobilisation of additional resources, convergence between government departments, institutions, employers and commercial bodies to ensure universal outreach of quality services and compliance with the existing policies and laws.

Local level committees could facilitate early learning and interaction with training staff, encourage interactions among young children belonging to different economic groups, castes and religion on a regular basis, reconstitute mothers' committees as parents' committees and monitor the quality of ECCE services, at the same time ensuring all children are protected against risks of abuse.

3.5.7 Regulate private sector services

The Government should consider a comprehensive regulatory framework to ensure consistent quality of ECCE services across public and private agencies. It should develop minimum norms and standards for all providers of ECCE, whether public or private. The framework should seek to create an enabling regulatory environment. More specifically, the ECCE Policy recommends the creation of National, State and District ECCE Councils to lay the regulatory framework of early childhood care and education in India. The National ECCE Council was set up only as an advisory and oversight body and gradually become an autonomous regulatory body for systematic improvements in the field of ECCE.[39]

An independent body, similar to the ECCE Council, may be set up to enable, inform, advocate and promote ECCE across public and private services, in India. Such a system is required for registration, accreditation and regulation, including monitoring of the adherence of basic norms and minimum standards by private service providers. CSOs and childcare cooperatives could be involved in the regulatory process based on norms and indicators established by this council.

Key messages

- There is substantial evidence that learning begins at birth. The holistic needs of health, nutrition, protection and stimulation during the early years facilitate cognitive and psycho-social development of children.

- Although India has the world's largest programme for young children, viz., ICDS, and a wide range of innovative ECCE models developed by NGOs, universalisation of ECD services is still a distant dream.
- The neglect of ECCE is a major critique of the ICDS since the 1980s, constrained by resource and capacity deficits. The neglect results in a cumulative burden that a child carries through schooling into adulthood.
- Various NGOs offer ECCE services to children who are unreachable by the services provided by the Government or the private sector. The NGO-run services are limited in their reach and impact, necessitating an urgent need for public systems and structures to provide quality ECCE to the most excluded children
- There is limited understanding of ECCE among parents, who tend to prioritise formal schooling.
- There are rural-urban differences, social category differences and wealth index differences in participation in the AWCs and private pre-school education centres.
- The mother tongue as the language of conversation and instruction enables easy comprehension while the young child can apply the innate ability to pick up sound patterns of other languages through gradual exposure.
- More investment in policy, legislation and planning, less so in monitoring and evaluation, and hardly any in implementation and quality enhancement, has led to the lack of a comprehensive perspective for good quality early education services.

Notes

1 Weisner et al., 1977; Also see, Samman et al., 2016.
2 Goldstein, 2012.
3 Oller et al., 1997.
4 Carpenter et al., 1998.
5 See Fernald et al., 1989; O'Neill et al., 2005; Aslin et al., 1998.
6 Mohanty, 2010.
7 Minority Rights Group International and UNICEF, 2009.
8 Oswalt, A. *Early Childhood Gender Identity and Sexuality*. Retrieved from www.gracepointwellness.org/462-child-development-parenting-early-3-7/article/12771-early-childhood-gender-identity-and-sexuality; date of access: 29 November 2019.

 9 Lancet, 2007.
10 Chaudhary et al., 2018.
11 UNESCO Institute of Statistics, 2017.
12 Retrieved from http://udise.in/Downloads/Publications/Documents/Flash_Statistics-2015-16_(Elementary).pdf; http://udise.in/Downloads/Elementary-STRC-2015-16/All-India.pdf; date of access: 29 November 2019.
13 Kaul et al., 2017.
14 Tripathy et al., 2014.
15 See www.indiaspend.com/in-2015-16-creches-served-more-children-than-a-decade-ago-but-achieved-limited-outcomes-59558/; date of access: 1 December 2019.
16 www.ncert.nic.in/departments/nie/dee/publication/pdf/deethemebased.pdf
17 Young Lives, 2017.
18 Sood, 2014; Singh, 2014.
19 Gupta, 2016.
20 Kaul et al., 2017.
21 Ibid.
22 Sianesi and Goodman, 2005.
23 MHRD, 2011.
24 Retrieved from http://planningcommission.nic.in/aboutus/committee/wrkgrp12/hrd/wg_elementary1708.pdf; date of access: 30 November 2019.
25 Law Commission of India, 2015.
26 Central Square Foundation, 2016.
27 Ministry of Human Resource Development (MHRD), Government of India, 2019.
28 Bronfenbrenner and Morris, 2006.
29 NCERT, 2006.
30 Kaul et al., 2017.
31 MWCD, n.d.
32 Kim and Umayahara, 2010.
33 Plan International, 2017.
34 Kaul and Bhattacharjea, 2019.
35 MWCD, n.d.
36 Reddy, 2017.
37 Kaul et al., 2017.
38 Government of India, MWCD.
39 Resolution, National Early Childhood Care and Education Council. dated 26 February 2014.

Bibliography

Abels, M., 2008. Field Observations from Rural Gujarat. In S. Anandalakshmy, N. Chaudhary and N. Sharma (Eds.), *Researching Families and Children: Culturally Appropriate Methods* (pp. 211–231). Sage, New Delhi.

Aslin, R.N., P.W. Jusczyk and D.B. Pisoni, 1998. Speech and Auditory Processing During Infancy: Constraints on and Precursors to Language. In D. Kuhn and R.S. Siegler (Eds.), *Handbook of Child Psychology: Vol. 2. Cognition, Perception and Language*. Wiley, New York.

Bateson, G., 1976. A Theory of Play and Fantasy. In J. Bruner, A. Jolly and K. Sylva (Eds.), *Play: Its Role in Development and Evolution* (pp. 119–129). Penguin Books, Harmondsworth.

Bronfenbrenner, U. and P.A. Morris, 2006. The Bio-Ecological Model of Human Development. In *Handbook of Child Psychology: Theoretical models of human development* (p. 793–828). John Wiley & Sons Inc.

Burke, K. (1966). *Language as Symbolic Action: Essays on Life, Literature and Method*. University of California Press, Berkley, CA.

Carpenter, M., K. Nagell and M. Tomasello, 1998. Social Cognition, Joint Attention, and Communicative Competence. *Monographs of the Society for Research in Child Development*. Vol 63. No 4 (Serial No. 225).

CECED, ASER and UNICEF, 2017. *The India Early Childhood Education Impact Study*. New Delhi.

Central Square Foundation, 2016. *Pre-primary Sections in Government Schools: Current Landscape and Recommendations*. New Delhi.

Chaudhary, N., S. Kapoor and P. Pillai, 2018. *Early Learning and Holistic Development: Challenges, Prospects and Way Forward*. Technical Background Paper for the Report, 2020. Mobile Creches, New Delhi.

Chaudhary, N. and S. Shukla, 2018. Family, Identity and the Individual in India. In G. Misra (Ed.), *Advances in Psychology* (pp. 142–188). Oxford University Press, New Delhi.

Devy, G.N., 2014. *The Being of Bhasha: A General Introduction*. Orient Black-Swan, Hyderabad.

Fernald, A., T. Taeschner, J. Dunn, M. Papousek, B. de Boysson-Bardies and I. Fukui, 1989. A Cross-Language Study of Prosodic Modifications in Mothers' and Fathers' Speech to Preverbal Infants. *Journal of Child Language*. Vol 16, pp. 477–502.

G.N. Devy dreams of 'multilingual territories' within monolingual states, 2018. Retrieved from https://www.livemint.com/Leisure/nt5QrPpHbdeTbml8j8fhmK/GN-Devy-dreams-of-multilingual-territories-within-monoli.html; date of access: 16 January 2020.

Grantham-McGregor, S., Cheung, Y.B., Cueto, S., Glewwe, P., Richter, L., Strupp, B. and International Child Development Steering Group, 2007. Developmental potential in the first 5 years for children in developing countries. The lancet, 369(9555), pp.60-70.

Goldstein, J., 2012. *Play in Children's Development, Health and Well-Being*. Toy Industries of Europe, Brussels, Belgium.

Government of India, MWCD. *National ECCE Curriculum Framework 2014*. Retrieved from https://wcd.nic.in/sites/default/files/national_ecce_curr_framework_final_03022014%20%282%29.pdf; date of access: 30 November 2019.

Gupta, S., 2016. Do Private Preschools add more 'value'? *Indian Statistical Institute*. Retrieved from https://www.isid.ac.in/~epu/acegd2016/papers/SwetaGupta.pdf; date of access: 16 January 2020.

In 2015-16, Anganwadis Served More Children Than A Decade Ago But Achieved Limited Outcomes. Retrieved from https://www.indiaspend.com/in-2015-16-creches-served-more-children-than-a-decade-ago-but-achieved-limited-outcomes-59558/; date of access: 1 December 2019.

Jagannathan, S., n.d. *The Role of NGOs in Primary Education: A Study of Six NGOs*. Retrieved from http://documents.worldbank.org/curated/en/76020146 8771257407/130530323_20041118114646/additional/multi0page.pdf; date of access: 24 November 2019.

Joshi, A. and A. Taylor, 2005. Perceptions of Early Childhood Teachers and Parents of Teacher—Parent Interactions in an Indian Context. *Early Child Development and Care*. Vol 175. No 4, pp. 343–359.

Kaul, V. and S. Bhattacharjea (Eds.), 2019. *Early Childhood Education and School Readiness in India: Quality and Diversity*. Springer.

Kaul, V., Bhattacharjea, S., Chaudhary, A. B., Ramanujan, P., Banerji, M., & Nanda, M., 2017. *The India Early Childhood Education Impact Study*. New Delhi: UNICEF.

Kim, G.J. and M. Umayahara, 2010. Early Childhood Care and Education: Building the Foundation for Lifelong Learning and the Future of the Nations of Asia and the Pacific. *International Journal of Child Care and Education Policy*. Vol 4. No 2, p. 1.

Law Commission of India, 2015. *Early Childhood Development and Legal Entitlements*. Report No. 259, August 2015. Retrieved from http://lawcommissionofindia.nic.in/reports/Report259.pdf; date of access: 30 November 2019.

Lewis, O., 1969. Culture of Poverty. In D.P. Moynihan (Ed.), *On Understanding Poverty: Perspectives from the Social Sciences* (pp. 187–220). Basic Books, New York.

Lombardi, J., 2015. A Foundation for Sustainable Development: Advancing Towards a New Era for Young Children and Families. A Good Start: Advances in Early Childhood Development. *Early Childhood Matters*. Vol 124, pp. 5–10.

Menon, S. and T.S. Saraswathi, 2017. Introduction. In T.S. Saraswathi, A. Madan and S. Menon (Eds.), *Childhoods in India: Traditions, Trends and Transformations* (pp. 1–20). Routledge, New Delhi.

Ministry of Human Resource Development (MHRD), Government of India, 2011. *CABE Committee on "Extension of the Right of Children to Free and Compulsory Education Act 2009 to Pre-school Education and Secondary Education."* Retrieved from https://mhrd.gov.in/sites/upload_files/mhrd/files/document-reports/RCFCE.pdf; date of access: 30 November 2019.

Ministry of Human Resource Development (MHRD), Government of India, 2018. *Samagra Shiksha Abhiyan*. Retrieved from http://samagra.mhrd.gov.in/about.html; date of access: 31 October 2019.

Ministry of Human Resource Development (MHRD), Government of India, 2019. *Draft National Education Policy 2019*. Retrieved from https://mhrd.gov.in/sites/upload_files/mhrd/files/Draft_NEP_2019_EN_Revised.pdf; date of access: 30 November 2019.

Ministry of Women and Child Development (MWCD), Government of India, 2013. *National Early Childhood Care and Education (ECCE) Policy*. Extract from the Gazette of India, Part 1, Sec 1, 12 October 2013. Retrieved from http://wcd.nic.in/sites/default/files/ecce_gazatte_notification_policy_comp.pdf; date of access: 12 August 2018.

Ministry of Women and Child Development (MWCD), Government of India, n.d. *National Early Childhood Care and Education (ECCE) Curriculum Framework*. Ministry of Women and Child Development, New Delhi.

Ministry of Women and Child Development, Government of India, 2015. *Rapid Survey on Children 2013-14: National Report*. Page 105. Retrieved from https://wcd.nic.in/sites/default/files/RSOC%20National%20Report%202013-14%20Final.pdf; date of access: 16 January 2020.

Ministry of Women and Child Development, 2017. *Integrated Child Development Services (ICDS) Scheme*. Retrieved from https://icds-wcd.nic.in/icds.htm; date of access: 16 January 2020.

Minority Rights Group International and UNICEF, 2009. *State of the World's Minorities and Indigenous Peoples 2009*. Events of 2008.

Mohanty, A., 2010. Language, Inequality and Marginalisation: Implications of the Double Divide in Indian Multilingualism. *International Journal of the Sociology of Language*. Vol 205, pp. 131–154.

Mufti, I., 2015. Education Department to Prepare List, Recommend EWS Children to Private Schools. *The India Express*, 17 July 2015. Retrieved from https://indianexpress.com/article/cities/chandigarh/edu-dept-to-prepare-list-recommend-ews-children-to-private-schools/; date of access: 1 November 2019.

Mullainathan, S. and E. Shafir, 2013. *Scarcity: Why Having Too Little Means so Much*. Henry Holt & Company, New York.

National Commission for Protection of Child Rights, 2017. *Know Violence in Childhood*. Retrieved from http://ncpcr.gov.in/showfile.php?lang=1&level=2&&sublinkid=1679&lid=1682; date of access: 4 November 2019.

National Council for Educational Research and Training (2015–16). *Patterns of Social Inequality and Exclusion*. Retrieved from http://ncert.nic.in/ncerts/l/lesy105.pdf; date of access: 11 November 2019.

National Council of Teachers of English, 2016. *Equity and Early Childhood Education: Reclaiming the Child*. Retrieved from https://secure.ncte.org/library/NCTEFiles/EquityEarlyEdBrief.pdf; date of access: 16 January 2020.

NCERT, 2006. *National Focus Group on Early Childhood Education*. Position Paper. Retrieved from www.ncert.nic.in/new_ncert/ncert/rightside/links/pdf/focus_group/early_childhood_education.pdf; date of access: 30 November 2019.

NIPCCD, 2014. *An Analysis of Levels and Trends in Infant and Child Mortality Rates in India*. New Delhi.

NITI Aayog, 2015. *A Quick Evaluation Study of Anganwadis Under ICDS*. Niti Aayog, Programme Evaluation Organisation, June 2015.

Oller, D.K., R.E. Eilers, R. Urbano and A.B. Cobo-Lewis, 1997. Development of Precursors to Speech in Infants Exposed to Two Languages. *Journal of Child Language*. Vol 24, pp. 407–425.

O'Neill, M., K.A. Bard, M. Kinnrl and M. Fluck, 2005. Maternal Gestures with 20-Month-Old Infants in Two Contexts. *Development Science*. Vol 8, pp. 352–359.

Oswalt, A. *Early Childhood Gender Identity and Sexuality*. Retrieved from www.gracepointwellness.org/462-child-development-parenting-early-3-7/article/12771-early-childhood-gender-identity-and-sexuality; date of access: 29 November 2019.

Plan International, 2017. Gender Inequality and early childhood development: A review of the linkages. Plan International, United Kingdom. Retrieved from https://plan-international.org/publication/2017-06-08-gender-inequality-and-early-childhood-development; date of access: 16 January 2020.

Reddy, R., 2017. Problems of Anganwadi Teachers in Urban Areas – A Study of Hanmakonda. *International Journal of Social Science and Economic Research*. 2(12): 5567–5578.

Roopnarine, J.L. (2014). Play as Culturally Situated: Diverse Perspectives on Its Meaning and Significance. In J.L. Roopnarine, M. Patte, J.E. Johnson and D. Kuschner (Eds.), *International Perspectives on Children's Play* (pp. 1–9). Open University Press/McGraw Hill Education.

Samman, E. et al., 2016. *Women's Work: Mothers, Children and the Global Childcare Crisis, a Summary*. Retreived from https://bernardvanleer. org/app/uploads/2016/07/Early-Childhood-Matters-2016_12.Pdf; date of access: 29 November 2019.

Sianesi, B. and A. Goodman, 2005. Early Education and Children's Outcomes: How Long Do the Impacts Last? *Fiscal Studies*. Vol 26, pp. 513–548.

Singh, R. and Mukherjee, P., 2017. Comparison of the effects of government and private preschool education on the developmental outcomes of children: evidence from young lives India. *Young Lives India*. Working Paper 167. Retrieved from https://www.younglives.org.uk/sites/www.younglives.org.uk/files/YL-WP167-Singh%20%281%29.pdf; date of access: 1 January 2020.

Sood, N., 2014. *Meaningful access and quality of preschool education in India.* Saarbrücken: Lap Lambert.

Suneja, S., 2018. *Ecology of Care of Children by Siblings.* Unpublished Doctoral Dissertation, Department of Human Development and Childhood Studies, University of Delhi.

Sutton-Smith, B., 1997. *The Ambiguity of Play.* Harvard University Press, Cambridge, MA.

Tripathy, M., S.P. Kamath, B.S. Baliga and A. Jain, 2014. Perceived Responsibilities and Operational Difficulties of Anganwadi Workers at a Coastal South Indian City. *Medical Journal of Dr. DY Patil University.* Vol 7. No (4), p. 468.

UNDP, 2017. *Decentralisation of ICDS Supplementary Nutrition Programme: Ensuring Timely and Quality Nutrition to All Beneficiaries in Odisha.* Retrieved from https://niti.gov.in/writereaddata/files/bestpractices/Decentralisation%20of%20ICDS%20Supplementary%20Nutrition%20Programme%20Ensuring%20timely%20and%20quality%20nutrition%20to%20all%20beneficiaries%20in%20Odisha.pdf; date of access: 5 November 2019.

UNESCO Institute of Statistics, 2017. Retrieved from https://data.worldbank.org/indicator/SE.PRE.ENRR.FE?end=2017&locations=IN&start=1971&view=chart; date of access: 29 November 2019.

UNICEF, 2012. *Care and Child Development Package.* Retrieved from www.unicef.org/earlychildhood/index_68195.html; date of access: 26 November 2019.

Weisner, T.S. et al., 1977. My Brother's Keeper: Child and Sibling Caretaking [and Comments and Reply]. *Current Anthropology.* Vol 18. No 2, pp. 169–190.

4   Prioritising the disadvantaged child

Poverty, social status with debilitating norms related to gender, caste, class and abilities, and geographies and habitats, often create conditions that deprive the young child of nurturing care and developmental opportunities in their critical and formative years. Exceptional conditions such as illnesses, disabilities, loss of the breadwinner and other crises within families further exacerbate the neglect and resulting development deficit.

This chapter explores a few categories of such children as they deserve urgent affirmative action. Children who grow up amidst poverty, and increasingly exposed to climate change induced vulnerabilities, belong to socially marginalised communities such as Scheduled Castes and Scheduled Tribes, the girl child, children with disabilities and those children who do not fit into the heteronormative framework of the society are particularly deprived of the opportunities for holistic development, nurturing care and protection. They are usually the hardest to reach by public services.

4.1   Children face extreme vulnerability in many ways

4.1.1   Poverty induces vulnerability and deprivation

Allen (2011) notes that adverse experiences in childhood have a detrimental impact, and adults who had adverse childhoods "showed higher levels of violence and antisocial behaviour, adult mental health problems, school underperformance and lower Intelligence Quotient (IQ), economic underperformance and poor physical health." The resulting negative outcomes may be viewed as a reflection of an inequitable society, deprivation of child rights and hindrance to the efforts of the State to improve overall development indicators or what may be termed as the 'last mile challenge.' **Reaching the furthest behind first holds the promise of inclusiveness, shared prosperity and sustainable development.**[1]

A young child from a socially marginalised household and community, with non-literate parents working in the informal sector, with limited endowments and entitlements, is less likely to experience nurturing care and avail of developmental opportunities. **Regional, caste and economic differences** need to be factored in the analysis of issues related to young children. The changing demographic landscape affects children right from the time they are born.

Starting with breastfeeding, immunisation, healthcare, nutrition to pre-school education, communities and parents make choices. These choices could adversely affect some children – especially girls and children born with disabilities. As the indexing exercise in Chapter 1 shows, the ecosystem in which the young child grows is not only influenced by the extent of income poverty but also factors like access to healthcare, gender equity, literacy, supply of safe drinking water and sanitation. When deprivations combine, they subject these vulnerable children to multiplied effects of discrimination, marginalisation and an unhealthy overall environment in which they develop.

Notwithstanding a period of rapid economic growth in India, about 33 percent of the population still lives in acute poverty (Agarwal, 2015) and continues to experience its ill-effects in the form of poor health, low levels of education and ultimately poor quality of life. Poverty is one thread that runs across all states and all communities in India. The standard of living has improved considerably over the last 15 years but inequality between socially advantaged and socially disadvantaged households, between rural and urban households remains evident (Singh et al., 2018).[2] A recent Oxfam report (2019) noted that India's top 10 percent population holds 77.4 percent of the total national wealth. **The worst affected by deprivations caused by poverty and inequality are young children.**

Quantitative data from sample surveys and several qualitative studies done over the last three decades show direct correlation between poverty and child health. The National Health Profile (2015) of the Government of India found that rural poverty was far more severe than urban across all states.[3] In Madhya Pradesh, 21 percent urban and 35.7 percent rural people lived below the poverty line. Other states with consistently poor child health indicators were Assam (38.9 percent rural and 28.3 percent urban); Chhattisgarh (44.6 percent rural and 24.8 percent urban) and Uttar Pradesh (30.4 percent rural and 26.1 percent urban). The YCEI (Table 1.2) highlights this linkage as well. Among states that perform low on the poverty index, including Arunachal Pradesh (0.488), Manipur (0.452) and Jharkhand (0.451), they are also the poorest three performers in the overall enabling environment for the young child. Chhattisgarh scores the lowest on the poverty index (0.404) but better on gender, health and education indices but still below the national average overall.

4.1.2 Young children are most susceptible to climate change impacts

SDG 13 targets to take urgent action to combat climate change and its impacts to which the young children are most susceptible. The world is expected to experience more of ocean acidification, ice-sheet melting, sea-level rise and so-called tipping points in climate effects much sooner than ever thought of.[4]

UNICEF (2015) estimated that over half a billion children globally live in areas that are prone to extremely high levels of floods and nearly 160 million children live in areas of high or extremely high droughts. Furthermore, 26 percent of the annual 6.6 million deaths of children under 5 in 2012 were due to environment-related causes and conditions.[5] According to yet another estimate, about 600,000 deaths in children under 5 is due to air pollution, which increases the risk of respiratory infection, adverse neonatal condition and congenital anomalies.[6]

Although environmental issues are global in nature, India ranks very low on air and water pollution levels compared to rest of the world (Chandra, 2015). India is highly prone to natural disasters such as floods, droughts, cyclones, earthquakes and landslides which have been a recurrent phenomenon. Out of 602 districts in the country, as noted in a 2011 study, 125 districts have been identified as most hazard prone areas in India (Vranda and Sekar, 2011). In the event of any natural calamities, children are more likely to be injured, more vulnerable to infections and malnutrition and are also exposed to greater danger through separation from their families or caregivers (Kamath, 2015). Moreover, infant and young children separated from their caregivers are at high risk of trafficking, abuse and exploitation as they are unable to communicate.

4.2 Children born in poverty confront multiple deprivations growing up

4.2.1 The cycle of poverty has a compounding impact on the young child

Chronic poverty of their households negatively impacts children in terms of nutrition, and access to quality ECD services. The consequences of inadequate nutrition, a lack of early stimulation and learning and exposure to stress last a lifetime. They lead to stunted development, low levels of skills needed for life and work, limited future productivity as adults, and transmission of poverty down the generations. Beyond this tragic impact on human life and potential, neglecting children fails to build the human capital needed for sustained economic prosperity.[7] Figure 4.1 shows the percentage of children under age 5 across various states of India, living in the poorest and richest wealth quintiles based on NFHS-4 data.

While the number of young children living in the poorest and richest household/s varies tremendously across state/s, about 25 percent of children under age 5 in India live in households belonging to the poorest quintile and only 14.7 percent live in households in the richest quintile. About or more than 50 percent of children under age 5 in Bihar and Jharkhand belong to

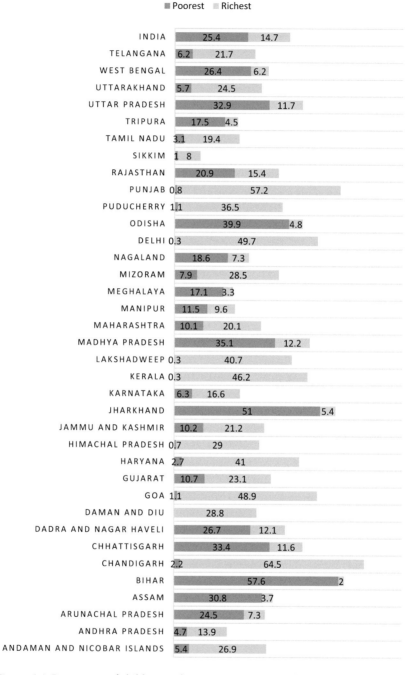

Figure 4.1 Percentage of children under age 5 in poorest and richest wealth quintiles in India

Source: National Family Health Survey-4, 2015–2016

the poorest households. In some states like Assam, Chhattisgarh, Madhya Pradesh, Odisha and Uttar Pradesh, more than 30 percent of children reside in the poorest households.

Impoverished communities often suffer from discrimination and end up getting caught in the vicious cycle of poverty which has a compounding impact on the lack and quality of care that a young child receives. Inter-generational poverty has long term consequences. From poor birth weight and neglect of early care, to recurring bouts of infections and diseases, it impacts children in multiple ways. Issues like hunger, illness and thirst are both causes and effects of poverty. They are often interrelated in such a way that one problem hardly ever occurs alone. Lack of access to water is a reflection of poverty, and being poor results in the inability to afford safe water and nutritious food. Poor health, lack of safe water or housing, child neglect and inability to study and earn a living fuel a cycle of poverty in which so many are trapped for life. Poor sanitation makes it easier to spread around old and new diseases, and hunger and lack of water make people more vulnerable to them. The YCOI and YCEI consider the overall impact of various factors to arrive at the indexing scores in each, primarily with this understanding that these multiple factors influence each other and go on to influence the overall outcomes and enabling environments for the young child.

Migration has been a coping strategy for households and communities facing uncertain livelihoods, poverty, natural calamities or conflicts. Pressures of rural poverty, increasingly unviable agricultural sector and underemployment, together with aspirations for a better life are driving men and sometimes entire families to move into towns and cities.

About 31 percent of India's population lived in urban areas in 2011, which has in all probability increased substantially with migration from rural and peri-urban areas. The Economic Survey, 2017, by the Ministry of Finance, estimated that inter-state migration in India was close to 9 million annually between 2011 and 2016,[8] while the Census 2011 pegged the total number of internal migrants in the country (accounting for inter- and intra-state movement) at a staggering 139 million. Uttar Pradesh and Bihar are the biggest source states, followed closely by Madhya Pradesh, Punjab, Rajasthan, Uttarakhand, Jammu and Kashmir and West Bengal; the major destination states are Delhi, Maharashtra, Tamil Nadu, Gujarat, Andhra Pradesh and Kerala.[9]

Many migrant families with low employment potential and opportunities are trapped in a vicious cycle of low daily wages, low productivity and chronic poverty. They are unable to secure children a good start to life as they tend to gravitate to slums where the living conditions are unhygienic and access to basic services is inadequate. In urban slums, sustainable access to safe water is related to improved water management practices, sanitation and hygiene. The perennial problem of open defecation has proved difficult to address even though the issue has been prioritised at the highest levels of the government. Municipal solid waste management (MSWM) in urban slums is a persistent challenge due to the rising population and the resultant infrastructural needs (Dube et al., 2014).

Migrants often leave their social support systems behind. While their earnings may increase in urban areas, the quality of life dips due to degraded environmental conditions of increasing pollution, lack of water and sewage, widespread exploitation and fragmentation of society. Lack of awareness and identity documents hampers their ability to avail of universal state benefits like subsidised food rations, free medical services or other social security entitlements.

The impact of migration on young children is immense though relatively less recognised. The parents are exploited, powerless and in distress as they try to get their bearings in increasingly harsh living conditions. While they seek work in the informal sector with grossly inadequate entitlements, young children are deprived of nurturing care. Box 4.1 brings forth one such story.

Box 4.1 Impact of migration

Falguni and her husband were faced with acute distress due to the intensive drought like conditions in their village and their inability to pay off the loans they had taken from the local *munshi*. A group of people were going to the city to work at a construction site, and they felt compelled to join.

In the city, a makeshift labour camp, loosely bricked and cramped houses without windows, cooking out in the open and standing in long queues to get water was their new reality. Reporting for work at sharp 9.00 in the morning, taking both her children with her to work – a four-year-old son and a six-month daughter-carrying bricks and cement for her husband in the hot sun was a new and not a pleasant experience.

One day her son developed fever, she took him to the local dispensary at the construction site. She was asked to get some tests done. Where should she go? And how? The site was too far from such facilities. Who would take care of her infant daughter whilst her son was sick?

(Bajaj, 2018)

4.2.2 Children living in slums face multiple risks

Census 2011 estimated that 65.5 million people in urban India live in slums. Of these, 8.1 million (12.3 percent of the total slum population) are children under 6 years of age. It is interesting to highlight that highest percentage of children (under age 6) residing in slums is found in the state of Bihar (16.8 percent) followed by Chandigarh (15.5 percent) and Rajasthan (14.8 percent). However, in absolute numbers of children growing up in slums, Maharashtra and Andhra Pradesh top the list with 1.4 million and 1.14 million respectively.

Although there are thriving communities in slums with strong social and economic networks, physical environments of slums present many challenges to residents, particularly children. Box 4.2 presents the state of an urban slum in Delhi and the unhygienic conditions therein. Children growing up in slums experience a childhood that often defies the imagination of both the 'innocent childhood' proponents and the 'universal childhood' advocates. The slums typically lack proper sanitation, safe drinking water, or systematic garbage collection; there is usually a severe shortage of space inside the houses where the children live and no public spaces dedicated to their use. These children do have a childhood, but it is of a different kind that sees them playing on rough, uneven ground, taking on multiple roles in everyday life and sharing responsibilities with adults in domestic and public spaces in the community.[10] Young children in the care of older siblings on streets and in slums are ubiquitous, but their issues have not merited adequate attention in the policy deliberations.

Compelled to respond to the urgent demands of earning/contributing for family survival in a new environment, women leave their toddlers locked in the house or with their older siblings who are withdrawn from school to undertake childcare. Alternatively, they sometimes take them for work but in either case, children face an insecure, unsafe and inappropriate environment not conducive for providing the essential ingredients for appropriate care. Feeding and other routines including interaction often get missed out leading to neglect and deprivation of the essential components required for optimum development.

The combination of a multitude of factors, when both parents have to work, with no extended or community support, leaves an indelible emotional and physical impact on the care and development of the young infants and children. Financial resource constraints and informal or uncertain livelihoods aggravate the pressure on parents, and particularly mothers who are often compelled to choose between childcare and employment or strike an uneasy balance. This has been the rationale for provision of maternity and paternity entitlements and childcare arrangements including crèches by the State.

According to a study by National Institute of Urban Affairs (NIUA) (2016), about 90 percent of migrant children did not have access to ICDS or any facilities at worksite, 65 percent suffered from various communicable diseases, while 80 percent did not have access to education and 40 percent worked as child labour.[11]

Box 4.2   A peek into the urban slums of Delhi reveals unhygienic living conditions

A survey of 1,200 familes in 2016 by Neenv – the Delhi chapter of FORCES – revealed an alarming picture of the life of young children in the urban slums of Delhi. The living conditions were unhealthy and unhygienic – open defecation, no running water or sanitation facilities, and open drains. Many children had not been immunised and were at high risk of infections and contagions. In the absence of any support systems for the care of their children, nearly 60 percent of women opted to stay at home instead of going out for work. Around 70 percent were not aware of the AWCs and the rest associated them with food distribution.

While family elders looked after 18 percent of the young children, elder siblings cared for about 14 percent of them. The role of elder siblings has been justified in the traditional construct of household economy but it is a cause of their deprivation from education, leisure and other basic necessities. About 9 percent of parents left their children alone at home when they went out for work, another 7 percent left them with the neighbours whilst the rest took their children to the worksites as they had no choice.

(Neenv Delhi FORCES, 2016)[12]

Many migrant children living in informal settlements and impoverished neighbourhoods are excluded from essential services and social protection and it is important that urban developers and policymakers give priority focus and attention to ensure survival, growth, development and protection of these vulnerable children. Alternative childcare support is deemed necessary when children are likely to be left alone without an adult caregiver and at high risk of neglect, violence, abuse, exploitation and trafficking. Crèches and day-care in urban poor slums deserve serious and urgent consideration in policy as alternative support systems, which can ensure safety, security and all-round development of young children. Table 4.1 shows the percentage of children under 6 in slums, those who are homeless and those who are working, across various states.

4.2.3 Children living on streets are deprived of quality ECD

India accounted for 1.77 million homeless people (Census 2011), of which 0.27 million or 15.3 percent were children below age six years. A Save the Children study (2012) of street children in cities of Uttar Pradesh, Bihar,

Table 4.1 Top 10 states by percentage of slum and homeless population and number of working children under the age of 6 in India

Slum children aged 0–6 years (in percent)	Homeless children aged 0–6 years (in percent)	Working children aged 5–6 years (numbers)
Bihar (16.8)	Dadra and Nagar Haveli (22.0)	Uttar Pradesh (250,672)
Chandigarh (15.5)	Rajasthan (20.7)	Bihar (128,087)
Rajasthan (14.8)	Haryana (19.8)	Maharashtra (82,847)
Meghalaya (14.4)	Punjab (19.1)	Andhra Pradesh (54,820)
Jharkhand (14.3)	Madhya Pradesh (18.7)	Madhya Pradesh (42,016)
Gujarat (14.3)	Jharkhand (18.6)	West Bengal (37,320)
Arunachal Pradesh (14.3)	Bihar (18.4)	Karnataka (33,489)
Jammu and Kashmir (14.2)	Chhattisgarh, 18.4)	Tamil Nadu (32,990)
Uttar Pradesh (13.8)	Meghalaya (18.4)	Rajasthan (29,939)
Haryana (13.6)	Gujarat (17.3)	Gujarat (29,871)

Source: Census of India, 2011

West Bengal and Andhra Pradesh found the highest proportion of under 6s among street children in Patna (32 percent), but their absolute number was the highest in Hyderabad. Another study by Action Aid (2013) of 25,625 boys and 10,938 girls below age 18 who lived on streets in Mumbai in 2013 found that 22.6 percent of the boys and 42.2 percent of the girls were below the age of 6. About 11 percent of the young children were beggars and 2 percent were rag pickers.

Young children living on streets literally grow up on their own with little parental support, as noted in Box 4.3. Their lives are at risk, and they miss on quality ECD. The available studies paint a dismal picture of their lives and living conditions. That they live on the streets is evidence of poverty and destitution, which is further compounded by harsh weather conditions, uncertain livelihoods and violence.

Box 4.3   Children living on streets experience parenting deprivation

A study based on interviews with 200 street children in Jaipur in Rajasthan found that 16 percent of them were in the 5–8 years age group, and only 29 percent were girls.[13] Most of them lived with their families on the streets while a few lived alone or with siblings. Parents worked late hours and several children also worked. Some of the children were engaged in begging.

Children narrated experiences of poverty, stressful family situations, working on the streets and close bonding with peers, drugs and substance addiction early in life, employers' demands and police brutality. For them, leisure was roaming the streets with other children and watching Bollywood films, however age inappropriate. The interviews indicated that girls earned less than boys and were more vulnerable to sexual exploitation and trafficking. Why girls in streets were fewer than boys can only be a topic of conjecture, but parenting in the street families was certainly ineffective.[14]

4.3 Socially marginalised communities face specific challenges

4.3.1 Scheduled Castes and Scheduled Tribes are among the most disadvantaged

Unequal distribution of income, goods and services pushes children born into ST and SC households in the category of most disadvantaged. Restricted access to basic services such as clean water, sanitation, nutrition, housing, education, healthcare and employment among these groups is due to a toxic combination of poor social policies and programmes, fewer occupation opportunities and lesser income (Vijayanath et al., 2010).

NFHS-4 data shows that for children (under age 5) living in poorest quintile households, about 27 percent were from SC households and 20.4 percent were from ST households while among richest quintile households, only 12 percent were from SC and less than 3 percent were from ST households. U5MR among SC and ST children (56 and 57 deaths per 1,000 live births respectively) has been higher than children belonging to other castes (39 deaths per 1,000 live births). The stunting levels are also higher. NFHS-4 found that the NMR among STs was 31.3, 33.0 among SCs, as against 23.2 among all others excluding SC, ST and other backward classes.

Higher prevalence of malnourishment and anaemia among children belonging to SCs and STs compared with those from the general category is indicative of the inability of development and welfare policies in addressing persistent backwardness of their communities satisfactorily. High child malnutrition is often attributed to lack of timely access to nutritious food and the barriers and bottlenecks to utilisation of health services by marginalised communities, especially those living in remote areas.

According to the NFHS-4, children (under 5 years) belonging to STs fared poorest in comparison to other categories. About 43.8 percent of them were stunted or short for their age, 27.4 were wasted or thin for their height, and 45.3 are underweight or thin for their age. This is the highest percentage share in all the three categories. Children belonging to SC communities fared better than ST children but poorly in comparison to the backward and general categories. About 42.8 percent were stunted, 21.2 percent were wasted and 39.1 percent were underweight.

The prevalence of anaemia among children is also higher among SC and STs. About 58 percent of children under 5 years are affected with anaemia in India. While 53.9 percent of children belonging to the general category were anaemic, the proportion of anaemic children belonging to STs, SCs and OBCs was higher at 63.1, 60.5 and 58.6 respectively. Table 4.2 shows the caste-wise malnourishment percentages among children under 5 years:

Table 4.2 Caste-wise malnourishment percentages among children under 5

	Stunted	*Wasted*	*Underweight*	*Anaemia*
Scheduled Castes	42.8	21.2	39.1	60.5
Scheduled Tribes	43.8	27.4	45.3	63.1
Other Backward Classes	38.7	20.5	35.5	58.6
Others (General)	31.2	19.0	28.8	53.9

Source: NFHS-4

Sudarshan and Seshadri point to the cumulative impact of the failure of convergence of services of various schemes and departments. When the departments and schemes work in silos, the desired impact cannot be achieved. They consider the failure of the AWCs to cater to the nutritional needs of children aged 6 months to 2 years to be a significant limitation of ICDS, especially as ST children in this age group are particularly deprived of adequate nutritious food due to household poverty and insecurities related to livelihood and land tenure for agriculture or harvesting of non-timber forest produce (Sudarshan and Seshadri, 2015).

The likelihood of the children migrating seasonally to cope with environmental and other shocks, marginalises them further as they end up living in under-resourced and unhygienic slums without ECD services.

Lower immunisation coverage of children belonging to ST communities adds to their vulnerability to infectious diseases as well as stunting and wasting. The immunisation coverage of ST children has consistently been lower than the national and rural Indian averages. NFHS-4 found that only 55.8 percent of ST children were fully vaccinated as against 61.3 percent in rural areas and 62 percent nationwide, and 9.2 percent of ST children were not immunised as against 6.4 percent in the rural areas and 6 percent nationwide.[15]

While issues related to availability, procurement, storage and maintenance of cold chain of vaccines affect the current system for immunisation, ST children appear to experience additional difficulties due to poor management, agenda-setting and prioritisation of tribal health problems within district administration and the state governments (Sudarshan and Seshadri, 2015).

The proportion of SC children in AWCs was higher than in the local population, and caste-based discrimination against mothers, children, AWWs and helpers declined from 14 percent in 2006[16] to 6 percent in 2016, and it was found to be higher in Rajasthan and Uttar Pradesh. The cases of caste discrimination included: upper caste women refusing to let their children accompany SC/ST helpers at the AWC, the upper caste Hindu helpers serving food to SC/ST children reluctantly, and the AWWs refusing to taste food cooked by SC/ST helpers. There were also cases of tribal women receiving lesser THR compared to upper caste women. Interestingly, the percentage of mothers who did not want children of different castes using the AWC increased from 2 percent to 9 percent.[17]

4.3.2 The girl child faces gendered forms of deprivation and neglect

Gender inequality is an important root cause of children's poor development in the early years.[18] In India, the girl child is often considered as a liability, whereas boys are given the exclusive rights to inherit the family name and they are viewed as additional status for their family (Jha and Nagar, 2015). In many parts of India, the birth of a girl child is not welcomed, this discrimination starts from even before the birth. She is killed as a foetus or later as an infant, which results in highly skewed child sex ratio in favour of boys in India. Indeed, declining CSR is a potent indicator of female disempowerment. Post-birth discrimination against girls is reflected in neglect in the intra-household distribution of food, nutrition and healthcare.

India currently faces declining sex ratio at birth (SRB) and adverse CSR as a result of systemic gender discrimination and ranks poorly in Human Development and Gender Index, as shown in Box 4.4. It is symptomatic of a patriarchal society that prefers sons over daughters and neglects girls at every stage and in various arenas.

Box 4.4   Benchmarking gender inequities and inequalities

India ranks 130 among 189 countries with a Human Development Index (HDI) value of 0.640 in the UNDP Human Development Report 2018. It marked nearly 50 percent increase from 0.427 in 1990 due to the achievement in poverty alleviation. Between 1990 and 2017, India's life expectancy at birth too increased by nearly eleven years, with even more significant gains in expected years of schooling. Indian school-age children can now expect to stay in school for 4.7 years longer than in 1990, whereas India's GNI per capita increased by a staggering 266.6 percent between 1990 and 2017.

However, India is ranked 95 with a score of 56.2 among 129 countries in the SDG Gender Index 2019 that measures global gender equality. The index takes into account 14 out of 17 SDGs that cover aspects such as poverty, health, education, literacy, political representation and equality at the workplace.[19] A score of 100 reflects the achievement of gender equality in relation to the targets set for each indicator. It means, for example, that 100 percent of girls complete secondary education, or that there is around 50–50 parity for women and men in Parliament. A score of 50 signifies that a country is about halfway to meeting a goal.[20]

The Human Capital Index (World Bank, 2018) has given India a score of 0.44 out of a total of 1.0, lower than the average for its income level countries. Simply put, children born in India today are likely to be only 44 percent as productive when they grow up, compared to a scenario if they enjoyed equal opportunities in education and health.

(*Human Development Report*, 2018;
Equal Measures 2030, 2019;
Human Capital Index, 2018)

India's SRB of 910 girls per 1,000 boys, or 955,000 'missing' girls, according to Census 2011, points to the serious problem of gender biased sex selection in India that portends serious socio-demographic consequences. The SRS (2013–2015) provides even more dismal data – 900 girls per 1,000 boys and lower than national average SRB in nine states (viz., Haryana, Uttarakhand, Gujarat, Rajasthan, Delhi, Maharashtra, Uttar Pradesh, Punjab, Jammu and Kashmir). Haryana had the lowest SRB of 831 girls per 1,000 boys. SRS data (2013–2015) for states with adverse SRB is presented in Table 4.3.

Table 4.3 Top 10 states with adverse SRB in India

Girls per 1,000 boys at birth (SRB)	
Haryana	831
Uttarakhand	844
Gujarat	854
Rajasthan	861
Delhi	869
Maharashtra	878
Uttar Pradesh	879
Punjab	889
Jammu and Kashmir	899
Assam	900

Source: Sample Registration System, 2013–2015.

In YCEI (Table 1.2), gender index has been computed through sex ratio data. Most of the states listed in Table 4.3 also score low on the overall YCEI, for instance Haryana (Rank 15), Maharashtra (Rank 17), Gujarat (Rank 20), Rajasthan (Rank 22), Uttar Pradesh (Rank 24) and Assam (Rank 25). The others score relatively better on other indicators, which allows a better overall ranking.

4.3.3 Transgender children face severe societal stigma

Growing awareness of diverse identities on the gender spectrum over the years has resulted in the acknowledgement, albeit muted, of transgender children. They are among the most marginalised categories of children, who are rendered invisible due to the stigma associated with people who do not identify with the heteronormative gendered identities. They grow up in an environment that is unwilling to recognise their identities, and tend to be more uncomfortable in their bodies since it does not fit their own sense of gendered identity, leaving them more vulnerable.[21] They grapple with acceptance issues and social ostracism throughout their lives.

Although children develop a clear concept of their gender identity as they grow older, they begin to grapple with some of the concerns early on. Parents and caregivers are more likely to identify early signals, which can be extremely disturbing for the family and community, and threatening for the young child.[22] The stigmatisation and ostracism of the transgender persons created a community that has lived on the margins of the mainstream society and looked out for their own through 'child-nabbing.'[23]

The issues related to children experiencing difficulties due to a mismatch of their behaviour with the social norms associated with their birth sex have been discussed among those who work with children even though the issue has not been subjected to an empirical enquiry. The acknowledgement of transgender people and granting of the legal status of 'third gender' in India[24] has made it possible to bring their issues out in the open.

Data on transgender children is almost non-existent. But a recent survey of 900 transgender persons in Delhi and Uttar Pradesh by the Kerala Development Society for the National Human Rights Commission in 2018 found that only 20 percent of them had completed primary school education, and only 15 percent of them in Delhi and 10 percent in Uttar Pradesh had been able to complete secondary education.[25] The stigma and trauma of nonacceptability, bullying, and abuse, restricts the mobility and schooling of these children early on, necessitating the need for gender sensitisation with a broader perspective and evidence based advocacy to address their specific issues.

4.3.4 Children with disabilities lack equitable and accessible services

Children with disabilities are in general more vulnerable to neglect, violence, abuse and exploitation. According to the 2011 Census, 1.24 percent of children in the under 6 age group in India were disabled, the various categories noted in Table 4.4. Among them, 20.4 percent had visual impairment, 23.3 percent had hearing impairment, 5.6 percent speech impairment, 9.6 percent physical impairment and 7.30 percent had multiple disability. About 1.4 percent (397,015) of SC children and 1.1 percent (176,110) of ST children below age 6 were disabled. Maharashtra identified the highest percentage (1.63 percent, 217,361) of children with disability.

Due to lack of accessible rehabilitation services, those born in remote areas and in poor families in particular have limited chances of getting early intervention services they deserve and become victims of gross neglect (Singh, 2013). **Research demonstrates that access to high quality early intervention services is critical to assist children with disabilities to reach their potential.** Early intervention services are crucial for children with disability, since the services can take advantage of the plasticity of the brain and provide opportunities for optimal development of the child's potential (ibid). Services are not ready to respond effectively and provide accessible and equitable services to children with disabilities. Children with disability aged 5–18 years who had attended the pre-school intervention programme comprised only 13 percent of the persons with disability.[26]

The AWCs with weak childcare component and capacity constraints do not provide a modicum of support to children with disabilities. The number of children with disabilities who receive meaningful support through ICDS and other pre-school programmes is negligible. The rate of acceptance is low due to poor motivation of AWWs who have little time for early stimulation and other educational development activities and prioritise other pressing problems over disability.[27]

4.4 Inadequate parental care impedes child development

4.4.1 Orphans lack due care

There is dearth of quantitative and qualitative information on orphans below the age of 6, and arrangements for their care in the extended family, children's homes and orphanages. According to an estimate, there are 20 million orphans in India, i.e., 4 percent of the child population.[28] The study highlighted that the states of Madhya Pradesh, Uttar Pradesh and Chhattisgarh are home to 6 million orphaned children under the age of 18. By 2021, these states will probably be home to 7.1 million orphans. The eastern region, encompassing Bihar, Orissa, Jharkhand and West Bengal, housed 5.2 million orphans and was likely to have 6 million orphans by 2021.

Table 4.4 Top 10 states by disability (%)

% children (0) with disability	% children (0–6) with visual impairment	% children (0–6) with hearing impairment	% children (0–6) with speech impairment	% children (0–6) with locomotor disability	% children (0–6) with disabled in mental illness	% children (0–6) disabled in Mental Retardation	% children (0–6) with multiple disabilities
Maharashtra (1.63)	Manipur (40.7)	Nagaland (33.7)	Goa (12.5)	Chhattisgarh (19.6)	Chandigarh (3.6)	Puducherry (13.3)	Dadra & Nagar Haveli (21.5)
Odisha (1.54)	Jharkhand (29.0)	Arunachal Pradesh (32.3)	Andaman & Nicobar (9.1)	Lakshadweep (18.2)	Daman and Diu (2.7)	Tamil Nadu (11.1)	Lakshadweep (19.5)
Bihar (1.52)	Bihar (27.3)	Uttar Pradesh (30.7)	Maharashtra (8.0)	Andaman & Nicobar (16.1)	NCT of Delhi (2.4)	Daman and Diu (8.8)	Kerala (16.4)
Punjab (1.42)	Rajasthan (22.9)	Punjab (30.2)	Dadra and Nagar Haveli (7.8)	Madhya Pradesh (13.7)	Andaman & Nicobar (2.3)	Kerala (7.5)	Sikkim (15.9)
Andhra Pradesh (1.39)	Odisha (22.3)	Haryana (29.4)	Andhra Pradesh (7.7)	Kerala (13.4)	Meghalaya (2.0)	Manipur (6.5)	Andaman & Nicobar (15.3)
Manipur (1.39)	Maharashtra (21.8)	Sikkim (28.8)	Kerala (7.5)	Chandigarh (13.2)	Mizoram (1.8)	Goa (6.5)	Mizoram (14.0)
J&K (1.38)	Arunachal Pradesh (21.6)	Meghalaya (28.8)	Sikkim (7.3)	Delhi (12.8)	J&K (1.7)	Karnataka (6.5)	Chhattisgarh (13.8)
Jharkhand (1.36)	Gujarat (21.0)	Bihar (28.7)	Chandigarh (6.9)	Rajasthan 12.6	Gujarat (1.5)	Arunachal Pradesh (6.2)	NCT of Delhi (11.9)
Uttar Pradesh (1.35)	Karnataka (20.8)	J&K (26.3)	Delhi (6.8)	Daman and Diu (12.4)	Goa (1.4)	Mizoram (6.2)	Chandigarh (11.9)
Karnataka (1.30)	West Bengal (19.9)	Jharkhand (25.5)	Mizoram (6.5)	Puducherry (11.9)	Sikkim (1.4)	Andhra Pradesh (6.0)	Himachal Pradesh (11.8)

Source: Census, 2011

According to the more recent NFHS-4, 3.2 percent of children under age 18 and 2.7 percent of children under age 15 were not living with biological parents, with 5 percent of children under age 18 orphaned with one or both parents dead.

Although there is a dearth of qualitative research on children with or without limited parental care, **institutionalisation needs to be viewed as the last resort.** There need to be well-designed checks and balances to ensure that childcare institutions provide young children with adequate care, stimulation, love and protection for their foundational development positively affecting their physical and socio-emotional development later in their lives.

4.4.2 Children in single-headed households face higher risks of parenting discrimination

Headship is a social factor that affects parenting and disadvantages young children of single parents. Single parents tend to be poorer than households where both parents are together. The percentage of single women heading households (widows, divorced, deserted) is higher than that for single men. Around 15 percent of households covered under the NFHS-4 were women headed.

A study of women headed households in Neyveli in Tamil Nadu found that women who were sole earners found it difficult to meet the expenses of education, clothing and other needs of their children. They caved in to the demands, even unreasonable, of their children at times. Furthermore, the drop-out rates tended to be higher among children of women headed households when compared to children of male headed households (Buvaneswari, 2008).

Young children are at a higher risk of gender and socially discriminatory parenting when it is mainly the mother or other women family members (e.g., a grandmother), or there is gender-discrimination in the physical, emotional, social and intellectual aspects of the parenting of the young child.

4.4.3 Children living in jails with their mothers suffer diverse deprivations

Children who are in jail with their mothers, who are either under-trial prisoners or convicts are another invisible group of vulnerable children who are often under the radar. According to the National Crime Records Bureau (NCRB) prison statistics, 1,681 children lived along with their mothers in prisons as on December 31, 2017.[29] The justice system provides for children under 6 to stay with their mothers who are under trial or have been convicted for legal offences. These children end up staying in jail not only because of their young age but also there is no one at home to look after them or to take care of them in absence of the mother.

The NCRB prison statistics for 2017 also showed that 417 children belonged to 365 convicted women prisoners, while 1,252 children were

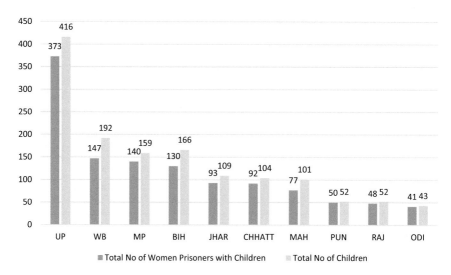

Figure 4.2 Top 10 states by number of women prisoners with children
Source: Prison Statistics of India, NCRB, 2017

with 1,077 women who were under-trial prison inmates (see Table 4.2).[30] The state of Uttar Pradesh had the highest number of children with imprisoned mothers – 416 children with 373 women – followed by West Bengal – 192 children with 147 women – and Bihar – 166 children with 130 women. Only ten states and UTs did not have women prison inmates with children.[31]

A jail does not provide a congenial environment to a child to experience a healthy, well rounded childhood due to the inherent violence, exclusion, punitive routines and lack of stable emotional relationships. Various laws stipulate that children living in prison should receive ECD. But a study by the National Institute of Criminology and Forensic Sciences in 2002 found that most of these children lived in difficult conditions and suffered from diverse deprivations related to food, healthcare, accommodation, education and recreation.

It is important that jail authorities ensure that pregnant women are provided with prenatal and postnatal care and the young child's nutritional, educational and psycho-social needs are met.

4.4.4 *Several disadvantaged groups continue to be overlooked*

Marginalisation of some social groups has been recognised but there are many, generally fewer in numbers but highly vulnerable to deprivation and exclusion. For instance, **the issues of children growing up in conflict zones** are hard to ascertain due to exceptional circumstances they are placed in. **Children of devadasis, sex workers, bar dancers are difficult to identify and** reach out to without perpetuating their extreme vulnerability. The umbrella term 'disadvantaged communities' needs to accommodate several categories but empirical data is lacking. Identification and situation assessment of such categories requires extensive enquiry into the notion of 'disadvantage.' The indicators of disadvantage need to focus on, but also look beyond, the categories based on caste, gender and poverty.

4.5 Key issues

4.5.1 Policies and programmes have failed in reducing discrimination

Government policies over the last two decades may have reduced the proportion of people living below the poverty line but the number of people living in poverty is still large and the inequities have increased significantly. The trickle-down effect has not taken place, and inequality and gaps in income and access to services have only helped widen the gap. The current practice of all-India programmes designed as one shoe fits all has clearly not worked.

Unless the poorest households (that also seem to experience the greatest shocks related to price rise, environmental hazards and crop failure) have adequate social protection and insurance, intergenerational transmission of poverty will continue to impact children living in these households (Singh et al., 2018).[32] Social security protection needs to be extended to such households in light of government of India's current commitment of *Sabka Sath, Sabka Vikas, Sabka Vishwas* as well as the SDG 1 related to ending poverty.

India is prone to several kinds of natural disasters and has begun experiencing the steady impact of climate change on the lives and livelihoods of people. The poor and marginalised living in some of the most eco-sensitive areas are among the worst affected. The government has about 200 laws dealing with environmental protection and environmental regulations that date back to the 1970s. However, none of them address the concerns of children, especially their protection before, during and after a disaster.

A more nuanced perspective to development planning is required, which takes into account discriminatory social norms and other barriers and bottlenecks. The inability to deliver the wherewithal for promotion of labour force participation of women has undermined efforts to empower them. Patriarchal mind-sets confine them to the role of primary caregiver and dearth of support services, such as crèches and day-care, hinder their ability to improve their financial condition and avail of other opportunities that come with it. Maternal entitlements are often beyond the reach of women who work from home or in the informal sector.

The MNREGA worksites and factories covered under the Factories Act of 1948, Mines Act of 1952, Plantation Act of 1951, Inter-State Migrant Workman Act of 1979, Building and Other Construction Workers Act

(BOCWA) of 1996, and the National Rural Employment Guarantee Act (NREGA) of 2005 are expected to provide crèche services to children of an overwhelming majority of poor rural and urban women who are engaged in paid and unpaid work. Infants left alone near construction sites, in rural roads related work and near factories are a common site in the absence of crèche services.

To stop female feticide in the country, the government enacted the Prenatal Diagnostic Techniques (Regulation and Prevention of Misuse) Act, 1994, to prohibit determination and disclosure of the sex of the foetus and any advertisements relating to prenatal determination of sex. The person who contravenes the provisions of this act is punishable with imprisonment and fine (MoHFW 2016). However, high gender inequality and persistent preference for the male child have fostered practices that circumvent the legal provisions or are conducted surreptitiously. A study showed that more than 90 percent of districts in India had higher female U5MR, and the four largest states (Uttar Pradesh, Bihar, Rajasthan and Madhya Pradesh) accounted for two-thirds of total U5MR among girls.[33] Effective implementation of the law needs to be accompanied by efforts to address the persisting 'son preference' that exists in Indian society. Two schemes designed by the Tamil Nadu government in 1992 deserve mention in the efforts to counter gender discrimination; Box 4.5 highlights the same.

Box 4.5   Government of Tamil Nadu schemes for the protection and development of girls

The Government of Tamil Nadu in 1992 introduced two schemes in 1992 to counter female infanticide and abandonment of the girl child. **The Cradle Baby Scheme** accepted for adoption female babies who would otherwise have been killed while **the Girl Child Incentive Scheme** gave incentives to mothers if the couple adopted permanent methods after the first two births, and if both were girls.

Nearly two decades after the Cradle Baby Scheme was introduced, Srinivasan and Bedi (2010) assessed its design and impact. Through a statistical analysis, they concluded that the scheme may have directly accounted for about 14 percent (370/2700) of the reduction in post-birth daughter deficit between 1996–1999 and 2003. They advocated for such a scheme with the caveat that encouraging parents to abandon female babies is not a substitute for tackling the crime of female infanticide and ensuring that families welcome the girl child.

A study by Women Power Connect and Campaign Against Sex Selective Abortion, however, found that mortality of babies in the cradle baby scheme is five times that of the average IMR in the state. The scheme is reportedly being extended to other states like Puducherry.

Campaigns against sex selective abortion observe that the scheme is a violation of Articles 7 and 9 of the CRC, which deal with the child's right to be cared for by her biological parents and requires the state to ensure that children shall not be separated from their parents, and, in case of separation from one or both the parents, the state should respect the rights of the child to maintain personal relationships with both parents.

A study in six blocks noted that the Girl Child Incentive Scheme picked up after 2001, but the impact on son preference was not much. The CSR actually declined in three of the six blocks after the scheme was introduced due to availability of technology for prenatal sex selection. The scheme failed in reducing the practice of dowry, which also showed an increase. The enrolment of girls to high school education improved not because of the scheme but because communities valued education and sought educated brides. About 60 percent of the beneficiaries opposed the rights of girls to inherit property indicating no impact on social attitudes. Parents continued to place restrictions on the mobility of girls and the times by which they should return home. They tried to marry them off after high school in the interest of 'family honour,' jeopardising their health and well-being due to the social pressure to conceive soon after marriage.[34]

The national *Beti Bachao Beti Padhao* scheme was initiated with the ambition of preventing gender biased sex selection, promoting the survival, protection, education and participation of the girl child (MWCD, 2016). Introduced initially in 100 districts with low CSR in 2014–2015, and expanded to another 61 districts in 2015–2016, the scheme is implemented by three ministries, viz., MWCD, MoHFW and MHRD through the District Collector. The scheme includes operationalisation of multi-sectoral District Action Plans, training of district level officials and frontline workers, public awareness activities such as street plays, signature campaigns, *Guddi Gudda* (girls-boys) boards, 'live your dream for one day' initiative (e.g., be a policewoman). Due to under-utilisation of the budgetary allocation and persistence of gender inequalities, the implementation of the scheme has come under scrutiny. Deep-rooted gender discriminatory norms may resurface once the scheme ends (OneIndia News, 2017).[35]

In order to provide care, protection and rehabilitation to children in streets, the National Commission for Protection of Child Rights (NCPCR) has developed a standard operating procedure (SOP) which includes a common framework for minimum standard of care and protection of children, access of such children to quality care and protection, access to foster care, sponsorship as per their requirements and also assurance that no child is forced to live on street (NCPCR and Save the Children, 2017). But if these SOPs are to deliver results, the district child protection units (DCPU) need to be active and keen to ensure effective child protection measures in their jurisdiction. But for the benefits to accrue meaningfully, it would also entail special provisions for the young child and capacity development of institutional care providers for ECD.

In order to respond to needs of children with disability, the Government referred to children with disabilities specifically in the National Plan of Action for Children, 2005, who had the right to survival, care, protection, security, dignity and equality for the development and full participation. It aimed to provide inclusive and effective access to health, education, vocational training and other specialised rehabilitation services for children with disabilities.

The National Policy for Children, 2013 and the Rights of Persons with Disability (PWD) Act, 2016 notified on 28 December 2016 to make it compliant with United Nations Convention on the Rights of Persons with Disabilities (UNCRPD), provide guidelines to ensure that all laws, policies, plans and programmes affecting children follow the principle of non-discrimination, full and effective participation and inclusion in society (MoSJE, 2015). Though the RPWD Act reflects a paradigm shift from viewing disability as a social welfare concern to a human rights issue, none of the policies on disability have been specifically designed for the under 6 age group.

Key to early intervention is assessment and management plan to ensure that the child is provided with appropriate interventions to bridge the developmental delays and remove the environmental barriers to maximise participation of the child both within and outside the family. **Neither ICDS nor National Rural Health Mission (NRHM) personnel are adequately trained to provide the necessary services through the PHCs and AWCs.**

According to a study, the AWCs are expected to conduct two surveys on young children with disability every year but according to the testimony of the AWWs, 30 percent of AWCs had never surveyed young children for disability and an additional 25 percent had not conducted a survey in the year of the study. The report did not examine the gender or social sensitivity of the messages communicated.[36]

Giving children who do not have parents or families to look after them into adoption by families that have the intense desire and means, with requisite checks and monitoring, is a better strategy than placing them in orphanages or other institutions. The Government of India established Central Adoption Resource Agency (CARA) in 1990 to simplify the process of adoption of orphaned or abandoned children and bring in greater transparency in the process. The Juvenile Justice (Care and Protection of Children) Act, 2015, made CARA a statutory body with the mandate to promote in-country adoptions and to facilitate inter-State adoptions in co-ordination with state agency, regulate inter-country adoptions, frame regulations on adoption and related matters from time to time.

Although there is demand for adoption of children without parental care, the existing system has been inefficient. According to CARA, there were 3,276 in-country and 651 inter-country adoptions in financial year 2017–2018. According to Child Adoption Resource Information and Guidance System (CARINGS), childcare institutions (CCIs) had only 1,766 children in their care across the country, whereas there were 15,200 prospective adoptive parents (PAPs). For every nine PAPs, only one child was available to adopt and while only 59 children were below the age of 2, 1,279 out of the total 1,766 children available for adoption has some form of disability.

4.5.2 Transformational potential of parenting remains untapped

The ECD services available to the most disadvantaged infants and young children are either poor in quality or unaffordable. Gender and socially transformative parenting, which could empower particularly vulnerable groups – such as street children, migrant children, children of sex workers, children of parents in marginal occupations, children living with disability or without parental care (and girls among them, and those belonging to SCs and STs) are just not available to them. Provision of quality ECD services to the most disadvantaged young children can help give them a good start in life and veer them towards more opportunities.

There is no evidence that mothers, across classes and types of families, follow better or more gender transformative and inclusive parenting practices than fathers. While gender disparities in access to food, nutrition and education may be lower in Kerala, Tamil Nadu, Maharashtra, the evidence does not support that parenting even in these states is devoid of gender and social bias. The spatial segregation of families across caste, class and religion also poses a barrier to inclusive parenting.

4.5.3 Comprehensive and good quality ECD services have abysmal public funding

ICDS is the most comprehensive system for delivery of ECD services in India but it is plagued by resource constraints. It covers 71.9 million children or about 45.3 percent of the total child population under 6 years of age of India. Although these children are more likely to be from the more disadvantaged communities in rural and urban areas, it is worrisome that those living in the most disadvantaged circumstances or located in remote regions are the hardest to reach. The remoteness and difficult terrain make it difficult for them to access ICDS services. Furthermore, **the package of services delivered through ICDS does not adequately address all the**

developmental needs of the young child. There is negligible or inadequate attention given to early childhood education and childcare component; the crèche component is missing. Special provisions to meet the unique developmental needs of the most discriminated young children is practically non-existent.

ICDS received INR 275.8 billion, i.e., 94.5 percent of the total budget of MWCD in 2019–20.[37] The allocation to the MWCD in the 2019–2020 was a meagre 1.05 percent of the total Union Budget. A multi-fold hike in the budget allocation for the MWCD as well as ICDS, along with improved social sector spending would create a safety net for the most disadvantaged communities and deliver quality ECD services to the hardest to reach young child. The required allocations are spelt out in Chapter 6.

4.6 Recommendations and action points

4.6.1 Strengthen ECD as an essential component of social protection

Universal provisioning of ECD programmes for children from birth till the age of six should be an essential component of the basket of social protection interventions. ECD has a crucial role in promoting physical and cognitive development, and school readiness among the young children belonging to most deprived communities and families. These programmes also have a major economic value for the individual, the family and the society in preventing the aggravation of disabling conditions. However, the principle of inclusion should be recognised and developed within the design and delivery in a comprehensive way by combining pre-school activities and early childhood healthcare. Plugging the gender/ socially transformative parenting deficit, as a right of the young child, could contribute to efficiency of the economy, egalitarian gender and social norms in society, and advancement of the rights of women, mothers and adolescent girls.

4.6.2 Improve data systems to reach the most disadvantaged children

State governments need to use data on the health and nutrition status of mothers and children as a powerful tool to identify geographical areas as well as specific disadvantaged groups where concerted action is required. Such data should be available in the public domain and online to enable researchers and health and nutrition experts to offer technical inputs. Available data suggests that the tribal areas in general due to their specific conditions and young children living there in particular need focussed attention. Schedule V areas need health, nutrition, childcare and pre-school education programmes tailored to meet local needs.

4.6.3 Sharpen focus on the urban young child

India's urban areas, especially its sprawling urban agglomerations, with their slum areas and areas where the socially disadvantaged are concentrated require greater attention with urgency. With moderate and severe malnutrition levels as significant in some urban ICDS projects as in some of the more severely affected rural ICDS projects, the municipal corporations and larger municipal councils need to play a stronger role in reducing urban child malnutrition, providing care and early education opportunities, and securing the protective environment. The *Zilla Parishads* could, however, look after smaller municipal council areas.

4.6.4 Ensure greater thrust on early screening and timely support to children with disabilities

Early intervention services should aim at securing the best interests of children with disabilities. There is an urgent need for ICDS and National Rural Health Mission (NRHM) to have specialist teams at cluster level to provide early intervention services, so that children with disabilities get a head start and are provided the maximum support tailored to meet their unique physical, social, emotional, communication and cognitive development needs. Early intervention services must adopt a combination of family centred and child-centred approaches. While the families are key to ensuring the best results, the offer of support including day-care facilities needs to factor in the specific needs of the child.

4.6.5 Promote adoption and guardianship

Given the prevalent mind-sets of adopting parents, CARA needs to simplify the process of adoption without undermining the rigorous screening of PAPs in the best interest of the child. Further it should make special efforts to provide the large majority of children with disabilities and other vulnerabilities with a loving home.

4.6.6 Implement child-focussed disaster risk management and reduction

Child-focussed disaster risk management and reduction, which factors in the vulnerabilities and needs of the young child, should be included in the disaster mitigation policy with sound investments in developing safe infrastructures, particularly well-located schools and health facilities with good road access. The interventions in the aftermath should include provisions of services for the young child, including nutritious food, health, care and safe spaces.

Key Messages

- Threats to early childhood development tend to cluster together, often in conjunction with poverty, social status, exclusion and gendered inequality. Exposure to one risk commonly means exposure to multiple risks and varied crisis in the family tends to contribute to widespread neglect of young children during their critical and formative years.

- While the number of young children living in the poorest and richest households vary tremendously across states, about 25 percent of children under the age of 5 in India live in households belonging to the poorest quintile and only 14.7 percent live in households in the richest quintile.

- Young children growing up on streets, in urban slums belonging to migrant families, experience extreme poverty and unhealthy living arrangements. Orphans, children living in single-headed households, or in jails with their mothers, transgender and intersex children, mostly become invisible despite their vulnerabilities.

- Unequal distribution of income, goods and services pushes children born into ST and SC households in the category of most disadvantaged. They are less likely to access basic health services due to a toxic combination of poor social policies and programmes and unfair occupation opportunities and income.

- Children with disabilities are more vulnerable to neglect, violence, abuse and exploitation. Access to high quality early intervention services is critical to assist these children to reach their potential; however, services are not ready to respond effectively and provide accessible and equitable services to such children from early childhood.

Notes

1 UN DESA, 2016.
2 Singh et al., 2018.
3 The National Health Profile (2015) used the Tendulkar methodology to estimate the percentage of people living below the poverty line in India.
4 A report of Intergovernmental Panel on Climate Change (IPCC) in "Climate Change Science Compendium 2009." Cited in Parks, 2009.
5 Prüss-Üstün et al., 2016.
6 Ibid.
7 UNICEF and World Bank, 2016.
8 OECD Economic Surveys: India 2017, n.d.
9 Census of India, 2011.
10 Chatterjee, n.d.
11 NIUA with support from Bernard van Leer Foundation, Status of Children in Urban India, Baseline Study 2016. Retrieved from https://smartnet.niua.org/sites/default/files/resources/statusl.pdf; date of access: 12 November 2019.
12 Neenv Delhi FORCES, 2016. Report prepared by DSSW and Mobile Creches.

13 Mathur, 2009.
14 Ibid.
15 NFHS-4, 2015–2016.
16 Dreze et al., 2006.
17 Kapoor et al., 2016.
18 Plan International, 2017.
19 SDG Gender Index, 2019.
20 This new index has been developed by *Equal Measures 2030*, a joint effort of regional and international organisations including African Women's Development and Communication Network, Asian-Pacific Resource and Research Centre for Women, Bill and Melinda Gates Foundation and International Women's Health Coalition. Retrieved from www.equalmeasures2030.org/products/sdg-gender-index/; date of access: 5 November 2019.
21 Hotchandani, 2017.
22 See Gander, 2019.
23 Hotchandani, 2017.
24 India's transgender community had no legal recognition until 2014. The Supreme Court judgement in the National Legal Services Authority (NALSA) and the Union of India case in April 2014 gave them the right to self-identification and provided for reservations across government and private sectors.
25 Iftikhar, 2018.
26 NSSO Survey, 58th Round (GoI 2005).
27 Madan, A. *Inclusive Education—An Elusive Goal in Early Childhood Education*. Retrieved from https://azimpremjiuniversity.edu.in/SitePages/pdf/Inclusive-edication-an-elusive-goal-in-early-childhood-education-Ankur-Madan.pdf; date of access: 9 November 2019.
28 Estimation by the SOS Children's Villages based on NFHS-3 and Census 2011 data.
29 NCRB, Prison Statistics India: 2017. Retrieved from http://ncrb.gov.in; date of access: 22 November 2019.
30 Ibid.
31 Ibid.
32 Singh et al., 2018, p. 20.
33 Guilmoto et al., 2018. Retrieved from www.thelancet.com/journals/langlo/article/PIIS2214-109X(18)30184-0/fulltext; date of access: 12 September 2019.
34 Women Power Connect and CASSA, 2015.
35 Retrieved from www.oneindia.com/india/how-beti-bachao-campaign-failed-to-live-up-to-its-claim-in-modis-home-turf-varanasi-2551080.html; date of access: 14 November 2019.
36 Kapoor et al., 2016.
37 Ministry of Women and Child Development, 2019.

Bibliography

Action Aid, 2013. *Marketing Street Children Matters: A Census Study in Mumbai City*. Action Aid, New Delhi.

Agarwal, P., 2015. *Reducing Poverty in India: The Role of Economic Growth. Institute of Economic Growth (IEG)*. Working Paper No. 349. Retrieved from www.iegindia.org/upload/publication/Workpap/wp349.pdf; date of access: 2 November 2019.

Allen, G., 2011. *Early Intervention: The Next Steps*. Retrieved from https://assets.publishing.service.gov.uk/government/uploads/system/uploads/attachment_data/file/284086/early-intervention-next-steps2.pdf; date of access: 16 January 2020.

Bajaj, M., 2018. *Childcare and the Childcare Worker*. Technical background paper for the Report, 2020. Mobile Creches, New Delhi.

Buvaneswari, M.G., 2008. Single Headed Households and Family Disorganisation at Neyveli Industrial Township. *Cauvery Research Journal*. Vol 1. No 2, January, pp. 117–120.

Chandra, M., 2015. Environmental Concerns in India: Problems and Solutions. *Journal of International Business and Law*. Vol 15. No 1, Article 1. Retrieved from https://scholarlycommons.law.hofstra.edu/cgi/viewcontent.cgi?article=1278& context=jibl; date of access: 7 November 2019.

Chatterjee, S., n.d. *Children Growing Up in Indian Slums: Challenges and Opportunities for New Urban Imaginations*. Retrieved from https://bernardvanleer.org/app/uploads/2017/10/ECM118_4_Challenges-and-opportunities-for-new-urban-imaginations-Sudeshna-Chatterjee1.pdf; date of access: 11 November 2019.

Dreze, J. et al. (Eds.), 2006. *Focus on Children Under Six*. Edition: Abridged Report. Citizens' Initiative for the Rights of Children Under Six, New Delhi.

Dube, R., V. Nandan and S. Dua, 2014. Waste Incineration for Urban India: Valuable Contribution to Sustainable MSWM or Inappropriate High-Tech Solution Affecting Livelihoods and Public Health? *International Journal of Environmental Technology & Management*. Vol 17. No 2–4, pp. 199–214.

Equal Measures 2030, 2019. Retrieved from https://www.equalmeasures2030.org/; date of access 25 November 2019.

Gander, K., 2019. Scientists Have Carried Out the Biggest Ever Study on Transgender Children—Here's What They Found. *Newsweek*, 18 November 2019. Retrieved from www.newsweek.com/transgender-kids-living-identity-develop-cis-children-1471729; date of access: 19 November 2019.

Guilmoto, C.Z., N. Saikia, V. Tamarkar and J.K. Bora, 2018. Excess Under-5 Female Mortality Across India: A Spatial Analysis Using 2011 Census Data. *Lancet Global Health*. Vol 6. No 6, pp. e650–e658. Retrieved from www.thelancet.com/action/showPdf?pii=S2214-109X%2818%2930184-0; date of access: 28 November 2019.

Hotchandani, K.R., 2017. Problems of Transgender in India: A Study from Social Exclusion to Social Inclusion. *International Research Journal of Human Resources and Social Sciences*. Vol 4. No 4, April 2017.

Human Development Reports, 2018. Retrieved from http://hdr.undp.org/en/2019-report; date of access 25 November 2019.

Iftikhar, F., 2018. 'Accept Us for Who We Are': Transgender Children Deprived of Normal School Life. *Hindustan Times*, 15 November 2018.

International Institute for Population Sciences (IIPS) and Macro International, 2007. *National Family Health Survey (NFHS-3), 2005–06: India: Volume II*. IIPS, Mumbai. Retrieved from http://rchiips.org/nfhs/NFHS-3%20Data/VOL-2/Front%20Matter.pdf; date of access: 19 November 2019.

Jha, P. and N. Nagar, 2015. A Study of Gender Inequality in India. *The International Journal of Indian Psychology*. Vol 2. No 3, pp. 2349–3429.

Judis, 2006. *Guidelines to Be Followed in Case of the Children of Women Prisoners Living in India—Judgement of Supreme Court of India*. Retrieved from www.wbja.nic.in/wbja_adm/files/Guidelines%20to%20be%20followed%20in%20case%20the%20children%20of%20women%20prisoner%20living%20in%20prison.pdf; date of access: 22 November 2019.

Kamath, S.S., 2015. Child Protection During Disasters. *Indian Pediatrics*. Vol 52, pp. 467–468.

Kapoor, A., D. Sinha and G. Meera, 2016. *Progress of Children Under ICDS: Revisiting the Focus Districts*. Centre for Equity Studies, New Delhi.

Madan, A. *Inclusive Education – An Elusive Goal in Early Childhood Education.* Retrieved from https://azimpremjiuniversity.edu.in/SitePages/pdf/Inclusive-edi-cation-an-elusive-goal-in-early-childhood-education-Ankur-Madan.pdf; date of access: 9 November 2019.

Mathur, M., 2009. Socialisation of Street Children in India: A Socio-Economic Pro-file. *Psychology and Developing Societies.* Vol 21. No 2, pp. 299–325.

Ministry of Health and Family Welfare (MoHFW), Government of India, 2016. *Pre-Conception and Pre-Natal Diagnostic Techniques (Prohibition of Sex Selection) Act, 1994—Standard Operating Guidelines for District Appropriate Authorities.* MoHFW and UNFPA, Government of India, New Delhi.

Ministry of Social Justice and Environment (MoSJE), Government of India, 2015. *First Country Report on the Status of Disability in India.* Department of Empow-erment of Persons with Disabilities, New Delhi.

Ministry of Statistics and Programme Implementation, Registrar General of India, GoI. *Census of India 2011.* New Delhi.

Ministry of Women and Child Development, 2016. *Beti Bachao Beti Padhao.* Retrieved from http://wcd.nic.in/bbbp-schemes; date of access: 12 August 2018.

Ministry of Women and Child Development, 2019. Demand No. 98, Retrieved from www.indiabudget.gov.in/budget/; date of access: 8 July 2019.

National Commission for Protection of Child Rights and Save the Children, 2017. *Standard Operating Procedure for Care and Protection of Children in Street Situ-ations.* Retrieved from http://ncpcr.gov.in/showfile.php?lang=1&level=0&linkid=102&lid=1306.

National Institute of Urban Affairs, 2016. *Status of Children in Urban India-Base-line Study, 2016.* New Delhi.

National Sample Survey Organisation, 2005. *Disabled Persons in India.* Report No. 485, NSS 58th Round. Ministry of Statistics and Programme Implementation, New Delhi.

NCRB, Prison Statistics India: 2017. Retrieved from http://ncrb.gov.in; date of access: 22 November 2019.

Neenv (Delhi Chapter – FORCES – Mobile Creches), 2016. *Survey Findings on the Situation of Young Children in Delhi – 'Situational Analysis of Children Under Six in Delhi'.* New Delhi.

NSSO, 2012. *Employment & Unemployment and Migration Survey: NSS 64th Round: July 2007–June 2008.* NSSO, Ministry of statistics and Program Imple-mentation, New Delhi.

OECD Economic Surveys: India 2017, n.d. Retrieved from www.oecd.org/eco/surveys/INDIA-2017-OECD-economic-survey-overview.pdf; date of access: 10 November 2019.

OneIndia News, 2017. *How Beti Bachao Campaign Failed to Live Up to Its Claim in Modi's Home Turf Varanasi,* 26 September 2017. Retrieved from www.one india.com/india/how-beti-bachao-campaign-failed-to-live-up-to-its-claim-in-modis-home-turf-varanasi-2551080.html; date of access: 22 November 2019.

Parks, N., 2009. UN Update: Climate Change Hitting Sooner and Stronger. *Environ-mental Science & Technology.* Vol 43. No 22, pp. 8475–8476.

Plan International, 2017. *Gender Inequality and Early Childhood Development: A Review of the Linkages.* Plan International. Retrieved from https://plan-international.org/publication/2017-06-08-gender-inequality-and-early-child-hood-development; date of access: 13 November 2019.

Prüss-Üstün, O.A., J. Wolf, C. Corvalan, R. Bros and M. Niera, 2016. *Prevent-ing Disease Through Healthy Environments: A Global Assessment of Burden of*

Disease from Environmental Risk. World Health Organisation, Geneva. Retrieved from www.who.int/iris/handle/10665/204585; date of access: 4 November 2019.

Save the Children, 2012. *Life on the Street—Street Children Survey in 5 Cities: Lucknow, Mughal Sarai, Hyderabad, Patna and Kolkata-Howrah*. Save the Children, New Delhi.

Save the Children, 2018. *Understanding the Benefits of Beti Bachao Beti Padhao Scheme*. Save the Children, New Delhi.

SDG Gender Index, 2019. Retrieved from https://data.em2030.org/wpcontent/uploads/2019/05/EM2030_2019_Global_Report_ENG.pdf; date of access: 4 November 2019.

Singh, R., 2013. Abuse and Neglect of Children with Disabilities: Under a Veil of Secrecy. In R.N. Srivastava, R. Seth and J. Niekerk (Eds.), *Child Abuse and Neglect: Challenges and Opportunities*. Jaypee Brothers, New Delhi.

Singh, R. and R. Kesarwani, 2018. *The Disadvantaged Child: Challenges, Prospects and Way Forward*. Technical Background Paper for the Report 2020. Mobile Creches, New Delhi.

Singh, R., P.P. Reddy and L. Beny, 2018. *Reaching the Last Child: Evidence from Young Lives, India*. Country Report. Young Lives, Oxford.

Srinivasan, S. and Bedi, A.S., 2010. Daughter elimination: Cradle baby scheme in Tamil Nadu. *Economic and Political Weekly*, pp.17–20.

Sudarshan, H. and T. Seshadri, 2015. *Health of Tribal People in India: A Linear Paper on Health for the National Tribal Human Development Report*. Ministry of Tribal Affairs, GoI, and UNDP.

UN DESA, 2016. *Leaving No One Behind: The Imperative of Inclusive Development*. Report on the World Social Situation 2016.

UNICEF and UNESCO, 2013. *Social Inclusion of Internal Migrants in India*. UNESCO, New Delhi.

UNICEF and World Bank, 2016. *Ending Extreme Poverty: A Focus on Children*. UNICEF and World Bank Group.

United Nations Children's Fund (UNICEF), 2015. *The Impact of Climate Change on Children*. Retrieved from https://www.unicef.org/publications/files/Unless_we_act_now_The_impact_of_climate_change_on_children.pdf; date of access: 16 January 2020.

Vijayanath, V., M.R. Anitha, S.N. Vijayamahantesh and G.M. Raju, 2010. Caste and Health in Indian Scenario. *Journal of Punjab Academy of Forensic Medicine & Toxicology*. Vol 10.

Vranda, M.N. and K. Sekar, 2011. (A298) Assessment of Psychosocial Impact of Flood on Children—Indian Experience. *Prehospital and Disaster Medicine*. Vol 26. No S1, pp. S83–S84. Cambridge University Press.

WHO, 2017. *Don't Pollute My Future–The Impact of Environment on Children's Health*. World Health Organization, Geneva.

Women Power Connect and Campaign Against Sex Selective Abortion (CASSA), 2015. *Impact of Government Initiatives on Enhancing Value of Girls*. Women Power Connect and Campaign Against Sex Selective Abortion, New Delhi/Tamil Nadu.

World Bank, 2018. *Human Capital Index and its Components*. Retrieved from https://www.worldbank.org/en/data/interactive/2018/10/18/human-capital-index-and-components-2018; date of access: 16 January 2020.

5 Childcare and the childcare worker

Neuroscientific research has iterated the significance of environmental inputs, stimulation and interaction in influencing the overall growth and maturity of infants and young children. Childcare meeting the holistic needs of babies and toddlers, encompassing stimulation during early childhood increases neural connections, securing attachments, contributing to learning and serving as an antidote to abuse and trauma that can have a lasting impact on their brains. The quality of childcare – be it by parents, family and others, including caregivers – largely determines young child's access to the wherewithal for physical development, early learning, safety and security. Although childcare is central to the holistic conception of ECD, multisectoral policies and programmes and multi-disciplinary research have for long neglected it in India.

This chapter discusses childcare, nurturing and protection, including arrangements such as crèches and day-care centres, the role of childcare providers within and outside home and the imperative of an ecosystem that encourages gender and socially transformative parenting, inclusion and social justice, and the safety and well-being of the young child. It further discusses the importance of childcare service provision in advancing women's entitlements, especially those working in the informal sector, by reducing the burden of care and enabling their participation in economic activities while supporting ECD.

5.1 Nurture and care during early childhood has been under-rated

5.1.1 The discourse on early childhood care is growing but still nascent

Way back in 1996 and 1997, articles in *Newsweek* placed some dramatic findings of neuroscience research in the public domain.[1] "A newborn's brain is composed of trillions of neurons. . . . The experiences of childhood determine which neurons are used, that wire the circuits of the brain. Those neurons that are not used may die."[2] 'Use it – or lose it!' headlined in *Newsweek* caught the popular attention of parents and policymakers to advocate for increased attention to early stimulation for infants and toddlers. The basic facts were compelling with popular interpretations going far beyond the existing evidence.

Research by Shonkoff and Phillips (2000) highlighted the rapidity of brain development through synapse formation or the construction of a dense network of neural connectivity on which cortical or intellectual activity largely depends, especially during the early years. It showed that the increase in synaptic density is 50 percent higher between birth to 2 years of age than in more mature adults. It starts declining gradually thereon between the ages of 2 to 16. This critical development of synaptic density grows through interaction and stimulation, which is a strong rationale for the provision of a nurturing and stimulating caregiver in early infancy.[3] Other studies have also demonstrated that maximal infant stimulation promotes optimum connectivity and that these connections are established far earlier than what was initially conceptualised.[4]

Current research findings increasingly demonstrate that secure attachments and communication contribute to enhanced learning in infants and young children. At another level, the claims about specific effects of abuse and trauma on the infant's brain[5] are also being further investigated to establish policy guidelines on 'nurturing care' for preventing neglect and violence during infancy.

Several countries have initiated programmes focussed on health and nutrition for children under the age of three, and foundational or readiness learning for children aged 3 to 6 with growing recognition of the importance of the early years. This dichotomy between two stages in early childhood, however, ignores the fundamental need of integrated and concurrent inputs for health, nutrition, safety, care and learning throughout the early years.

The current debate on early childcare is also centred on the specific environmental inputs required for optimal development of the infant's maturing nervous system. While arguing for certain non-negotiables like holistic and responsive care for optimal human development, research also clarifies that this can be achieved through a wide range of family settings, childcare practices and pedagogical approaches.

In India, the dominant narrative positions the family as the best place for a young child to grow up in and a child's home as a haven for its care and development. This understanding has relegated the perspectives on the young child within the political and policy domains to the background as it is primarily seen to be the responsibility of the family with minimal role to be played by the State. Therefore, the importance of childcare as a concept has neither been internalised nor accepted at a policy level because the young child is seen from the lens of a family, specifically as a woman's responsibility in which the State has little or no role to play.

5.2 Home-based childcare is crucial but increasingly challenging

5.2.1 Family may not always be able to provide the best childcare

Owing to the natural environment it provides and the emotional bonding of the child within this, **the family is the best place for a child to grow up in. It is the primary caregiver and influencer for a child's learning and overall development.** The presence of caring and nurturing adults who are able to stimulate them, especially from birth to the age of 3, contributes to increased neural connections and facilitates emotional bonding, self-confidence and development of relationships. This can also be laid by loving and responsive interplay during physical care of a child and activities such as bathing, dressing, feeding and playing.

The single most common factor for children who develop resilience is at least one stable and committed relationship with a supportive parent, caregiver, or other adult. These relationships provide personalised responses, scaffolding and protection that buffer children from developmental disruption. They also build key capacities – such as the ability to plan, monitor and regulate behaviour – that enable children to respond or adapt to adversity and thrive.[6] This combination of supportive relationships, adaptive skill-building and positive experiences is the foundation of resilience.

However, diverse challenges of poverty, inaccessibility to financial and material resources, disenfranchisement and weak social networks, may result in the inability of a family to provide an optimal caring environment for ECD. These acute challenges within family settings necessitate assistance and support from the State to facilitate the required care to a child.

In principle, children from better socio-economic families under normal circumstances have a higher probability[7] of receiving warm, responsive, linguistically rich[8] and protective relationships during critical periods of their development. Functional families, where economic security as well as a close connect between members exist, are more likely to provide nurturing care as they have the means and opportunities to take advantage of the systems to support them.

But families differ in varying degrees in their endowments and entitlements, social and spatial mobility patterns and factors such as migration. Further, there are multiple circumstances that can affect their capability and adequacy to provide optimal care to a child. As the YCEI (Table 1.2) shows, states which perform poorly in terms of the poverty index (like Arunachal Pradesh, Manipur, Chhattisgarh, Jharkhand) also perform poorly in terms of the overall YCEI. Arunachal Pradesh, Manipur and Jharkhand are the bottom three performers in the Index, since the socio-economic status has a direct relation to the kind of care families can provide the young child with.

Globalisation and market forces have also altered family functioning even if its organisation may not have changed. The resulting dynamics have presumably destabilised some traditional boundaries within and outside the family network and strained the relationships between sexes, responsibility for childcare and eldercare, thereby affecting the family life. The transformations in the economic, political and technological realms have impacted the ability of families to control their economic and social well-being. Many families are compelled to look for self-reliance at a time when fewer options are available and strained social support systems are contributing to exclusion of certain groups.[9]

The globalised world order has widened economic disparities between and within societies. In India, rural distress, economic compulsions and aspirations for a better life are driving men and sometimes whole families to move into towns and cities, where about 31 percent of the population resides (Census, 2011). The deficit in transformative parenting where parents play an equal, and appropriate role in bringing up their children, is also acute especially in the informal and unorganised sector due to the failure of state, markets, community and households. Parents affected by intersecting marginalities are constrained in terms of exposure to positive and non-stereotypical parenting or the time and resources to spend on such parenting.

According to the Periodic Labour Force Survey (PLFS), urban workers put in 56 hours a week at work compared with 48 hours of work by a rural worker. While urban male workers worked 58–59 hours, urban women worked 41–42 hours on an average.[10] Both men and women work long hours, but they are often not eligible for any social security benefit. About 49.6 percent of regular wage earners/salaried employees, 49 percent men and 51.8 percent women, in the non-agriculture sector were ineligible for any social security benefit. While earnings go up, the quality of life suddenly dips due to degraded environmental conditions of increasing pollution, lack of water and sewage, widespread exploitation and fragmentation of society, affecting young children the most.

The multiple challenges that are faced by urban migrant families, or issues due to extreme poverty, lack of education, social exclusion or in families where both parents are working, result in a severe impact on young children and their development, thus requiring provision of childcare support through appropriate State interventions. This necessitates the availability of trained childcare workforce to provide support and services at home as well as in institutional settings. **Trained, qualified, recognised and motivated ECD workforce is the backbone for early childhood programmes** and as a state-regulated intervention, can be brought in to provide due care especially where families lack the required resources and enabling environments.

5.2.2 Toxic stresses and violence against the young child are neglected

In addition to the challenges stemming from the inability of families to provide childcare and the lack of redressal from the State, there are issues of violence that can come up within families as infants and young children are exposed to direct abuse by primary caregivers and other family members or can be hurt inadvertently in incidents of domestic violence. There is a broad consensus among government agencies, NGOs and activists, who have been working for elimination of violence against children, that child sexual abuse is mostly perpetrated by people close to them and is not limited to any caste or class.[11] The young child is often unable to communicate and the families tend to deny the occurrence of such acts, which contributes to difficulties in addressing the problem by involving law enforcement agencies.

Children who live in homes where their mothers are being beaten or abused are more vulnerable to violence than children who live in homes where this is not the case. The Global Report on *Ending Violence in Childhood* (2017) notes, "Children who grow up in abusive homes where they experience both physical and emotional abuse by their caregivers are likely to also be experiencing other forms of abuse, elsewhere, or at the hands of other perpetrators." It further notes that while violence against children has the potential to occur in rich as well as poor households, the risk increases owing to stress from poverty, which tends to sap parents' energies and undermine their mental health.[12]

There are also issues related to the exposure of children to and through digital technologies, especially where parents are unable to attend to them owing to their preoccupation in other chores. A growing body of empirical studies on the subject identifies the complex and dangerous ways it is affecting children, including young children.[13] Several cyber security experts point to the practice of young children being handed over mobile phones to entertain themselves by parents or caregivers busy with other things. As young children acquire proficiency in using the device, they are exposed to a plethora of age inappropriate content. Innocent exploration or a click of wrong button over pop-ups can expose them to sexually explicit or extremely violent imagery.[14]

Child sexual abuse materials (CSAM), including pictures, videos and animation in the cyberspace is a major global challenge.[15] The phenomena of 'sharenting' or excessive exposure of the images of infants and young children on social media by their parents and guardians, increases the risk of identity theft, humiliation, privacy violations and future discrimination, and raises concerns about developmental issues related to autonomy and consent.[16] The practice of livestreaming images of young children made to perform sexual acts is a worrying new trend globally.[17]

The WHO has recommended that infants and 1-year-olds should not spend any time at all looking at electronic screens. The screen time for children aged 2, 3 and 4 should be limited to just an hour every day and lesser the better for reducing sedentary behaviour (TV viewing, watching videos, playing computer games), which leads to obesity and impede motor and cognitive development and psychosocial health.[18]

Inadequate empirical research on environmental factors, which may contribute to violent behaviours, has not allowed a body of preventive measures

to emerge. It has been noted that protective relationships can help in addressing toxic stresses, which accumulate with strong, frequent or prolonged adversity, such as physical or emotional abuse, chronic neglect, caregiver substance abuse or mental illness, exposure to violence and/or the accumulated burdens of family economic hardship and can disrupt the development of brain architecture and other organ systems, and increase the risk for stress-related disease and cognitive impairment, well into the adult years.[19] Toxic stresses and strains in the social fabric, due to factors such as poverty and marginalisation of rural and urban communities and residence in areas affected by conflict, strife and natural disasters, can be fertile grounds for overt and covert violence.

The work of Mobile Creches with urban migrant families indicates the challenges they face due to extreme poverty, livelihood insecurity, long working hours, lack of education, poor health and social exclusion and unsafe neighbourhoods. Domestic violence is rife with women and children as victims. Safety of their infants and young children is a common concern of women who are engaged in wage labour in the informal sector. Either they leave their children behind or take them along, the well-being of children is compromised. Many of them complain of the inadequate and poor quality of services offered at the local AWC. A well-equipped AWC with trained workers and suitable timings is the kind of support they need for ECD and security of their children.[20]

5.2.3 The role of caregivers is gendered

The importance of childcare as a concept faced resistance in the policy and public domains largely because the young child has been seen from the lens of a family. The sanctity accorded to the family in Indian ethos has perpetuated the belief that the parents and other senior members of the family know and do the best for the child.

This formulation can be faulted on several grounds. It overlooks the patriarchal social norms, close relationships and role expectations guided by age and sex that generally characterise Indian families. It considers the mere existence of relationship rather than the quality of interactions with young children by focussing on the plethora of people including parents, older siblings, other members of the immediate or extended family who ostensibly look after the young child. Although it places the responsibility of childcare squarely in the domain of females – mainly the mother, and thereafter other family members such as grandmothers, aunts and older siblings – it does not factor in the gender-based differentials in household resource allocation. In societies with son preference like India, irrespective of who parents, young girls have lesser access to healthcare, early learning, education and nutrition and opportunities to play than young boys.

And if the household can afford one, a hired domestic help – usually a young girl or woman from a poor and needy family – is drawn into childcare. The ubiquitous domestic help in most Indian middle and upper class families is crucial for the functioning of the household. Infants and young children are often entrusted in her care, but her responsibility is usually confined to minding, cleaning and feeding. They may have a nurturing mind-set, but they lack the knowledge and skills required for quality childcare, such as interacting with the child through songs, lullabies, playing, 'reading' picture stories and other activities for age appropriate stimulation.

In India, the parenting approach falls more into discriminatory and ameliorative categories and less into transformative ones with the former showing persistence in terms of differential social aspects of parenting and a bit of support from fathers while the latter is a transformation from the conventional gendered parenting on equal terms.[21] Though fathers do help when women are working, their input is far from equal. Social norms in many societies, including India, have for long entrusted fathers with the role of main breadwinners and, if need be, the mothers with the responsibility for generating supplementary income.

Fathers are expected to be disciplinarians while mothers have to be caring and nurturing. But what it is to be a parent varies across countries, contexts and time and the expectations from fathers and mothers have changed over time. However, in recent times, the role of father in nurturing and caring for their children is assuming importance as it provides a different dimension of stimulation and care which is good both for the child as well as for the father. There is greater recognition that with the exception of breastfeeding, fathers can nurture their children just as much as mothers, and mothers too can be breadwinners. Parents can also be single, non-heterosexual and non-biological.

Although some traditional practices may be harmful and traditional wisdom may be found wanting, there is also a lot in conventional practices that is valuable, and which should be retained through concerted efforts for favourable developmental outcomes and culturally meaningful experiences of childhood and family life. Research with indigenous communities highlights the potential of developmentally assistive and healthy beliefs and practices in the continually evolving child development policy framework.

5.2.4 *Women's triple burden is disempowering*

The care of infants and young children has always been in the domain of the family, but it is essentially the mother who is primarily responsible. **The pressure on women, the traditional care providers, is increasing manifold with the disintegration of the traditional joint family or extended family support system and emergence of nuclear households.** In view of livelihood insecurity and heightened aspirations, they are venturing outside the home for wage employment while still bridled with the responsibilities of household chores and childcare. The triple burden on women especially those from poor households working in the unorganised sector, with severely lacking maternity entitlements and social protection, finds them bogged down by unequal access to the market and lower wages, in addition to the responsibility of childcare and the household.

Driven to earn with weak support systems, their ability to provide quality nurturing and stimulating care is compromised and is usually the first casualty. This neglect does not attract any attention because other concerns assume priority, and lack of knowledge of its importance, feeds into the assumption that 'children grow up on their own' and only need feeding and physical care.

Studies have found a strong link between fertility and labour market outcomes including participation, employment and wages provided to women with higher fertility leading to lower participation.[22] The disproportionate responsibility on women for childcare also results in less time for paid work, thus undermining their equal right to decent work and social security as well as bringing forth the lack of provisions for childcare in informal work settings that results in women dropping out of the labour force.[23] Women with access to day-care have been known to earn at least 50 percent more, and 70 percent of older children have been found to have started going to school for the first time, as they did not have to look after their younger siblings in the absence of their working mothers.[24]

While mothers are primarily responsible for the care of children up to the 3 year age group, older children are roped into childcare thereafter. According to a study by FORCES in 2013, the proportion of children involved in childcare increased to 23 percent for the 3–6 years age group.[25] The trade-offs between caring for their children and providing economically for them is difficult, a reflection of the limited choices they have rather than any paucity of love and affection.

When older sisters are entrusted with the responsibility of childcare while the mother is occupied with other chores within the household, or working outside, they are deprived of developmental opportunities. They miss out on school in order to look after the younger sibling and the quality of childcare suffers as they themselves are children without sufficient maturity. A child who is left unattended, or in the care of a sibling is much more likely to be undernourished and prone to illness and developmental deprivation.[26]

According to the Socio Economic and Caste Census (SECC), most of the 12.8 percent of rural households headed by women have a monthly income of less than INR 5,000. According to the Census, in about 23 million female headed rural households, 10.11 percent earned less than INR 5,000 a month and only 0.89 percent earned more than INR 10,000 a month. Overall, 14 million households are 'considered for deprivation.' The grading of deprivation is based on the condition of housing, landlessness, absence of an able-bodied adult member, any adult male member or a literate adult.[27] Such calculations do not factor in women's unpaid labour contribution to the care functions within the households.

An Overseas Development Institute (ODI) report in 2016, *Women's work: mothers, children and the global childcare crisis*, identified a 'care gap' in most countries. Noting the adverse effects of a lack of care on children when mothers are pushed to their limits by the demands of caring and providing for their families, it recommended policy and programmatic changes to support women with childcare services, so that they can overcome stress and participate in economic development.[28]

Alternative support through trained childcare workforce is particularly necessary in situations where children are likely to be left alone without an adult caregiver. A challenge worth addressing would be to provide for full day quality childcare by trained and well-remunerated workers who have knowledge of the science and techniques of ECD as well as the aptitude and motivation to work with young children. Quality childcare services, while ensuring all-round development of young children together with their safety and security, hold the promise of providing women with time, space and opportunities to exercise their agency, utilise developmental opportunities and empower themselves.

5.3 Provision of childcare services is grossly inadequate

5.3.1 The State's role has been peripheral in the childcare discourse

The idea of the State having a duty and social responsibility towards citizens for childcare beyond the conventional spheres of law and order, defence, transport and infrastructure is of relatively recent origin and revolutionary. While recognising that all children have a right to be brought up by their parents (Article 7), the CRC obligates the State to provide a conducive environment for parenting, and to intervene when parents are in conflict with the law, are not alive, are abusing the child or are unable to live with each other (Article 9).

Recognising the important role of parenting in nurturing, educating and socialising children, which is also critical for the progress towards the SDGs, the United Nations observes June 1 every year as the Global Day of Parents. Implicit in the SDG 4 *"Ensure inclusive and equitable quality education and promote lifelong learning opportunities for all"* is the reinforcement of States' responsibilities in ensuring access of young girls and boys to quality early childhood development, care and pre-primary education by 2030. And implicit in SDG 5 *"Achieve gender equality and empower all women and girls"* is the imperative of sharing and recognition of unpaid care work to lessen the burden on the mother and promote the well-being of the child. However, the SDGs and their targets and indicators do not use the term parenting, leave alone transformative parenting. [See Annexure 3 for the targets and indicators under SDGs 4 and 5 globally and in India.]

Targets on malnutrition, child mortality, early learning and violence that outline an agenda for improving ECD are embedded in the SDGs and provide opportunities for eliciting commitments and investments. Global institutions like UNICEF, the World Bank Group, UNESCO and WHO have already expressed their commitment to the ECD agenda. United Nations' Global Strategy for Women's, Children's and Adolescents' Health 2016–2030 synthesises the new vision under the objectives of Survive, Thrive and Transform, whereas the Nurturing Care Framework (NCF), developed by the WHO in collaboration with other organisations, builds on the foundation of universal health coverage, with primary care at its core, as essential for all sustainable growth and development.

The NCF provides strategic directions for supporting the holistic development of children, from pregnancy up to age of three, through multiple sectors – including health, nutrition, education, labour, finance, water and sanitation and social and child protection, to address the needs of the youngest children, to achieve the results envisioned in the SDGs. It defines nurturing care as

> conditions created by public policies, programmes and services. These conditions enable communities and caregivers to ensure children's good health and nutrition, and protect them from threats. Nurturing care also means giving young children opportunities for early learning, through interactions that are responsive and emotionally supportive.[29]

In terms of the State's obligations to the young child, India can rightly claim that ICDS has been in existence since 1976 with the ambition of providing a package of maternal and child health related interventions, including supplementary nutrition and ECCE. However, its nutrition component has overshadowed other objectives, the early childhood education is weak, and childcare is negligible. While it is seen to be the role of AWWs to take care of the varied aspects of children's everyday development, including health and nutrition as well as early learning in a meaningful way, when it comes to childcare over an extended period of time each day – matching with the work timings of mothers – the AWCs exclude such children by design. While it is reported of initiatives by states like Tamil Nadu and Karnataka of increased timings for AWCs to cater to the demand of day-care, especially for children of women working in the informal sector, the question of an additional trained worker remains unaddressed.

The **National Policy for Children, 2013,** mentioned three aspects related to parenting, viz., (1) all children have the right to grow in a family environment, in an atmosphere of happiness, love and understanding; (2) children are not to be separated from their parents, except where such separation is necessary or in their best interest; and (3) families are to be supported by a strong social safety net in caring for and nurturing their children.

The **National ECCE Policy, 2013,** was a watershed moment recognising the rights of children under 6. It was for the first time that a policy gave due recognition to the holistic needs of the young child, acknowledging the "synergistic and interdependent relationship between the health, nutrition, psycho-social and emotional needs of the child," and also laying the framework for under 3s. In addition, the policy also duly considered the fact that families require supportive measures to ensure the overall growth and development of the child. The policy emphasises play-based and child-friendly techniques that could ease the way of children into formal schooling. However, even as the policy focusses on early learning, it falls short of defining the provisions of care for those under 3 who do not go to pre-schools. It also does not address the issue of day-care required by mothers working in the informal sector. Likewise, it mentions the need to strengthen the various structures under ICDS but is vague when it comes to the question of addressing malnutrition and the diet it envisages.[30]

The **Draft National Women's Policy, 2016,** does not mention the term parenting or the need for gender sensitive parenting, but it recommends better implementation of the Maternity Benefit Act, including the provision for nursing breaks to improve the health and emotional well-being of infants. It mentions that children of migrant women/ parents should have access to education in destination places but fails to specify access to early childhood education, especially of girls living in the streets, daughters of sex workers and daughters of parents in conflict with law. It does however refer to the need to sensitise parents about the importance of pre-primary education of girls and free women's time by expanding the chain of crèches.

Although there are legislation and policy frameworks pertaining to parenting, the issue of childcare in general and day-care in particular have not received the attention they deserve. And as a result, the conditions for utilising the gender and socially transformative potential of parenting of the young child have neither been explored nor created.

Employers in the sectors that hire high numbers of migrant, contractual workers, are obliged to provide working women with day-care facilities for their children under various labour laws. Factories Act, 1948, the Mines Act, 1952, the Plantation Act, 1951, the Inter-State Migrant Workman Act of 1980, Building and Other Construction Workers Act (BOCWA) of 1996, and NREGA, 2005, make provision of crèches mandatory. *Annexure 5* lists all the relevant legislation that mandates the setting up of such facilities.

However, these laws focus on provision of crèches for women workers rather than all workers and are inconsistent in terms of the minimum number of women workers required to mandate the facility. The lack of recognition of the criticality of ECD and the foundational needs of the child in the legal provisions, and non-availability of guidelines to set up crèches at the worksites multiply the difficulties in providing childcare services of a certain quality. Lack of notified rules under the labour laws and absence of guidelines for crèches has meant that even when there are legal provisions for under 6 children of women working across many informal sector jobs, awareness is low, the demand for childcare entitlements is invisible and the neglect of young children is pervasive.

The Maternity Benefit Act, 1961 (amended in 2017) was instituted in order to ensure women received their maternity entitlements and were not hindered by childbearing or childcare responsibilities to participate in the workforce. The 2017 amendment brought about three significant changes to this Act. One, the leave entitlement duration was increased from 12 weeks to 26 weeks. Two, the provision of leave was also introduced for adoptive and surrogate mothers. Three, every establishment with 50 or more employees was mandated to establish a crèche facility. The Act lays down the minimum guidelines for the establishment of crèches, as noted in Box 5.1.

The MWCD guidelines for crèches provide a comprehensive set of standards to facilitate the setting up of good quality crèches. They provide sample immunisation schedule, meal charts, and growth monitoring requirements as per WHO standards, provision of essential materials, developmental checklists and a list of activities for varied age groups.

Box 5.1   Maternity Benefit Act, 2017, delineates National Minimum Guidelines for Crèches

Building upon the National ECCE Policy, 2013, and in a bid to facilitate the setting up, managing of and standardising crèche facilities within work spaces of full-time employees as well as daily wage, temporary, consultant and contractual personnel, in establishments recognised under the Maternity Benefit Act, the MWCD has developed minimum norms and standards for running crèches for children aged six months to six years.

The guidelines envisage the location of the crèche at or near the workplace, or within 500 meters in the beneficiaries' neighborhood for easy access. They recommend 8–10 hours of functioning per day by the crèche in view of the need for childcare while parents' work for roughly 8 hours per day. Regarding infrastructure, they recommend a ground floor concrete structure, well-lit and ventilated with child friendly toilet facility, ramps and handrails for easy access, and enough space for children to rest, learn and play. They call for demarcation of areas for under 3s and 3–6s for eating, sleeping, cleaning, breastfeeding activities.

The guidelines further lay down standards with respect to the crèche environment, equipment for nutrition, medical aid, play, safety and protection of children, health practices including regular visits by medical practitioners, hygienic and well-balanced nutrition practices including serving of three meals a day, crèche transactions like age-appropriate activities, skills and flexible curriculum with disciplinary techniques that do not involve corporal punishment or verbal abuse. There are also standards and norms regarding hygiene and sanitation practices – both environmental and personal – to ensure that cleanliness of the crèche and the personal hygiene of the child is maintained and preventive measures like washing hands are practiced to minimise the spread of germs and infection.

Source: MWCD[31]

While these guidelines have the potential to ensure the minimum quality of childcare for children of employees in the formal sector, they again bring to the light the stark absence of any guidelines and the State's absolute neglect of childcare provisions in the informal sector, whether at the national or the state level.

The first crèche scheme launched in 1975, Crèches for Working and Ailing Mothers Scheme, was limited in its financial norms and rigid schematic patterns.[32] And yet it was a strong recognition of the importance of childcare during early years and the significance of state enabled childcare care for working mothers. The National Crèche Fund was introduced in 1994, in response to the Shram Shakti report recommendations. In 2002, both programmes were combined to launch the Rajiv Gandhi Crèche Scheme with revised norms. This was further rechristened as the National Crèche Scheme in 2017, with one significant change in the programme pattern – the monitoring responsibility lies with state WCD. State departments can opt to run crèches directly or through NGO implementing partners.

The **National Crèche Scheme** (NCS) intends to provide a safe place for mothers to leave their children aged 6 months to 6 years while they are at work. It offers flexible timings and affordable services for children of women working in the informal sector in rural and urban areas. The services include supplementary nutrition, healthcare inputs like immunisation, polio drops, basic health monitoring, sleeping facilities, early stimulation (for children below 3 years) and pre-school education for children aged between 3–6 years.

The mechanism of the NCS being a grant-in-aid scheme to be run and managed by NGOs, monitored by the state WCD, has stayed with minor budgetary and superficial reviews over the years. Ten percent of annual running costs are expected to be borne by the implementing NGO, while central and state funds cover 90 percent of the costs, making it a deterrent for implementing NGOs to come forward for running crèches and day-care services under this scheme.

The already poor allocations for the scheme declined from Rs 200 crores in 2017–2018 (BE) to only INR 50 crore in 2019–2020 (BE).[33] Even when the budgeted allocations were higher, the actual spending was very low, with the revised budget estimates being INR 65 crores in 2017–2018 and INR 30 crores in 2018–2019. As reported in the Hindustan Times (2019),[34] "the number of facilities under the National Crèche Scheme has reduced from over 23,000 in 2015 to around 7,000 this year," translating into "one crèche per 21,000 children." Only 7,930 crèches were functional across the country in 2019.[35]

As the only crèche scheme for children of women working in the informal sector, the NCS has severe limitations in budget allocations, implementation, and administration, especially when it comes to a sustained solution for young children and working mothers in rural and urban poor areas.

5.3.2 Parental entitlements in the interest of childcare are lacking

Providing support to a woman to discharge her triple role in a society that is so strongly patriarchal is indeed a challenge. The role of women has not been sufficiently recognised or compensated, albeit there is increased articulation of the imperative of childcare support by the state and other agencies.

Working and actually witnessing the challenges faced by women in their daily struggles, various women's studies researchers and activists found support in the Shram Shakti Report way back in the 1988.[36] Their groundwork enabled rigorous pressure to be exerted for setting up a national commission to monitor the situation of women working in the unorganised sector. The Shram Shakti Report of the National Commission on the Status of Women connected the low social, economic and health status of women to the demands of childbearing/rearing during her most productive years and made a strong case for the state to provide systems and make adequate investments for childcare services. It contributed significantly to the widening of the notion of childcare beyond the confines of a home to a social policy.

The stated goals of the NCS include the improvement of the health and nutrition status and physical, cognitive, social and emotional development of children from marginalised families and education and empowerment of their parents and caregivers for better childcare. But while the crèche workers are expected to motivate parents for immunisation and health and nutrition counselling if their child's growth is not adequate, ECCE is clearly neglected. While the scheme mentions training of crèche workers on the appreciation of parents' involvement in crèche programmes, the training content does not have a component on parents' education on ECCE. Parental education on ECCE is also not part of their tasks.

There is a crèche monitoring committee, but representation by parents is not mentioned. Unlike the guidelines on the ECCE Framework, there is no reference to breaking gender or social stereotypes and barriers. There is no reference to reaching children marginalised by caste, class, religion, ethnicity, disability or those living with sex workers, on the streets or in prisons.

The Maternity Benefit Act, 1961, provided women employed in factories, shops or commercial establishments with ten or more employees certain period of leaves before and after childbirth. The Maternity Benefit (Amendment) Act, 2017, has increased the maternity leave and introduced provisions relating to working from home and a crèche facility (see Box 5.2). Since the Maternity Benefit Act including the Amendment Act is applicable to every organisation with fifty or more employees, its impact is fairly wide.

One of its important features is its gender transformative approach towards childcare as the conditionality about minimum employees is not restricted to women alone. However, while the amendment sought to provide entitlements that were more beneficial to the women employees, it imposes the entire cost of these benefits squarely on the employers, "which could lead to a negative trend in hiring women in meaningful roles" (Mathew, 2019).[37] This gendered benefit of paid leave could result in employers running the risk of incurring additional costs if they hire women.

Box 5.2 Maternity Benefit Act, 1961, and Maternity Benefit (Amendment) Act, 2017

Key provisions

- The employer must intimate every female employee in writing or electronically at the time of her appointment regarding all benefits available to them under the Maternity Benefit Act.
- Women who have completed 80 days in the 12 months immediately preceding the date of her expected delivery is entitled to maternity leaves for a maximum of 26 weeks of which not more than eight weeks shall be preceding the expected date of her delivery. However, the woman can also take the entire 26 weeks of leave post the delivery.
- Women having two or more surviving children shall be allowed maternity leave of 12 weeks of which not more than six weeks should be before the expected date of her delivery.
- Women are allowed six weeks' leave in case of miscarriage or a medical termination of pregnancy.
- Women adopting a child up to three months or opting for surrogacy are entitled to 12 weeks of maternity leave from the date of adoption or commissioning.
- The employer can neither dismiss a woman for seeking maternity leave nor can they serve a termination notice to her during the

course of the leave that expires before the leave ends, nor can they change the terms of service to her disadvantage during the leave. The employer may agree to allow her to work from home depending on the nature of work assigned to her even after she has availed of the maternity benefit.

• It is mandatory for establishments for 50 or more employees to set up crèche facilities that mothers are entitled to visit up to four times a day or to two nursing breaks per day.

(Ministry of Labour and Employment, 2017)

Although women working in the organised or formal sector are entitled to salary equivalent to six months for two children under the Maternity Benefit Act, their counterparts in the unorganised or informal sector have no such guarantee.

Pradhan Mantri Matru Vandana Yojana, previously known as *Indira Gandhi Matritva Sahyog Yojana*, inaugurated in 2017, provides partial cash compensation for the wage loss to enable pregnant and lactating women to take adequate rest before and after delivery of the first living child. The assumption is that the cash incentive would result in improved health seeking behaviour among them. The centrally sponsored Conditional Maternity Benefit Programme commits only INR 5,000 and that too for the first child and is reportedly plagued by implementation challenges.[38] This is a major criticism of the scheme purported to cover the vast majority of working mothers in the informal jobs sector.

5.3.3 Childcare component in ICDS is negligible

ICDS centres have, for decades, functioned as feeding and distribution centres with very little attempts made to strengthen the other components, especially the pre-school and community counselling aspects. It has partially helped to improve malnutrition rates to some extent, and some of the southern states like Tamil Nadu and Karnataka have actually set an example on how to maximise the returns from this programme. Extended timings, better infrastructure for the centres, higher honoraria and training of the AWWs have all contributed in great measure to making ICDS work in these states.

However, one of the major conceptual flaws in the design of the programme is the different areas of focus for the different age groups. The comprehensive holistic needs for both the age groups were sacrificed as it got translated into 'immunisation' and 'take home rations' for the under 3s and supplementary nutrition and a non-functional pre-school programme for the 3–6 year-olds. The absence of planning for 'care' in the design of the programme, whereby a child's safety, protection, early bonding and early stimulation could take place, was one of the major underlying reasons of failure for India to take advantage of the great investments that the nation had made in this flagship programme.

The programme ignored the emerging need for care which was required as a result of the demographic changes taking place across the rural, tribal and urban parts of the country. It has also suffered due to weak governance and administrative systems which contributed to large scale corruption and mismanagement. More importantly, it fails to give due importance to the role of the ICDS worker by involving her in other activities like the census, specific campaigns and schemes. The *Anganwadi* worker (AWW) and helper are the basic functionaries of the ICDS who run the *Anganwadi* Centre (AWC) and implement the programme in coordination with the functionaries of the health, education, rural development and other departments. But the programme failed to acknowledge their work by continuing to give them an honorarium and training them inadequately. This led to the creation and proliferation of a private sector waiting to make the most of the State's failure to respond to the growing aspirations of parents.

However, after a promising thrust in the 12th Five-Year Plan of converting 5 percent of AWCs into *Anganwadi*-cum-Crèches (AWCCs), the state, in 2018, has moved back from its larger vision. Few states like Rajasthan, Madhya Pradesh and Delhi rolled out the AWCC as a pilot in identified districts. Yet, funding blocks, lack of clarity from the Centre about continuation of the initiative, operational challenges and states' reluctance to allocate additional resources led to the gradual closing down of the AWCCs in these states and a missed opportunity for young children of women workers engaged in informal work both in rural and urban areas.

Box 5.3 Mobile Creches plays a pioneering role in providing alternative childcare services

Mobile Creches is a pioneer in the movement for crèche or day-care services for young children of working mothers. It has trained workers, supervisors and officials in the government and voluntary sector over the years. In recent years it has worked towards operationalising crèches in about 200 AWCs, which served as AWCCs, in Madhya Pradesh, Rajasthan and Delhi in partnership with the state governments. The communities and government officials were orientated to the concept of AWCC through training and demonstration so that they can play a supportive role.

Getting the established systems to contribute to effective and efficient AWCCs been a major stumbling block. At a positive level, the centres open on time, attendance levels of children have increased, and the trained workers work with motivation and enthusiasm notwithstanding the delays in honoraria, rations and other logistical support. In Madhya Pradesh, the AWWs and helpers reported that the understanding of the importance of proactive interventions in the lives of young children gave them a mission, and they remained in contact with their trainers due to the quality of training and bonding during the process.[39]

This pilot initiative was appreciated by many policymakers but due to lack of political will and popular demand, they have not shown commitment to scaling up the model. The absence of scientific evidence on the impact of 'care' and the strong patriarchal system prevalent in India have hindered the creation of political demand from the parents and communities for alternative care arrangements. The government's decision to replace the pilot programme with the National Programme for Day-care and Crèches to be run by the NGOs or through the ICDS, does not address the existing and potential demand for childcare support and crèches.

5.3.4 *The implementation of day-care provisions in the labour laws is weak*

One of the most glaring limitations of the legal provisions for crèche services is the conditionality that a minimum number of women must work at the site if the facility is to be provided. The rules framed for implementing crèches under labour laws are weak, with the entire financial and organisational burden falling on the employer, who tries to escape through multiple loopholes available in the existing laws. A major lacuna of the crèche provisions under the labour laws is its focus on the number of women workers employed and silence on the children's need for a safe, caring and stimulating crèche and day-care centre.

The gendering of the rules actually works to the disadvantage of women, who are at higher risk of being excluded from opportunities to work. A study by the Institute of Development Studies (IDS) UK, in 2017, found about 95 percent of the women were not even aware of the legal provision for crèches and had never availed of such a facility.[40] The unsatisfactory implementation is reflected in the absence of norms for the quality of service which allow a basic crèche with an untrained childcare worker that provides custodial care and the lack of data on the coverage of such crèches with the Ministry of Labour.

The private sector is rather heterogeneous in its approach to childcare provisions. **The corporate bodies, mandated by the MBA (amended 2017) to provide for crèche facilities, have made some cautious inroads into** providing crèche facilities mainly to attract and retain their employees. They have adopted different models in response to the needs of their employees. The crèches in this sector are run by third parties, or self-managed, or have tie-ups with other companies. They are set up at the workplace or near the residences of workers to prevent them from travelling long distances with their children.[41] Some corporates also provide flexible working hours and extended childcare leave. However, the small-scale and the mid-sized enterprises tend to evade their statutory obligations of minimum wages and social protection obligations. The crèche is usually not a priority on their agenda, and they find ways to escape the mandatory requirements.

5.3.5 Proliferation of private services shows uneven quality with limited outreach

Spontaneous and informal arrangements for childcare are mushrooming in response to changing family dynamics, especially in the growing urban and peri-urban areas, and the non-availability of crèches and day-care. Parents generally demand custodial care for the safety of their children and in any case most of these arrangements are unable and ill-suited for ECD service delivery, especially to children below 3. For instance, women in many urban slums pay their neighbours a sizeable amount for basic custodial care of their young children, who are deprived of play, learning or bonding opportunities and are at risk of neglect, violence or even abuse. It is very difficult to regulate such informal arrangements.[42]

Then there are unregulated pre-schools and day-care centres that pressurise children to read and write way ahead of their developmental readiness while neglecting the integrated elements of care, health, nutrition and love. A count of such informal or even registered play schools, crèches and nurseries is not available but such arrangements are extremely popular with local communities.

It is hard to monitor the quality of informal arrangements and public and private childcare service providers with respect to the space, infrastructure, adult-child ratio, safety, health, nutrition, infant stimulation and early education standards laid down in the ECCE quality framework. In the absence of uniform norms and minimum standards for public and private childcare services, and the absence of a regulatory body for the same, the regulation by the State is non-existent. The training and ensuing competencies are also widely different among childcare workers engaged in the private sector.

5.4 Good practices can provide policy pointers and lessons

5.4.1 Some state-level initiatives in childcare are noteworthy

Government of Chhattisgarh's Phulwari initiative: The state government initiated Phulwari in Sarguja district in 2012 to address high levels of malnutrition. The focus is on mobilising community support for mothers in ensuring child feeding and care and improving household availability of food through cultivation of rice, kitchen gardens, horticulture and backyard poultry. The scheme draws upon the resources from *Gram Panchayats* and *Mitanin* programme instead of providing for a centre or paid manager and workers.

A **Phulwari** is a nutrition and childcare centre which is set up on a space offered by a local resident and is managed by mothers collectively. The *Gram Panchayats* provide them cash assistance to provide three hot cooked meals to children aged 6 months to 3 years and one meal to pregnant and lactating women. Every day, two mothers volunteer to take care of children at the Phulwari for 6–7 hours while others go for work. The *mitanins* facilitate and support the process, including maintenance of accounts and records. The state government decided to replicate the Phulwari initiative across all the eighty-five tribal blocks of the state.

5.4.2 *Civil society initiatives have shown creative ways of collaboration*

Over the last five decades, **Mobile Creches** has demonstrated that it is possible to provide quality care to children of vulnerable sections of the population through creative partnerships with different stakeholders, with limited infrastructure and resources. Its programme is holistic with components that can be replicated in other situations with minor refinements. It works with government, CSOs, communities and employers, running centres on construction sites and slums to provide a comprehensive set of childcare services to children in the absence of their parents who are at work. The holistic programme, which seeks to provide emotional and physical security to children, is run by frontline workers who are trained, motivated for ECD and monitored for their performance through systems and processes based on quality norms. Mobile Creches has contributed to capacity building of childcare workers, supervisors and decision makers in the government and voluntary sector. Their strategy of involving all the stakeholders in the initial orientation workshops has paid dividends in terms of close coordination and synergetic action for improved outcomes.

Action Against Malnutrition (AAM) has developed a community-based collaborative model. Its crèches, staffed by two workers from the community, provide children with a safe and conducive environment while their mothers work. The caregivers are provided extensive training on childcare, especially identifying and taking specific nutritional interventions to help severely malnourished, growth faltered and sick children. Although the focus is on promoting the interface of the community groups with the government programmes like ICDS, and frontline workers like ASHA and Mitanin, the caregivers are trained and encouraged to incorporate specific developmental play activities with children. A consortium of organisations has helped with the design, facilitation, training and technical support for monitoring child health. This model enables community involvement in the management of the crèche and some of the significant elements can be adapted for other programmes.

Alternative care arrangements have necessitated for new ways of thinking about care which are grounded in local communities and sensitive to the context-specific needs. Often, a striking absence from mainstream crèche facilities are elements of care, and simultaneously promoting initiatives for capacity-building of parents for them to be involved in childcare. Both these components are integral to the **SEWA** (Self Employed Women's Association) childcare model. SEWA was an early starter in recognising the link between women's work, social security entitlements and quality childcare services as it provided a flexible, community-led network of crèches to its members. In partnership with the government, SEWA has worked to help policies and programmes better adapt to the specific needs of women workers in the informal sector.

Others like **Centre for Learning Resources** (CLR) and **Pratham** have focussed on collaboration with the ICDS. They employ different strategies involving technical support to showcase how the quality of existing programmes can be improved.

5.5 Key issues

5.5.1 *Imperative of quality childcare has not been duly recognised*

Global efforts towards poverty reduction and women's financial empowerment have acknowledged the importance of early childcare arrangements such as crèches, day-care services and play schools. They can provide the infant, toddler or pre-schooler with the care necessary for them as well as facilitate the entry and continuation of women in the labour force in the organised and unorganised sectors. It would unlock their employment potential, increase productivity and prospects of higher earnings, and may even reduce stress resulting from accumulated burden of multiple roles and responsibilities, disadvantages and hardships experienced at their households.

Public sector provisions such as basic infrastructure, childcare and elderly care facilities and affordable private sector services can improve the lives of women who shoulder the care and domestic work burden and are forced out of the workforce. When women do not have an income, their decision-making power within the household and mobility are considerably reduced. Too much unpaid work by women devalues the work they do in the paid market. Their work is assumed to be less significant and the occupations that women are crowded into get badly paid.

It is an appealing proposition that childcare at home and institutional settings would provide young children, especially the 6 month to 3 year olds, nurturing care along with adequate nutrition, healthcare and other wherewithal for a firm foundation for life, and older siblings would be released from childcare responsibilities to access education and a brighter future. Three groups, viz., the young child, the girl child and the woman, all of whom need urgent interventions for their safety, health and development, stand to gain from a well-functioning system of childcare. The investment in quality childcare benefits society by improving the present and potential productivity of two generations and disrupting the intergenerational transmission of poverty.

However, most parents are unaware of the importance of early childcare arrangements for infants and toddlers. Women in the informal sector who bear a disproportionate burden of work both within and outside the household need maternity entitlements and childcare provisions. But their voices have not been amplified sufficiently in the policy arena because patriarchal social and institutional norms have confined childcare to the domain of maternal responsibility and resisted the attempts to widen the scope of roles and responsibilities.

Lack of articulated demand has hampered the supply of alternative childcare arrangements. Furthermore, parents are unable to visualise good quality alternative care or crèche services due to their scarcity. The AWCs or private day-care facilities do not exactly inspire confidence. The lack of a deep understanding of the principles of child development and the systems and protocols required to run crèches and childcare facilities restrict the opening of such facilities and fail to allay public scepticism about the quality of care and safety of young children.

5.5.2 Resource constraints are major impediments to setting up of crèches

A good ECD programme requires human resources of high calibre for formal childcare inclusive of parental support, responsive parenting programmes and home-based support. The combination of aptitude, training and responsibility of the workforce in institutionalised early childcare setups contribute to improved outcomes for young children. The ASHAs and AWWs do not command sufficient respect as professionals especially when childcare is perceived to be just feeding and cleaning of babies. The lack of importance that state structures assign to the frontline workers and payment of honorarium instead of regular wages for their work makes their work be seen as not dignified. Meanwhile, the risks and levels of responsibility involved are much higher as the childcare workers are expected to demonstrate empathy as well as verbal and non-verbal cues to communicate with a developing infant and toddler and high levels of alertness to prevent mishaps.

The varied requirement for crèches, as noted in Box 5.4, has multiple financial resource implications. Trained human resource is required with an adult-child ratio as per the set norms; capacity building and motivation of the human resource are fundamental to the childcare programme vision. Adequate and appropriate infrastructure needs to be in place for space, equipment, safety concerns, water and sanitation. Maintaining an optimum quality of integrated inputs in health, nutrition, and early education, as well as better systems for monitoring, supervision, regulation and enforcement require financial investments. Further, ensuring parental involvement, community participation and responsibility to be inclusive especially with regard to disadvantaged children, creating awareness about the critical life period also requires sufficient budgets. However, the financial restraints do not permit the investment in the required infrastructural, human resource and quality interventions.

Box 5.4   A quality crèche or day-care should include certain key dimensions

The following standards define the governance and management for delivery of quality childcare services at scale.

- **Location and infrastructure:** The centre or crèche should be easily accessible, structurally safe and preferably on the ground floor with clean and spacious surroundings. The centre should be well ventilated with provisions for clean water, sanitation and electricity. Space deemed adequate per child is 12 sq. feet.
- **Space and arrangements:** The classroom should be bright, cheerful and equipped with child-accessible displays of learning material that encourage a wide variety of age-appropriate activities for learning, playing and resting.
- **Equipment and materials:** Sturdy, safe and easy to maintain furniture, age appropriate play equipment in adequate quantity, and provisions for supplementary nutrition, cleaning, personal hygiene, sleeping and medical aid should be readily available. Low-cost, easily available and environment friendly material should be preferred.
- **Human Resources:** Trained personnel should be deployed with the recommended adult child ratio of 1:8 for under threes and 1:15 for 3–6 year olds, paid not less than the minimum wages, and receive ongoing mentoring support and opportunities for skill upgradation.
- **Nutrition practices:** All children should receive fresh, nutritionally balanced and culturally acceptable supplementary diet spread over three times a day, including a hot cooked meal for lunch.

The food should be prepared, stored and served following strict hygiene procedures.

- **Classroom curriculum and transactions:** Age and developmentally appropriate activities should take care of all the domains of development and encourage self-confidence. Varied activity corners for a free or structured and small or large group activities should be created.
- **Safety, health and hygiene practices:** Each child should be age appropriately immunised and undergo regular medical check-ups. Washing hands, wiping noses, sanitising toys and such measures should be promoted to minimize the spread of germs. Safety and protection systems should be in place, with strict supervision to minimise hazards within and outside the centre.
- **Monitoring, supervision and stakeholder participation** are essential at multiple levels and robust systems can be developed to ensure the best interests of the children, community and other stakeholders. Linkages of families with the local facilities can be forged to facilitate and synergise convergence.

Source: MWCD, 2013, 2014[43]

Most existing services are being delivered without adequate guidelines and regulatory mechanisms. It is easier to hold ICDS than the private ECCE centres accountable, due to the existing ICDS monitoring mechanisms. If socially transformative ECCE services are to be realised, it makes the need for regulation across public and private services even more important.

5.5.3 *Ultimately the focus should be on caring and nurturing ecosystems*

Gender and socially transformative parenting needs to be promoted proactively as a prerequisite to design, delivery and utilisation of good quality ECD services. It would require improvement in the legal and policy framework, with its implementation and targeting of children affected by multiple identities through culturally relevant, appropriately designed responsive parenting education programmes.

Acute deficit in parenting is particularly evident in the case of the girl child, street children, migrant children, children of sex workers, children of parents in marginal occupations, children with disability, orphans, SC and ST children and children living in conflict areas. Spatial segregation of families across caste, class and religion also poses a barrier to inclusive parenting. Plugging this parenting deficit is a right of the young child, can lead to more egalitarian gender and social norms in society and further the rights of women, mothers and adolescent girls, and contribute to efficiency of the economy.

In addition to the mothers, every effort should be made to engage with fathers to involve them proactively in parenting. The role of fathers in the gender-based division of parenting responsibilities is important but less explored. The time they spend with young children, the activities they engage in, and their style of parenting are crucial. There are some linkages like the more time fathers spend with children, the less violent they are. A beginning has been made as enough fathers are concerned about the happiness of their children and love their children enough to do something about it, leaving room for intervention. Getting both mothers and fathers on board could create positive ripple effects and improve the uptake of knowledge regarding good child rearing practices.

5.6 Recommendations and action points

5.6.1 *Recognise childcare as a profession*

There is an urgent need to professionalise the childcare sector through due recognition by the State, of the childcare workers by replacing the current system of paying honoraria to paying adequate remuneration and improving working conditions for them. ECD professionals should be fully trained, adequately paid, and supported with appropriate working conditions, equipment, learning opportunities and guidance. Recognised training institutions, following an approved curriculum and pedagogy, must be made widely available.

The childcare providers should belong to the same community or background as the young children, to the extent possible, to facilitate ease of communication, as they understand the local, regional context, community dynamics and the cultural traditions. The child is most comfortable in local dialects and cultural traditions during early years.

Skills, knowledge and attitude of service providers largely determines the quality of services. Regular wages commensurate to their qualification and designations could attract qualified staff. Public and private service providers need to make efforts to keep their morale and motivation levels high in addition to in-service capacity development interventions. Coaching, mentoring and supportive supervision have been found to enhance workers' willingness to work with diligence. Clarity on roles, protocols and system support also contribute to the discharge of quality services. And last but not the least, regular feedback sessions could enable exploration of the quality of their work and other creative possibilities.

5.6.2 *Improve the training design*

Wide disparity in qualifications, and the nature and duration of training of childcare workers has implications on the inequitable quality of programmes. Most of them are not aligned with the curricular recommendations made by NCTE, the body overseeing quality of training for ECE teachers. The training framework needs to be re-visualised if the ICDS is to provide quality ECCE to the age group from birth to 6 years, and most importantly for the under 3s. Quality childcare also entails building capacities to prevent and address abuse of infants and young children.

Experiential and participatory methodologies like role plays, preparation of teaching materials, exposure visits and reflective discussions need to be incorporated as the probability of trainees being semi-literate remains high. **The training should be designed to provide them hands-on-experience and equip them with skills for community outreach and interaction with parents and community leaders.** Participatory techniques help the trainees to arrive at theoretical concepts through discussion without being told directly in a dry and didactic manner. Extended periods of practice and reflection should in due course enhance their learning.

On-site supportive supervision, collective sharing and problem solving are useful strategies that have shown appreciable results in strengthening the training. Refresher/in-service training at regular intervals can take place through digital media to update them to new research and best practices taking place across the world. Face-to-face trainings can be planned every five years to facilitate mutual learnings as also to sustain motivation and energy.

In-service training, building upon the capacities and experiences of the existing childcare workers across the country must be duly recognised by training institutions. Policies and systems must enable existing working cadres across childcare services to pursue learning and career development opportunities to gain knowledge, develop competencies and remain motivated. It is equally important for these policies to promote and ensure quality preservice trainings based on minimum eligibility criteria, curricular framework, duration and opportunities for regular refresher courses. The training programmes must focus on balancing theoretical knowledge with practice experiences, using face-to-face, distance education, MOOC and other appropriate methods to create a professional ECD cadre.

The supervisory cadre too should ideally come in with some field experience and the ability to link up with the local resources and stakeholders. Their training would entail not only the understanding of the principles of child development but also administration, organisation and management of systems. They should increasingly assume the role of a mentor and be the first port of problem solving for the childcare workers.

To ensure quality childcare, apart from the caregivers, senior level personnel responsible for planning, quality oversight and programme design to ensure desired outcomes and impact would be necessary. Post-graduate education (advanced diploma or Master's degree) in the core subject complemented with skills of analysis, strategic planning and research would be an added advantage. An understanding of the wider concerns on gender, child rights, understanding of the sociological dimensions of poverty and political dimensions of policymaking would be desirable and thus should be incorporated in the initial and refresher training design.

5.6.3 Strengthen ICDS with a strong childcare component

There is a need for a State supported system for crèche services and other complementary childcare services to ensure that all families are enabled and empowered to rear and nurture children with the required care and attention. **Since the ICDS is already in place and has created infrastructure and systems in almost every village, hamlet and urban slum, it must be utilised to respond to the growing demand for crèches and day-care services** as it has high potential to provide childcare support across India, especially to the most vulnerable populations.

Tribal communities living in remote areas, families living on streets or dependent on irregular wages from work at construction sites, mines, brick kilns and other such hazardous workplaces, prisoners, sex workers and people living with HIV are among the hardest to reach by public services. Extension of the outreach of ICDS beyond 48.2 percent would be crucial for making available childcare services to such disadvantaged communities. As was originally proposed in the restructured ICDS mission 2012, 10 percent of AWWs (later 5 percent of AWWs were approved) should be converted into AWCCs with adequate budgets, better implementation and monitoring mechanisms.

This would entail conversion of the existing AWCs into AWCCs to serve women working in the informal sector, appointment of an additional trained crèche worker and helper at every AWCC, provision of space, additional equipment and financial support for the full day-care for under 3s and 3–6-year age groups and extension of the timing of AWCCs to support parents who have special requirements. Children of sex workers and parents in the entertainment industry may need crèche through the night. The network of AWCCs could be expanded in due course in accordance with demand for such services.

Childcare must be reimagined as a mandate for all children requiring care, whether at the worksite or in neighbourhoods, to support working parents. It is not enough for the State to provide the access to nutrition and healthcare services; it must enable care within the home and outside of it in institutional settings through proper training, professionalisation and investment at multiple levels. Equally important, crèches can play a positive role in being enablers of women's participation in the workforce.

In addition, the design of ICDS deserves a revisit in the context of more recent developments like the RTE and NNM, and the imperative of

responding to the diversity of local needs. A universal design cannot serve the distinct priorities of regions and social groups. For example, provision of breakfast in addition to lunch in tribal areas may alleviate malnutrition and centres that are open from 7:00 in the morning to 5:00 in the evening can provide day-care to children of many women engaged in wage labour in the informal sector.

Decentralised and localised design would entail rejuvenated community-based monitoring and support structures and allocation of higher financial resources, as most state governments currently lack the financial resources for overhauling and rolling out this promising programme efficiently and effectively. Various models for childcare centres, such as those developed by Mobile Creches and SEWA cooperative childcare centres which operate longer hours, could be replicated and/or adapted.

Human resource management: The conflicting and overlapping roles and responsibilities of childcare or crèche worker need to be addressed within the framework for strengthening ICDS. There will be implications in terms of remuneration, performance standards and accountability. Their current roles and responsibilities need to be rationalised if they are to assume the additional responsibility of childcare and provide quality services. Two trained workers and two helpers should be employed to work in two shifts. The minimum wages must be fixed and the timings of AWWs could be extended for two shifts of six hours each. This could also help accommodate children from 6 months to 3 years.

Human resource development: The training design, content and methodology should stem from the recognition that a comprehensive set of interventions can address the specific needs of infants and young children. The content should incorporate adequate knowledge of health, nutritional, cognitive and socio-emotional needs of young children across the entire continuum of birth to 6 years. The training design should facilitate generation of public awareness and participation of parents and communities. It should incorporate appropriate community communication techniques like puppets and other folk media to promote traditional practices and sharpen their communication skills to influence childcare practices.

Guidelines: In view of the increasing reports of neglect and ill-treatment of young children in institutionalised settings, clear guidelines for prevention of violence, abuse, exploitation and trafficking need to be followed with rigour. This would entail training of the frontline staff, including the AWWs, and dialogue with parents and communities for preventive measures, identification of survivors, reporting protocol and provision of medical, legal and counselling services.

5.6.4 Reimagine and strengthen the National Crèche Scheme

As the only centrally sponsored scheme for crèches and day-care services, the NCS has great potential to provide much required childcare services to children under 6 of working mothers, especially women working in the unorganised sector, in urban and rural India. In order to meet the demand for safe and quality childcare support for some of the most vulnerable children, and to supplement the recommended AWCC programme, the NCS needs serious programmatic and budgetary revisions.

A fundamental recommendation to reimagine the scheme, would be for the state to run the NCS, to the maximum extent possible, under its own state department systems, as opposed to providing for it as a grant-in aid scheme for local NGOs.

A revised NCS by the MWCD should increasing budgetary allocation to provide for at least two workers and a helper for a unit of 25 children (as per the adult child ratio for under 3s and 3–6 year-old children in the ECCE policy guidelines). There should be flexibility at the district level to run crèches with ten to twenty-five children in a single unit, as per the urgent requirements of the local communities. Further, investment in adequate training and periodic refresher trainings are required to build capacities, motivate and monitor the childcare workers. The honorarium for workers and helpers is pitiably low and must be enhanced to meet minimum wage norms of states.

The current scheme lacks provision for costs related to the renting of adequate and safe spaces, the purchase of safe cooking fuel and transportation for food, and a special diet for under-weight children. Nutrition costs per child must follow the ICDS norms. These costs should be considered in the budget. While the allocation for rent needs to be benchmarked differently for rural, urban and metropolitan areas, cost indexing for nutrition funds is recommended every two years.

While the scheme talks about involving parents, offering parent counselling, there are no budgetary provisions for community awareness and prioritising community monitoring practices – most importantly, parental support in the form of counselling, education and other forms of home-based support.

Finally, in the re-imagination of the NCS, it must stand on the values of non-discriminatory, inclusive, unconditional, accessible services to all children, especially the most marginalised and excluded young children and their working mothers. It should be particularly available as a safe provision for children with disabilities, children in conflict areas, disaster prone zones, remote tribal habitations, hilly areas and those places that are the hardest to reach. It must make special provisions to include single working mothers, female headed households, survivors of violence and other forms of abuse, homeless women and other marginalised groups and individuals.

5.6.5 Support parents for childcare entitlements

The policy and legal framework for childcare needs to be strengthened to ensure provision of childcare centres and crèches at all workplaces, public works and construction sites across the country.

The provisioning for universal maternity entitlements is an important social security element that needs to be implemented for ensuring close proximity of the mother and child for emotional bonding and breastfeeding. The MBA should be amended to widen its scope to workplaces, formal as well as informal, which engage more than fifty workers. In view of the growing number of private service providers, a regulatory framework needs to guide their facilities and services.

5.6.6 *Promote gender and socially transformative parenting*

Parental counselling programmes conducted through a professional cadre of workers could create a supportive environment at home, foster gender and socially transformative parenting, and facilitate their role in demanding accountability for local services. **Periodic parenting practice surveys and monitoring of the link between drop out of girls at secondary level, and shift in parenting responsibilities to them** could provide valuable information for the design of interventions. These recommendations could be integrated into the National ECCE Policy, 2013, and Curriculum Framework, with necessary allocation of budget and trained staff.

Key Messages

- The significance of environmental inputs, stimulation and interaction influencing the overall growth and well-being of infants and young children has been strongly iterated by neuroscientific research. However, even as childcare is central to the holistic conception of ECD, multi-sectoral policies and programmes, multi-disciplinary research has long neglected it in India.
- The dominant narratives position the family as the best place for a young child to grow up in, relegating the perspectives on the young child within the political leadership and policymakers to the background as it is primarily seen to be the responsibility of the family with a minimal role to be played by the State.
- Diverse challenges may result in the family being unable to provide an optimal caring environment for the holistic development of the child, necessitating assistance and support from the State to enable them in providing the required care to a child.
- The lack of recognition of childcare as professional work, and therefore the consequent lack of recognition of childcare workers, ICDS workers as trained, qualified individuals delivering critical service to the nation is a major issue. This lack of recognition severely impacts the overall perception with regard to childcare.
- There is a mushrooming of unregulated pre-schools and day-care centres that pressurise children to read and write way ahead of

their developmental readiness while the integrated elements of care, health, nutrition and love take a backseat. The regulation by the State is non-existent in the absence of uniform norms and minimum standards for childcare services.

- There is an urgent need to professionalise the childcare sector through due recognition by the State, of the childcare workers by replacing the current system of paying honoraria to paying adequate remuneration and improving working conditions for them.

Notes

1 Begley, 1996. Also see, Begley, 1997.
2 Ibid.
3 Shonkoff and Phillips, 2000.
4 Bruer, 2000.
5 Teicher, 2002.
6 Resilience, Center on the Developing Child Harvard University, n.d.
7 Ranjani, *Gender and Social Inclusion in Parenting of the Young Child in India*, pp. 6–7; Ramachandran, 2018, p. 8.
8 Perkins et al., 2013.
9 Trask, 2011.
10 Period Labour Force Survey 2017–18.
11 MWCD, 2007; Also see Choudhry et al., 2018.
12 Know Violence in Childhood, 2017.
13 Gottschalk, 2019.
14 Sharma, 2019.
15 ECPAT International, 2018.
16 Retrieved from www.forbes.com/sites/jessicabaron/2018/12/16/parents-who-post-about-their-kids-online-could-be-damaging-their-futures/#627dd8ce27b7; date of access: 9 October 2019.
17 See United Nations, 2015.
18 WHO, 2019.
19 Retrieved from https://developingchild.harvard.edu/science/key-concepts/toxic-stress/; date of access: 11 October 2019.
20 Neenv Delhi FORCES, 2016. Report prepared by DSSW and Mobile Creches
21 Ranjani, *Gender and Social Inclusion in Parenting of the Young Child in India*.
22 Ospina et al., 2017.
23 Moussie, 2016.
24 Chatterjee, 2018.
25 FORCES, 2013.
26 Raj et al., 2015.
27 Masoodi, 2015.
28 Overseas Development Institute (ODI), 2016.
29 WHO et al., 2018.
30 Matharu, 2015.
31 For more, see National Minimum Guidelines for Setting Up and Running Creches Under Maternity Benefit Act 2017, n.d.

32 Rajiv Gandhi Crèche Scheme: The Mobile Creches Experience, 2011. Supported by Plan India. An internal document capturing the ground level experiences of implementing the RGCS in different settings.
33 Retrieved from https://pib.gov.in/Pressreleaseshare.aspx?PRID=1580461; date of access: 22 November 2019.
34 Why the Centre Must Invest More in the National Crèche Scheme, 2019.
35 Data given in response to Question in the Rajya Sabha; UNSTARRED QUESTION NO-3797 asked by Mr Nadimul Haq.
36 Shramshakti: Report, 1988.
37 Mathew, 2019.
38 Pradhan Mantri Matru Vandana Yojana (PMMVY), 2017; Also see: Johari, 2019.
39 Kak and Govindaraj, 2018.
40 Sengupta and Sachdeva, 2017.
41 IFC, 2017.
42 Mobile Creches, 2019.
43 These prerequisites for quality childcare services are taken from the *Quality Standards Framework* of ECCE Policy that identifies key principles, indicators and good practices needed for ensuring quality ECCE services.

Bibliography

Bajaj, M., 2018. *Childcare and the Childcare Worker*. Technical Background Paper for the Report, 2020. Mobile Creches, New Delhi.
Begley, S., 1996. Your Child's Brain. *Newsweek*, 18 February 1996. Retrieved from www.newsweek.com/your-childs-brain-179930; date of access: 4 November 2019.
Begley, S., 1997. How to Build a Baby's Brain. *Newsweek*, 28 February 1997. Retrieved from www.newsweek.com/how-build-babys-brain-174940; date of access: 4 November 2019.
Bruer, J.T., 1999. *The myth of the first three years: A new understanding of early brain development and lifelong learning*. Simon and Schuster, New York.
Chatterjee, M., 2018. As India Rethinks Labour Rules, One Item Not on the Agenda: Childcare Facilities for Women Workers. *The Scroll*. Retrieved from https://scroll.in/article/905727/as-india-rethinks-labour-rules-one-item-not-on-the-agenda-childcare-facilities-for-women-workers; date of access: 28 November 2019.
Choudhry, V., R. Dayal, D. Pillai, A.S. Kalokhe, K. Beier and V. Patel, 2018. Child Sexual Abuse in India: A Systematic Review. *PLoS One*. Vol 13. No 10, p. e0205086, 9 October 2018.
ECPAT International, 2018. *Trends in Online Child Sexual Abuse Material*, April 2018. ECPAT International, Bangkok. Retrieved from www.ecpat.org/wp-content/uploads/2018/07/ECPAT-International-Report-Trends-in-Online-Child-Sexual-Abuse-Material-2018.pdf; date of access: 8 October 2019.
FORCES, 2013. *Needs Assessment for Creches and Childcare Services*. Commissioned by the MWCD.
Gottschalk, F., 2019. *Impacts of Technology Use on Children: Exploring Literature on the Brain, Cognition and Well-Being*. OECD Education Working Paper No. 195. doi:10.1787/8296464e-en. Retrieved from www.oecd.org/officialdocuments/publicdisplaydocumentpdf/?cote=EDU/WKP%282019%293&docLanguage=En; date of access: 25 February 2019.

IFC, 2017. *Tackling Childcare: The Business Case for Employer-Supported Childcare*. Retrieved from www.ifc.org/wps/wcm/connect/topics_ext_content/ifc_external_corporate_site/gender+at+ifc/priorities/employment/tackling_child-care_the_business_case_for_employer_supported_childcare; date of access: 22 November 2019.

Johari, A., 2019. Indian States Are Failing to Help Mothers—And UP Is the Worst. *The Scroll*, 21 November 2019. Retrieved from https://scroll.in/article/944357/indian-states-are-failing-to-help-mothers-and-up-is-the-worst; date of access: 22 November 2019.

Kak, M. and R. Govindaraj, 2018. *Evaluating Integration in the ICDS: Impact Evaluation of an AWC-Cum-Creche Pilot in Madhya Pradesh*. World Bank Group, Washington, DC. Retrieved from http://documents.worldbank.org/curated/en/49395153 7776051558/Evaluating-Integration-in-the-ICDS-Impact-Evaluation-of-an-AWC-cum-creche-pilot-in-Madhya-Pradesh; date of access: 14 November 2019.

Know Violence in Childhood, 2017. *Ending Violence in Childhood: Global Report 2017*. Retrieved from http://globalreport.knowviolenceinchildhood.org; date of access: 5 November 2019.

Masoodi, A., 2015. Census Reveals Gloomy Picture of Life in Female-Headed Households. *Live Mint*, July 2015. Retrieved from www.livemint.com/Politics/RjAdjOgWkNMqHGI1DqX8tJ/Census-reveals-gloomy-picture-of-life-in-female-headed-house.html; date of access: 12 October 2019.

Matharu, S., 2015. Education Policy for Kids Under Six. *Down to Earth*, 17 August 2015. Retrieved from www.downtoearth.org.in/news/education-policy-for-kids-under-six – 38054; date of access: 4 November 2019.

Mathew, J., 2019. How Can the Maternity Benefit Act Increase Female Workforce Participation? *EPW Engage*. Retrieved from www.epw.in/engage/article/how-can-maternity-benefit-act-increase-female; date of access: 27 November 2019.

Ministry of Labour and Employment, 2017. Retrieved from https://labour.gov.in/annual-reports; date of access: 25 November 2019.

Ministry of Statistics and Programme Implementation, Registrar General of India, GoI. Census of India 2011. New Delhi.

Ministry of Women and Child Development (MWCD), Government of India, 2007. *Study on Child Abuse: India 2007*.

Ministry of Women and Child Development (MWCD), Government of India, 2013. *National Policy Children-2013*. Retrieved from http://india.gov.in/national -policy-children 2013; date of access: 22 November 2019.

Ministry of Women and Child Development (MWCD), Government of India, 2016. *The National Policy for Women 2016, Articulating a Vision for Empowerment of Women: Draft*. Retrieved from http://wcd.nic.in/sites/default/files/national_ecce_curr_frame-work_final_03022014%20%282%29.pdf; date of access: 24 November 2019.

Ministry of Women and Child Development (MWCD), Government of India, 2017. *Rajiv Gandhi National Creche Scheme for the Children of Working Mothers*. Retrieved from https://wcd.nic.in/sites/default/files/Revised%20RGNCSScheme_210515.pdf; date of access: 25 November 2019.

Ministry of Women and Child Development, n.d. *Quality Standards for Early Childhood Care and Education (ECCE)*. Retrieved from http://www.nipccd-earchive.wcd.nic.in/sites/default/files/PDF/Quality%20Standards%20for%20ECCE.pdf; date of access: 16 January 2020.

Mobile Creches, 2019. *Reimagining Childcare and Protection for All.* Mapping Vulnerabilities of Children of Informal Women Workers in Delhi. Draft Report.

Moussie, R., 2016. *Child Care from the Perspective of Women in the Informal Economy.* UNHLP. Retrieved from www.wiego.org/publications/childcare-perspective-women-informal-workers; date of access: 21 October 2019.

Murthy, R.K., 2018. Parental Care and the Young Child. Technical background paper for the Report 2020. Mobile Creches, New Delhi.

National Minimum Guidelines for Setting Up and Running Creches Under Maternity Benefit Act 2017, n.d. Retrieved from https://wcd.nic.in/sites/default/files/National Minimum Guidelines.pdf; date of access: 5 November 2019.

Neenv (Delhi Chapter – FORCES – Mobile Creches), 2016. *Survey Findings on the Situation of Young Children in Delhi—'Situational Analysis of Children Under Six in Delhi'.* New Delhi.

Ospina, E.O. and S. Tzvetkova, 2017. *Women's Employment 2018.* Retrieved from https://ourworldindata.org/female-labor-force-participation-key-facts; date of access: 4 October 2019.

Overseas Development Institute (ODI), 2016. *Women's Work: Mothers, Children and the Global Childcare Crisis.* Retrieved from www.odi.org/publications/10349-women-s-work-mothers-children-and-global-childcare-crisis; date of access: 13 October 2019.

Perkins, S.C., E.D. Finegood and J.E. Swain, 2013. Poverty and Language Development: Roles of Parenting and Stress. *Innovations in Clinical Neuroscience.* Vol 10. No 4, pp. 10–19.

Plan International, 2017. *Gender Inequality and Early Childhood Development: A Review of the Linkages.* Plan International. Retrieved from https://plan-international.org/publication/2017-06-08-gender-inequality-and-early-childhood-development; date of access: 13 November 2019.

Pradhan Mantri Matru Vandana Yojana (PMMVY), 2017. Retrieved from https://wcd.nic.in/sites/default/files/PMMVY%20Scheme%20Implemetation%20Guidelines%20._0.pdf; date of access: 8 November 2019

Raj, A., L.P. McDougal and J.G. Silverman 2015. Gendered Effects of Siblings on Child Malnutrition in South Asia: Cross-Sectional Analysis of Demographic and Health Surveys from Bangladesh, India, and Nepal. *Maternal and Child Health Journal.* Vol 19. No 1, pp. 217–226.

Ramachandran, V., 2018. *From the Womb to Primary School: Challenges, Policies and Prospects for the Young Child in India.* Technical Background Paper, p. 8. Mobile Creches, New Delhi.

Ranjani, M.K. *Gender and Social Inclusion in Parenting of the Young Child in India.* Technical Background Paper, pp. 6–7.

Resilience, Center on the Developing Child Harvard University, n.d. Retrieved from https://developingchild.harvard.edu/science/key-concepts/resilience/; date of access: 20 November 2019.

Sengupta, S. and S. Sachdeva, 2017. *From Double Burden of Women to a "Double Boon": Balancing Unpaid Care Work and Paid Work.* Policy Brief. IDS, Brighton. Retrieved from www.ids.ac.uk/publications/from-double-burden-of-women-to-a-double-boon-balancing-unpaid-care-work-and-paid-work/; date of access: 21 November 2019.

Sharma, P., 2019. Kids Addicted to Electronic Screens Susceptible to Obesity, Diabetes. *India Today*, 27 April 2019. Retrieved from www.indiatoday.in/mail-today/

story/kids-addicted-to-electronic-screens-susceptible-to-obesity-diabetes-1511877-2019-04-28; date of access: 25 June 2019.

Shonkoff, J.P. and Phillips, D.A., 2000. *From neurons to neighborhoods: The science of early childhood development.* National Academy Press, Washington DC.

Teicher, M.H., 2002. Scars that won't heal: The neurobiology of child abuse. *Scientific American,* 286(3), pp.68–75.

Trask, 2011. Retrieved from www.un.org/esa/socdev/family/docs/egm11/Traskpaper. pdf; date of access: 1 October 2019.

UNDESA, 2018. *SDGs Global Indicator Framework for the Sustainable Development Goals and Targets of the 2030 Agenda for Sustainable Development.* Retrieved from https://unstats.un.org/sdgs/indicators/indicators-list/; date of access: 22 June 2018.

United Nations, 2015. *Study on the Effects of New Information Technologies on the Abuse and Exploitation of Children.* United Nations Office on Drugs and Crime, Vienna. Retrieved from www.unodc.org/documents/Cybercrime/Study_on_the_ Effects.pdf; date of access: 10 October 2019.

WHO, 2019. *Guidelines on Physical Activity, Sedentary Behaviour and Sleep for Children Under 5 Years of Age.* Retrieved from https://apps.who.int/iris/handle/10665/311664; date of access: 29 March 2019.

WHO, UNICEF and World Bank Group, 2018. *Nurturing Care for Early Childhood Development: A Framework for Helping Children Survive and Thrive to Transform Health and Human Potential.* WHO, Geneva. Retrieved from https:// apps.who.int/iris/bitstream/handle/10665/272603/9789241514064-eng.pdf; date of access: 19 November 2019.

Why the Centre Must Invest More in the National Creche Scheme. *Hindustan Times,* March 2 2019. Retrieved from https://www.hindustantimes.com/columns/why-the-centre-must-invest-more-in-the-national-creche-scheme/story-k4I3ZD-VnjwWQbVnUB5O6EP.html; date of access: 23 November 2019.

6 Fiscal allocations and expenditure for child development

6.1 The fiscal experience highlights gaps in public spending

For India to adequately provide for the developmental needs of its children, especially young children, the fiscal space for this critical age group needs to expand significantly. In this chapter, we examine the status and trends in public expenditure and gaps where public spending needs to be enhanced.

For the year 2019–2020, the total budget of MWCD stood at INR 296.6 billion. Of this budget, ICDS has been allocated INR 275.8 billion, i.e., 94.5 percent of the ministry's budget.[1] As a percentage of the total Union Budget, this allocation in 2019–2020 to MWCD is a meagre 1.05 percent of the total central government's budget.

Children under 6 years of age constitute 13.1 percent of the total population (Census, 2011). In numbers, this translates into 158.8 million children. ICDS covers 71.9 million children of these children, or 45.3 percent of the total child population under 6 years of age in India. All the children under 6 years of age are eligible to receive ICDS benefits irrespective of their family income. Many of those who do not participate in the scheme are children from families that are either better off than the most disadvantaged or children located in remote regions thereby making it difficult for them to access ICDS services.

This Report has highlighted the primacy of the role of the State to invest in the well-being of the young child. This investment is the right of each child. Such investment improves the quality of human capital of the nation, widens individual choices and guarantees the necessary quality of life of its people. The returns on such investment are also significantly higher than any other comparable spend.

This chapter takes a holistic view of the universe of public schemes and programmes that directly and indirectly impact the well-being of children under 6 years of age, into a framework of the childcare ecosystem. Following this, the expenditure committed to the set of schemes and programmes within each component of the childcare ecosystem has been assessed. An attempt has been made to estimate the spending per child from the assembled expenditure data. Further, trends in allocation and expenditure have been analysed to identify the budgetary requirements for a system that could satisfactorily and effectively serve the needs of children under 6 years. The analysis is based on annual expenditure data from 2014–2015 to 2019–2020.[2]

6.1.1 *There is a lack of financial commitment to the needs of the social sector*

To contextualise the expenditure analysis, two measures are used – total social sector spending per year as a percentage of India's GDP; and as a percentage of the Union Budget. The social sector spending comprises the budgets of MWCD, Ministry of Consumer Affairs, Food and Public Distribution (MCAFPD), Ministry of Drinking Water and Sanitation (MDWS), Ministry of Health and Family Welfare (MoHFW) and Ministry of Human Resource Development (MHRD). This gives a measure of Government of India's financial commitment to needs of the social sector.

The chapter addresses the following questions which are key for a fuller understanding of policy attention backed by public expenditure for the young child in India:

1   What is the money that is currently spent by the government of India annually on a typical child under 6 years of age? This is the cumulative per child expenditure of all the centrally sponsored schemes that apply to this category of children, in addition to those that apply to pregnant, nursing and lactating mothers.
2   What is the total annual budget of the ministries that are responsible for servicing various needs of this group of children? This includes the MWCD, MoHFW, MCAFPD, MDWS and MHRD.
3   What is the coverage of key schemes like ICDS Umbrella and those that provide child protection services?
4   How do the budgets and allocations vary and how have they moved over a five-year period, 2014–2015 to 2018–2019?
5   What is the total social sector spending by the government of India, of which the budget for children under 6 years of age is a subset? In this context, there is need to contextualise the total social sector spending as a percentage of the annual budget of Union of India and as a percentage of India's GDP, in order to assess the adequacy of social sector spending vis-à-vis the need for essential services in India.
6   What are the trends in utilisation of funds, coverage of beneficiaries, needs and funding gaps at the state level with respect to the childcare ecosystem?

The analysis relies on publicly available data sources, primarily central government budgets, to answer these questions and present the findings. Based on analysis of the data sources and findings, suggestions are made on budget increases and specific action areas that would improve the status of young children.

Four key observations emerge from the analysis:

1   **Insufficient budgets:** The budget allocations across all aspects of children's needs (nutrition, education, healthcare, care and protection) are grossly inadequate to address the requirement and these needs.
2   **Low management capacity:** In cases where the schemes have sufficient budget allocations, the performance of the schemes is hampered by lack of state capacity to fully and productively utilise the budget.
3   **Lack of balance in childcare budgets:** The analysis suggests that nationally and across states, budget interventions made by the governments in child development are not balanced across areas. While budgets for nutrition are sizeable, reproductive and child health, childcare and protection remain poorly financed and even the allocated budgets in these critical areas are not fully utilised. Interlinkages between schemes in nutrition, health, education and childcare are necessary for the interventions to make significant and lasting impact. In several cases government schemes work in silos.
4   **Poor data availability:** Critical information that can inform design, progress and new interventions in childcare, seems to be difficult to gather at state and district levels. There are no publicly available databases which record multi-dimensional data on children at district level and the money that is being spent on them for various needs. This Report has, therefore, had to be primarily based on national level data (ministry budgets, allocations to states and coverage under schemes). A significant challenge to an assessment of this nature is the inadequacy in the collation of data by a designated office at the state level and limited availability of state-level data in the public domain.

6.1.2 Overall expenditure within the childcare ecosystem is negligible

The comprehensive childcare ecosystem approach, shown in Box 6.1, has been adopted in the chapter which includes aspects of childcare necessary for ideal child growth, care and protection. It assigns all the government schemes, primarily centrally sponsored schemes (CSS) and examines the expenditure within the components of childcare ecosystem as well as cumulatively, to arrive at an indicative figure for allocation made by the central government towards each child in India.

It needs to be noted that the Report assumes universal application of government schemes and the computation of per child expenditure is obtained by dividing the total allocation with the population of children under 6 years of age in India. It can be argued that the chapter underestimates per capita expenditure by universalising the beneficiary numbers. To reference the available money to current beneficiary number may not be a realistic indicator of government resources that are available for childcare needs.

If the government was to provide for all eligible children, then what will be the effective amount of money available per child? The trends show in various tables that there is very little increase in budgets year on year. So, when there is a surge in number of children needing the services, it does not seem likely that a proportionate increase in budget will be made. An alternative method is to go by the reported beneficiaries for each of these schemes.

For the analysis, budget documents of relevant ministries were studied, and fund releases and flows were examined for the period 2014–2019, for schemes pertaining to the childcare ecosystem. This included central government allocations as well as expenditures reported by state governments where available. However, there is a further challenge when it comes to access and coverage. It emerges from the possibility of two types of errors, the inclusion of children from better-off households and the exclusion of those from the worse off ones.

6.1.3 *Lack of data availability poses challenges*

The data for the analysis is drawn from Union Budget documents – Annual Financial Statement and Expenditure Budget Vol. II, and Demand for Grants as available on India Budget portal of the Government of India. Another important source is the Reserve Bank of India's (RBI) data on state finances. Sub-national trends analysis draws on data made available by RBI in addition to these sources, responses to questions in Lok Sabha catalogued by *IndiaStat* database are used to analyse spending and beneficiary numbers. Given the data constraints, this analysis is a reasonable estimate of all the spending directly and indirectly related to children under 6 years of age. Wherever disaggregated data is not available, aggregated figures have been included. Thus, an overestimation in some cases is possible. In some cases, as in healthcare spending figures, there is likelihood of under-estimation because data for all children-targeted programmes and schemes is not available. In years where Revised Estimate is not available, Budget Estimate has been taken as the basis.

6.2 Trends indicate continuing under-allocation

6.2.1 *There is inadequate allocation and under-utilisation of funds*

The funding of vulnerable children, especially in the under 6 age group, has been woefully inadequate. **Trends indicate that the situation of under allocation (as a percentage of the Union budget) is likely to worsen.** Inadequacy in coverage and budgetary allocation is observed across all schemes. However, budgetary expenditures are particularly low for supplementary nutrition for

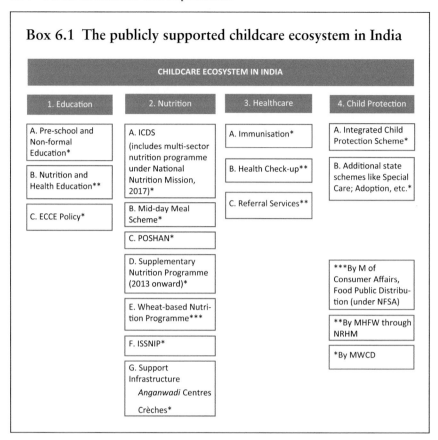

Box 6.1 The publicly supported childcare ecosystem in India

Table 6.1 Centrally sponsored schemes, intended groups and ministries

Schemes	Intended group	Ministry
i. ICDS ii. RCH – II, NRHM iii. JSY iv. *Pradhan Mantri Matru Vandana Yojana*	Pregnant and Lactating Mothers (PALM)	MWCD MoHFW
i. ICDS ii. RCH – II iii. Rajiv Gandhi National Crèche Scheme	Children 0–3	MWCD MoHFW
i. ICDS ii. RCH – II iii. Rajiv Gandhi National Crèche Scheme iv. Nirmal Bharat Abhiyaan v. National Rural Drinking Water Programme (NRDWP)	Children 0–6	MWCD MoHFW MDWS
i. *Samagra Shikha Abhiyaan* (SSA) ii. Mid-day Meals (MDM)	School-going children aged 6–14	MHRD

the under 6 age group and pregnant and lactating mothers (categorised as PALM under ICDS), healthcare, ECCE, childcare and protection [including for the Integrated Child Protection Services scheme (ICPS)]. It has been further noted that even the allocated moneys in Reproductive and Child Health (RCH) and ICPS are not fully utilised. Poor allocations have long term adverse impact as low utilisation often leads to lower budget allocations in subsequent years.

6.2.2 Per child expenditure in India is low

Considering the universal application of the childcare system and services to children under 6 years of age, an analysis of the public spending towards child nutrition, healthcare, education and other necessary protection services indicates that India spent INR 1,723 per child in 2018–2019, as shown in Table 6.2. The population of children under 6 years of age is 158.8 million. Of these, ICDS covers 71.9 million children as calculated from the total number of beneficiaries across the states. **This spend needs multi-fold enhancement if the scheme is to reach the entire eligible population and to extend to the education component as well.**

In addition to the Union budgets, some states spend substantial amounts of money on nutrition-based programmes from state funds. However, a clear analysis of this component of spending from state resources requires reliable and disaggregated data. For example, Karnataka provides eggs and milk to

Table 6.2 Calculation of total national budget per child per year from 2014–2015 to 2018–2019 (INR)

	2014–2015	2015–2016	2016–2017	2017–2018	2018–2019
1. Nutrition	1,132.3	1,022.1	954.9	1,187.6	1,336.0
2. Education	Accounted under Nutrition in this estimation (as NECCE)				
3. Healthcare	416.1	447.7	389.9	469.1	345.2
4. Child Protection	24.0	24.4	35.9	38.6	42.0
Grand total	**1,572.4**	**1,494.3**	**1,380.7**	**1,695.3**	**1,723.1**
Population of children from birth to age 6 (in million)	163.7	164.7	166.4	168.1	172.8
Total Spending for children in 0–6 age group (in INR million)	257,454.8	246,107.4	229,797.7	284,959.9	297,796

Source: www.indiabudget.gov.in/previous_union_budget.php[3]

children in AWCs out of its own resources. It also tops up the honorarium paid to AWWs, constructs new AWCs and toilets and has even started 450 new urban AWCs from its own resources entirely.

In education, **budgets over the last four years have not increased**. Similarly, in healthcare, RCH budget has declined. Budgets under ICPS for child protection are minimal.

6.2.3 Revised nutritional norms for supplementary nutrition are inadequate

To understand India's nutritional support to children and mothers, the following tables indicate the financial norms and nutritional norms that serve as reference scale for ICDS. The current cost norms for benefits per child, for severely malnourished children and for Pregnant and Lactating Mothers (PALM) were set in 2017. The Tables 6.3 and 6.4 indicate the rate at which per child cost is being factored in the budgeting for nutrition by the Government of India.

Table 6.3 Financial norms for supplementary nutrition under ICDS

Beneficiaries	Previous norms (per beneficiary per day) w.e.f. October 16, 2008	Revised cost norms (per beneficiary per day) as per phased roll-out w.e.f. 22 October 2012 up to November 2017	Present norms (per beneficiary per day) w.e.f. November 2017
Children (6 months to 72 months)	INR 4.00	INR 6.00	INR 8.00
Severely malnourished children (6 months to 72 months)	INR 6.00	INR 9.00	INR 12.00
Pregnant women and lactating mothers	INR 5.00	INR 7.00	INR 9.50

Source: MWCD Annual Report 2017–2018[4]

Table 6.4 Nutritional norms in ICDS

Revised nutritional norms in ICDS (w.e.f., 24 February 2009)		
Beneficiaries	Calories (Cal)	Protein (g)
Children (6–72 months)	500	12 to 15
Severely malnourished children (6–72 months)	800	20 to 25
Pregnant women and lactating mothers	600	18 to 20

Source: MWCD Annual Report 2017–2018

With these norms, the total annual spending in 2017–2018 on children under 6 years of age stood at INR 157.5 billion and INR 57 billion for pregnant and lactating mothers. As a part of the SNP, the total spending (at the rate of INR 6 per child and INR 7 per woman) is estimated to be INR 215.5 billion in 2017–2018. The appropriateness of these cost norms with respect to the price of procuring food which can deliver the required nutritional norm is also an issue. For instance, the price of food that can provide 12–15 g of protein is likely to be significantly more than INR 6.

6.2.4 MWCD budget 2017–2019 to 2019–2020 has been inadequate but shows a trend increase overall

Of the total Union Budget of India in 2019–20, MWCD has been allocated INR 296.6 billon. This is 1.05 percent of the Union Budget. **As a percentage of India's GDP, MWCD's budget accounts for 0.19 percent.** The following table indicates the trend in MWCD's spending on ICDS from 2017–2018 to 2019–2020. Among the major changes, National Nutrition Mission and Child Protection Services have seen a very high increase in the budget. However, the National Crèche Scheme continues to remain grossly underfunded. The expenditure on various schemes within ICDS is shown in Table 6.5.

Table 6.5 Expenditure on schemes within ICDS by MWCD from 2017–2018 to 2019–2020

Expenditure budget of MWCD for ICDS from 2017–2018 to 2019–2020 (INR in million)

Umbrella ICDS	2017–2018	2018–2019	2019–2020 (BE)	Difference in budget (2017–2018 to 2019–2020)	Change from 2017–2018 to 2019–2020 (%)
Anganwadi Services (Erstwhile Core ICDS)	1,515.500	1,789.000	1,983.4	467.900	30.87
National Nutrition Mission (including ISSNIP)	89.300	306.100	340.0	250.700	280.84
Pradhan Mantri Matru Vandana Yojana	204.800	120.000	250.0	45.200	22.05
Scheme for Adolescent Girls	45.000	25.000	30.0	–15.062	–33.43
National Crèche Scheme	4.879	3.000	5.0	0.121	2.48
Child Protection Services	63.800	92.500	150.0	86.219	135.18
Scheme for welfare of working children in need of care and protection	0.000	0.001	0.0	0.000	0.00

Source: indiabudget.gov.in, MWCD Budget SBE98[5]

6.2.5 Social sector spending has decreased

The allocation in core areas of spending has decreased not only under ICDS but across all social sectors. **Social sector spending across relevant ministries has decreased,** as Table 6.6 shows. This is seen across the board – the decrease is by both Centre and states.

1 As a percentage of Union Budget

MWCD figure as percentage of Union Budget appears to be going up. This is because the budget included a small increase in cost norms for ICDS and in honorarium. Adding another table with the absolute numbers, changed sharing patterns (increased share to be borne by the states) and *Ayushman* allocation makes the picture look different.

2 As a percentage of GDP

Further, as may be seen, social sector spending as a percentage of national GDP has remained flat at around 2.6 percent of GDP over the period 2014–2015 to 2019–2020, as noted in Table 6.7.

States' social sector expenditure (SSE) averaged 5.4 percent of GDP in India in the pre-global financial crisis period, rising since 2010–2011 to about 8.0 percent of GDP in 2017–2018 (RE). Increased per-capita state overall social sector expenditure was associated with a decrease in mortality for both boys and girls aged 1–4 years. In boys aged 1–4 years, an increase of 10 percent in per-capita overall social sector expenditure was associated with a 6.8 percent reduction in death rate, while for girls the corresponding reduction was 4.1 percent.

6.2.6 Trends show increased allocation to nutrition and education, under-allocation to RCH and ICPS

- **Nutrition:** In 2016, ICDS covered about 45 percent of the population under 6 years of age. It provided supplementary nutrition to over 101 million beneficiaries and pre-school education to over 34.5 million beneficiaries. There were 1,349,153 AWCs in the country at the end of 2016. Plan allocation in the 11th Five-Year Plan was INR 440 billion, which increased 2.8 times to INR 1,235.8 billion in 12th Plan.[7]
- **Education:** Under *Samagra Shiksha Abhiyan*, the budget increased to INR 329,980 million in 2018–2019. The National ECCE programme has seen a significant increase in allocation over 2014–2015 as may be seen in Table 6.8.
- **Reproductive and Child Health:** As Table 6.9 shows, the budget for RCH which is a part of NRHM has decreased. It is also evident that the state governments are not able to utilise the approved budget. Not only are

Table 6.6 Social sector spending in India across ministries as percentage of Union Budget

	2014–2015	2015–2016	2016–2017	2017–2018	2018–2019	2019–2020*
GDP in mn INR (MOSPI)	105,276,740	113,861,450	121,960,060	130,108,430	139,606,345.4	150,076,821.3
Total Union Budget (percentage of GDP)	15.80	15.68	16.22	16.46	17.60	18.55
MWCD (percentage of UB)	1.27	0.58	0.88	1.03	1.01	1.05
MCAFPD (percentage of UB)	6.97	7.03	7.15	7.20	7.16	6.99
MDWS (percentage of UB)	0.92	0.35	0.71	0.93	0.91	0.65
MOHFW (percentage of UB)	2.36	1.80	1.93	2.28	2.22	2.27
MHRD (percentage of UB)	4.98	3.87	3.66	3.72	3.46	3.37
Total Social Sector Spending or the sum of all ministries (percentage of UB)	16.49	13.62	14.33	15.17	14.76	14.33

*Budget Estimate
Source: GDP data from Ministry of Statistics and Programme Implementation, Govt. of India; Ministry budgets from *indiabudget.gov.in*[6]

Table 6.7 Social sector spending in India across ministries that administer social and welfare functions, as a percentage of India's GDP, from 2014–2015 to 2019–2020

Social sector spending as a percentage of GDP

	2014–2015	2015–2016	2016–2017	2017–2018	2018–2019	2019–2020
GDP in mn INR (MOSPI)	105,276,740	113,861,450	121,960,060	130,108,430	139,606,345.4	150,076,821.3
Total Union Budget as % of GDP	15.80	15.68	16.22	16.46	17.60	18.55
MWCD as %GDP	0.20	0.09	0.14	0.17	0.18	0.19
MCAFPD as % of GDP	1.10	1.10	1.16	1.19	1.26	1.30
MDWS as % of GDP	0.15	0.05	0.11	0.15	0.16	0.12
MHFW as % of GDP	0.37	0.28	0.31	0.38	0.39	0.42
MHRD as % of GDP	0.79	0.61	0.59	0.61	0.61	0.63
Total social sector spending (Sum of all ministries) as % of GDP	2.61	2.14	2.32	2.50	2.60	2.66

Source: GDP data from Ministry of Statistics and Programme Implementation, Govt. of India; Ministry budgets from *indiabudget.gov.in*

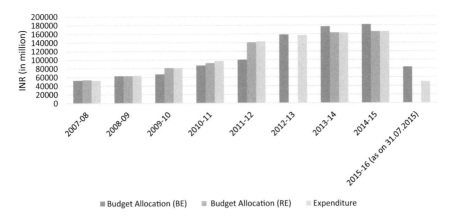

Figure 6.1 Budget allocation and expenditure under ICDS Scheme during the Eleventh Plan and the first two years of the XII Plan

Source: MoWCD; ICDS Scheme expenditure data published on www.indiastat.com/

Table 6.8 Expenditure across states for implementation of National ECCE Policy from 2014–2015 to 2017–2018

State-wise fund released/expended for implementation of National ECCE Policy under ICDS in India (2014–2015 to 2017–2018)

Year	Expenditure (in million INR)
2014–2015	2319.574
2015–2016	1260.110
2016–2017	3898.430
2017–2018	4059.489

Source: www.indiastat.com/

budgets small, but the utilisation data across states and state-wise over the period 2009–2010 to 2015–2016 also shows that state governments have not been able to utilise the approved budget under the State Programme Implementation Plans (SPIPs). There is an average under-utilisation of 41.7 percent of the approved budget. This is a significant indicator of lack of adequate focus on reproductive and child health among the states.

Further, Table 6.10 shows significant under-utilisation of the allocated funds under RCH.

• **Child Protection:** Considering the large population of children under 6 years of age and the need, the Integrated Child Protection Scheme (ICPS) appears to be grossly underfunded, as shown in Table 6.11.

Table 6.9 Reproductive and Child Health (RCH) budget of MoHFW from 2013–2014 to 2017–2018

Year	RCH budget (in million INR)
2013–2014	68,122.5
2014–2015	73,741.9
2015–2016	64,897.7
2016–2017	78,849.9
2017–2018	59,666.0

Source: MoHFW budget[8]

Table 6.10 Utilisation of approved budgets under the State Programme Implementation Plan for child health programme from 2009–2010 to 2015–2016 as a total budget of all the states

Year	SPIP approved	Expenditure reported	Difference between expenditure and approved	Unutilised (%)
2009–2010	11322.80	9719.61	1603.19	14.16
2010–2011	26420.60	13537.71	12882.89	48.76
2011–2012	21107.00	10402.47	10704.53	50.72
2012–2013	46104.99	1117.45	44987.54	97.58
2013–2014	32584.35	22332.48	10251.87	31.46
2014–2015	32604.00	24399.00	8205.00	25.17
2015–2016	29999.00	20657.00	9342.00	31.14

Source: MoHFW data[9]

Table 6.11 Funds released to states under Integrated Child Protection Scheme

Year	Funds released in million INR
2009–2010	426.37
2010–2011	1147.14
2011–2012	1769.31
2012–2013	2590.93
2013–2014	2657.81
2014–2015	3937.62
2015–2016	4389.21
2016–2017	5084.80
2017–2018	5246.99
2018–2019*	1096.58

*Budget Estimate
Source: ICPS data[10]

Table 6.12 Performance of ICPS from 2009–2010 to 2017–2018

Year	No. of states that have signed MOUs	Budget allocation (in million INR)	Amount sanctioned (in million INR)	No. of beneficiaries
2009–2010	17	500	426.3	36,780
2010–2011	34	1000	1,151.3	92,379
2011–2012	34	1800	1,775.4	50,118
2012–2013	34	2730	2,538.4	75,052
2013–2014	35	2700	2,657.8	74,983
2014–2015	36	4500	4,484.3	91,769
2015–2016	36	4500	4,973.0	76,634
2016–2017	36	6100	5763.0	87,119
2017–2018	36	6480*	4172.7	-

*Budget Estimate
Source: MWCD, Government of India[11]

The performance of the scheme as may be seen in Table 6.12 shows that the coverage of beneficiaries remains very small.

6.3 Sub-national trends show variations in management capability and spending

Approximately, INR 431 million is spent per day on providing nutrition to 71 million children across India as of March 2018. This figure is calculated by assuming a conservative INR 6 per child that the Centre spends on nutrition. At the sub-national level, **most of the states have not demonstrated management capability of spending the allocated money from the Centre.** States with high malnutrition rates among children seem particularly incapable of spending central funds. The states with least utilisation capacity are also the states that have poor status of children – for example Bihar and Rajasthan. At the same time, Karnataka and Chhattisgarh seem to utilise their allocation as well as add a substantial budget of their own to total spending.

To understand the situation of the young child in the Indian states, it is relevant to see the distribution of approximately 80 million young children who benefit from ICDS (Figure 6.2). Uttar Pradesh has the highest number of young children served by ICDS, though in percentage terms only 48.2 percent of the total number of children receive ICDS benefits. Maharashtra, Bihar, Madhya Pradesh and West Bengal together have 32 percent of the children. These five states account for 50 percent of the young children who benefit from ICDS. The inability of these states to undertake public expenditure finds a correlation with poorer outcomes for the young child and also reflects the general governance deficits in social policy implementation and the general mindset. Uttar Pradesh, Bihar and Madhya Pradesh are

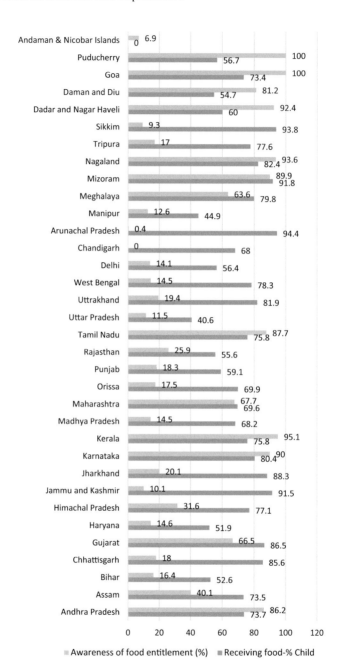

Figure 6.2 Status of Supplementary Nutrition Programme (SNP) in India, 2018

Source: Supplementary Nutrition Programme data[12]

among the poor performers in YCEI (Table 1.2) as well, with performance below the all-India average.

The status of Supplementary Nutrition programme in India also varies highly across states. Figure 6.2 shows the awareness about food entitlements and food benefits received by children in each state. We see a mixed pattern, of states with high percentage of children receiving food vs awareness and vice versa. This has to do with the nature of the pressure from below. Lack of awareness results in low pressure from the potential beneficiaries, low expectations and, hence, low utilisation.

6.3.1 High variations in coverage and child spend impact outcomes

States with the highest population of children under 6 do not even cover half of the total children. Bihar and Rajasthan's coverages are below the national average. Both these states are also ranked as poor performers in YCOI (Table 1.1) and YCEI (Table 1.2). Table 6.13 compares the coverage of children in five states and indicates the per child spending in these states. Annually, West Bengal spends INR 246 per child and Madhya Pradesh spends INR 994 per child. Table 6.14 depicts the situation in the top 11 states based on coverage. As may be seen in Tables 6.13 and 6.14, there is high variation, and clearly the outcomes of children in these states will be different.

6.3.2 Social spending in states reflects low fiscal priority

Study of state finances and their budgets affirm the broader observation of inadequate focus on social sector needs of which young children and their well-being is a part. Analysis of state budget documents analysed by the Reserve Bank of India show that in the year 2017–2018, based on budget estimates, only NCT Delhi and Chhattisgarh spent more than 50 percent of their total disbursement on social sector (see Annexure 6, Table A.6.28).

Table 6.13 States with highest population of children under 6, their ICDS coverage and money available for each beneficiary[13]

States according to highest to lowest 0–6 population (Census of India, 2011)	Coverage of ICDS (in percentage)	ICDS money/ beneficiary (in INR)	ICDS money/ child (of total 0–6 pop) (in INR)
Bihar	26.6	1,629.5	535.3
Madhya Pradesh	62.6	1,302.2	993.9
Rajasthan	24.9	1,723.6	571.5
Uttar Pradesh	48.2	1,353.3	829.3
West Bengal	57.8	349.8	245.9

Table 6.14 Top 11 states based on coverage of children under ICDS and their respective expenditure[14]

States	Total beneficiaries 0–6	Total beneficiaries 0–6 + PALM	0–6 population	Coverage (%)	Expenditure by the state in 2016–2017 (INR million)	Centre Allocation 2017–2018 in mn	ICDS money/ beneficiary (in INR)	ICDS money/ child (0–6 pop) (in INR)
Bihar	4,940,640	6,104,018	18,582,229	26.6	9,543.4	9,946.3	1,629.5	535.3
Chhattisgarh	2,013,902	2,469,528	3,584,028	56.2	5,535.4	4,439.9	1,797.9	1,238.8
Jharkhand	2,634,116	3,392,958	5,237,582	50.3	5,064.6	4,757.4	1,402.2	908.3
Karnataka	4,036,695	5,092,165	7,161,033	56.4	13,788.4	7,654.9	1,503.3	1,069.0
Madhya Pradesh	6,607,796	8,051,031	10,548,295	62.6	12,091.6	10,483.9	1,302.2	993.9
Maharashtra	5,312,961	6,317,563	13,326,517	39.9	2,416.6	10,135.6	1,604.3	760.6
Odisha	3,918,422	4,643,551	5,035,650	77.8	10,478.0	6,905.9	1,487.2	1,371.4
Rajasthan	2,616,106	3,482,900	10,504,916	24.9	5,934.4	6,003.1	1,723.6	571.5
Uttar Pradesh	14,334,752	18,216,779	29,728,235	48.2	33,296.6	2,4652.6	1,353.3	829.3
Uttarakhand	607,332	776,827	1,328,844	45.7	2,670.1	3,718.1	4,786.2	2,798.0
West Bengal	6,117,637	7,438,321	10,581,466	57.8	Not reported by the state	2,601.9	349.8	245.9

The average social sector expenditure as a percentage of total disbursements by states is 42.5 percent, with a low of 30.5 percent to a maximum of 56.6 percent in the year 2017–2018. Uttar Pradesh, with one of the highest numbers of young children, spends about 37 percent on the social sector. The trend for states from 2001–2002 to 2017–2018 may be seen in Table A.6.28 in the statistical tables.

Eight of the eleven items within the social sector expenditure are related directly to the well-being of young children. States spending more than 50 percent of total disbursement on social sector are also the ones with better outcomes of nutrition, health and protection of its young children. However, in overall terms, **we see lower fiscal priority for social sector spending in states as at the national level.**

6.4 International comparisons show India's potential untapped

Among similar placed income countries, India performs poorer on outcome-based indicators like percentage of children who suffer from wasting, severe wasting, stunting and underweight nutritional status. From the Joint Malnutrition Estimates data jointly published by UNICEF, WHO and the World Bank, the chapter examines trends for change in key nutrition indicators during a similar time period in India, China, Bangladesh and Brazil. These countries have been considered for comparison because they nearly started at the same level and their development status was also similar at the start, however, along the decades the change in nutritional status of children varied significantly. This offers a useful contrast to understand India's efforts in tackling malnutrition.[15]

The Figures 6.3, 6.4, 6.5 and 6.6 dramatically show the much more rapid improvement across four health and nutrition indicators in China in comparison to the progress in India and highlights the need to vastly increase the spend to close this gap. Even Bangladesh and Brazil have shown improved performance. China had contained the percentage of children below 10 percent for all the nutritional status indicators by 2013. Brazil managed to achieve this by 2007. Bangladesh has performed better than India in controlling wasting and severe wasting. The preference of this outcome-based comparison is due to the fact that reliable public spending data across these countries is difficult to obtain.

6.5 Key issues

6.5.1 *Spending per child shows widespread funding gaps*

In order to lessen the impact of poor socio-economic condition of households, it is necessary that at least adequate nutrition and early childhood care is provided of a reasonable quality so as to not add to the burden

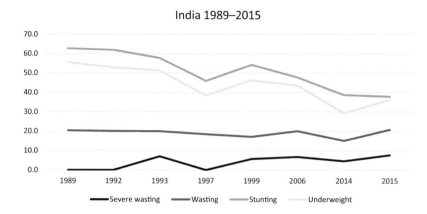

Figure 6.3 India's standing with regard to stunting and wasting[16]

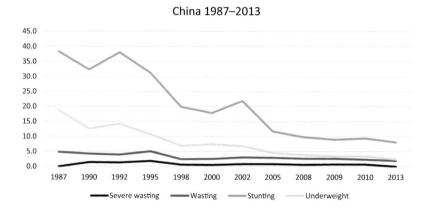

Figure 6.4 China's standing with regard to stunting and wasting[17]

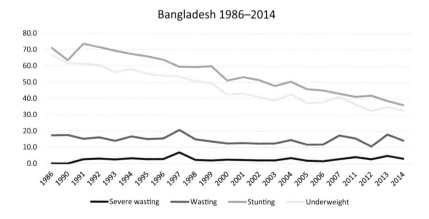

Figure 6.5 Bangladesh's standing with regard to stunting and wasting[18]

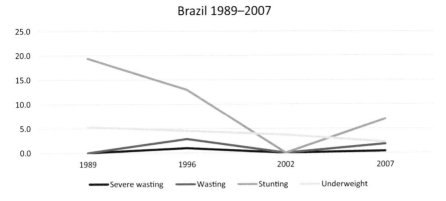

Figure 6.6 Brazil's standing with regard to stunting and wasting[19]

on families due to poor developmental outcomes of malnourished children. Therefore, a major funding gap is seen in the spending per child in India. ICDS must assume universal application of the services under the umbrella, and therefore at the existing and revised cost norm of INR 8 per child (6–72 months) per day and INR 9.50 per day for PALM beneficiaries, the ICDS will need to double its spending to about INR 800 billion, to cater to both the revised norms and to account for universal application. This report has already highlighted the high percentage of stunting, wasting and under-weight children. To address this, **direct spending on nutritional programmes will have to increase significantly.**

The following areas and issues need particular attention:

1   In view of large variances in outcome indicators, states and districts showing poor performance need special attention and enhanced funding beyond the standard norm to enable these areas to catch up. Social audit mechanisms in poorly performing states also need to be strengthened to ensure that funds allocated actually reach the intended beneficiaries.
2   The National Nutrition Mission initiative needs to be scaled up, bet-ter targeted on achieving improved nutrition and health outcomes and provided increased budgets.
3   Budgetary gaps in ICDS that have been identified in this Report need to be plugged.
4   There are many identified bottlenecks in learning and lack of social spaces for the child. Budgets towards ECCE including for the more organised pre-primary institutions as well as the ECCE component need to be enhanced multi-fold.
5   Budgets need to be specifically provided for each of the disadvantaged child categories, including children with disabilities, the SC/ST child, children living in slums, etc. The girl child needs to be made a priority area in the child budget.

6 Specific provisions for dealing with child abuse and neglect are presently miniscule. The provisions for ICPS are grossly inadequate for making a significant impact.

7 National Crèche Scheme and *Anganwadi* centres cum crèches have negligible budgets at present and need a multi-fold hike in outlays.

8 There is no specific programme to address the adverse sex ratio at birth and female infanticide. Special programmes in a mission mode with an effective mass communication strategy need to be launched.

6.5.2 There are huge spending gaps across various sectors

Effective implementation of direct interventions for child development together with the performance of other inter-connected sectors and issues have a positive impact on outcomes for children. Specifically, adequate budget provision in the following areas is needed:

- **Childcare:** As noted earlier, budget provisions towards childcare and protection are miniscule at present. Specifically, provisions for crèches, including *anganwadi*-cum-crèches, are negligible and need multi-fold enhancement.
- **Poverty reduction:** Poor households are unable to provide an enabling environment for their child's well-being. There is a close inverse correlation between child indicators and poverty of households. Budgetary provisions for schemes that have a direct attack on poverty, such as NREGA, need to be enhanced.
- **Female literacy:** Child outcomes in households that have educated household members, especially female members, have a very positive impact. Budget for girls' education need to be adequately provided.
- **Public health:** The functioning of the public healthcare system is a critical factor for the physical well-being of the child and budgets under NRHM and RCH need to be substantially increased.
- **Water supply and sanitation:** Safe drinking water for each household and properly designed and implemented sanitation and waste disposal system needs much higher levels of funding. The focus needs to go beyond provision of toilets to each household.

6.6 Recommendations and action points

6.6.1 Increase social sector budgets

In view of the inter-connections between sectors, especially health, education, water supply and sanitation, poverty and rural employment, **social sector budgets that have remained flat at around 2.6 percent of GDP should be enhanced immediately to at least 4 percent of the GDP.** Without adequate financial resources, improvements in child well-being, cognitive development, as well as care and protection would be extremely challenging.

As percentage of union budget, childcare and welfare needs to immediately get enhanced from the present 1 percent to at least 5 percent. The immediate aim should be to extend the current nutritional and financial norm per child to the entire under 6 years age group population in every state. A national benchmark, which can be emulated by states, in terms of minimum allocation for providing 'childcare ecosystem service' per child must be developed. This is the level of expenditure states must reach annually, by aggregating all available resources, to provide for the under 6s. Table 6.2 shows that the total spending per child at the national level was INR 1723 in 2018–2019. As stated earlier, this extension of current financial norm to all the children will mean enhancing the budget of ICDS from INR 276 billion to INR 800 billion at least.

6.6.2 Professionalise childcare services

For 1.4 million sanctioned AWCs, at present there are an estimated 55,187 supervisors. Of these, 36.2 percent of the sanctioned supervisor posts are vacant. In terms of other staff, 7.5 percent of AW Worker posts and 10 percent of AW Helper posts were vacant in 2018.[20] These need to be filled up on priority.

The AWWs and ASHAs should be treated as professionals and made full time paid workers to enable them to discharge their assigned roles in the manner required.

AWWs are at present treated as part-time, 'voluntary' workers but are expected to manage the AWCs as well as undertake critical household outreach activities. The participation of children under 3 years of age in the activities in the AWCs is quite low, and home visits by the AWCs for counselling their families are crucial. Despite the increase in the honorarium of AWWs in recent years, their average remuneration at the national level is estimated at INR 4,500. The honorarium is higher in some states but lower in other states. Given the full-time nature of the role and the fact that household visits need the worker to make herself available beyond standard working hours, it is recommended **that AWWs should receive a monthly remuneration of INR 10,000, which should be benchmarked to the wholesale price index (WPI) and increased on a pro-rata basis for each rise in the WPI.**

ASHA is the first port of call for any health-related demands of deprived sections of the population, especially women and children, who find it difficult to access health services. They are expected to mobilise the local community and facilitate their access to reproductive and child health and related services (e.g., immunisation, ante- and postnatal check-ups, supplementary nutrition, sanitation) being provided by the government at the AWC, PHC and sub-centres. However, they are paid even lower remuneration in comparison to AWWs. In addition to a monthly honorarium of INR 1,800, they receive performance-based incentives for promoting universal immunisation, referral and escort services, other healthcare programmes and construction of household toilets. Given the wide and varied role that the ASHA is expected to perform at the village level, a living wage and remuneration in keeping with her role is justified. It is recommended that the **ASHA worker should receive a fixed monthly remuneration of INR 8,000 in addition to the performance incentives, with the remuneration being pro rata revised with increases in WPI.**

Additional budget requirement

If the salaries of workers – AWW and ASHA – are increased to the amount indicated earlier which would be the first step to treat them as full time professional childcare workers, it is estimated that the additional budget requirement on the ministry will be INR 167.7 billion. The calculation in Table 6.15 assumes the sanctioned strength of workers.

Budgets and sustainability

India's GDP is estimated to be INR 1,500 billion. The total budgetary outlay of the Central Government is INR 220 billion. About 4 percent of GDP for the social sector would require an outlay of INR 60 billion which would mean enhancing the outlay to 25 percent from the present level of around 14–16 percent at present. This is required to redress the long years of neglect of the social sector. Within this, the child budget of INR 12.5 billion annually would amount to 20 percent of the social sector outlay. This would provide adequate provision for all the funding gaps including for professionalisation of childcare services.

The returns on this social investment and child-centred programmes would exceed budgetary spends on any alternate government infrastructure or welfare programmes. According to the World Bank, every U.S. dollar spent on nutrition-specific interventions provides a return on investment

Table 6.15 Additional expenditure requirement on account of increased salaries

	Current salary (INR)	Proposed salary (INR)	Hike	Total sanctioned workers	Total expenditure (INR billion)
Anganwadi worker	4,500	10,000	5,500	1,400,000	77.00
ASHA	1,800	8,000	6,200	900,000	66.96
Total additional budget required per annum (INR billion)					167.76

of up to $35 through increased cognitive and physical development and improved health.[21]

6.6.3 Transform AWCs to anganwadi-*cum-crèches in priority areas*

The AWCs should be converted progressively into *anganwadi*-cum-crèches. This will require the additional support of a helper plus an additional crèche worker in addition to the AWW. The nutrition component will also need to cater to a full meal in addition to the supplementary nutrition component presently being provided. The additional nutrition cost is estimated at INR 10 per child per day. The additional helper is costed at INR 7,000, while the crèche worker is budgeted at INR 10,000 per month.

In phase 1, it is proposed that 100,000 *anganwadi*-cum-crèches may be established. About 80 percent may be established in rural areas in the states with the poorest child indicators – viz., Odisha, Bihar, Uttar Pradesh, Madhya Pradesh, Rajasthan, Chhattisgarh and Jharkhand. The balance may be established in urban slums in selected towns and cities, where the AWC is located in a properly constructed building.

- **Budget requirement:** Cost estimation based on certain norms brings forth that the annual budget requirement to support 100 thousand *anganwadi*-cum-crèches is INR 30.36 billion (see Table 6.16). It is expected that the benefits of the crèche scheme in terms of the well-being and care of children belonging to poor urban and rural households would have multiplier beneficial impact on the economy. Other funding possibilities at the *panchayat*/local level should also be explored for the expansion of the network of crèches.

6.6.4 Strengthen ECCE component under ICDS

The ECCE component at the AWC level is weak due to inadequate training of AWWs and supervisors and inadequacy of local play and appropriate

Table 6.16 Additional budget of upgrading AWCs to *anganwadi*-cum-crèches

	Proposed salary (INR)	Total workers	Total expenditure (INR billion)
Anganwadi helper	10,000	100,000	9.60
Crèche worker	8,000	100,000	12.00
Additional nutrition per child (20 children/crèche)	12		8.76
Total budget for *Anganwadi*-cum-Crèche per annum (INR billion)			30.36

Table 6.17 Annual budget requirement (in billion INR)

S. No	Purpose	Additional budget required (in billion INR)
1	Supplementary Nutrition as per revised norms and universal application	524.00
2	*Anganwadi* Worker salary	77.00
3	Helpers	30.24
4	Crèche Worker	12.00
5	Crèche Helper	9.60
6	ASHA Workers	66.96
7	Learning Material	4.20
8	Training Budget	10.00
9	NNM	60.00
10	Special assistance to regions/states with poor child development indicators	200.00
	Total	994.00

materials for the pre-school. The overall budget and the budget for the training component need to increase significantly to cover training cost and material cost annually. The additional budget requirement for learning material is estimated at INR 4.2 billion per annum, while the training budget additional requirement is estimated at INR 10 billion per annum. Table 6.17 lists the overall additional requirements.

Key Messages

- The childcare ecosystem in India comprises of education, nutrition, healthcare and protection of children, and in tandem they work towards nurturing and comprehensive development of the young child. Investment by the State as its primary role in the well-being of the young child is critical because it is his or her right, which a progressive State must uphold.
- Effective implementation of direct interventions for child development together with the performance of other inter-connected sectors and issues has a positive impact on outcomes for children. Specifically, there is need for adequate budget provisions in poverty reduction, female literacy, public health, water supply and sanitation.
- The budget allocations across all aspects of children's needs (nutrition, education, healthcare, protection) are insufficient to address the requirement and demand for these needs. Even in cases where the schemes have sufficient budget allocations, the performance is hampered by lack of State capacity to utilise the budget.

- Interventions made by the governments, nationally and across states in child development are ad-hoc. The widest intervention is made in nutrition whereas reproductive and child health remains poorly targeted, as seen in low utilisation rate of allocated budgets.
- The paucity of data is a major issue; critical information that can inform design, progress and new interventions in childcare is difficult to gather at state and district levels. There are no publicly available databases which record multi-dimensional data of children at the district level and the money that is being spent on them for various needs.
- A major funding gap is seen in the spending per child in India. ICDS must assume universal application of the services under the umbrella, and therefore even at the current cost norm, the ICDS will need to enhance its spending to INR 800 billion.

Notes

1 MWCD, 2019a.
2 Total budget of MWCD for the year 2019–2020 used for the analysis is the same as indicated in Statement of Expenditure document of the ministry (SBE98 and SBE99 documents of Government of India's www.indiabudget.gov.in website). There has been no revision made to the budget estimate (BE). The '2019–20 BE' in SBE98 is indicated as 'Budget 2019–20' in SBE99 document.
3 The calculations are based on figures from expenditure budgets of respective ministries available at this website. Spending under each component is multiplied by population of children between 0–6 as indicated in Census 2011 to calculate total spending for children in 0–6 age group, annually.
4 Retrieved from https://wcd.nic.in/annual-report; date of access: 30 November 2019.
5 Retrieved from www.indiabudget.gov.in/previous_union_budget.php; date of access: 30 November 2019.
6 See www.indiastat.com/database.
7 Annual Report 2015–16 of the MWCD.
8 Retrieved from www.indiabudget.gov.in/previous_union_budget.php; date of access: 30 November 2019.
9 Retrieved from www.indiastat.com/; date of access: 30 November 2019.
10 Ibid.
11 Ibid.
12 Ibid.
13 Computation of ICDS money per beneficiary and ICDS money per child is based on ICDS data published on www.indiastat.com/.
14 Ibid.
15 The estimates assume the following definitions of the indicators of malnutrition, as per WHO Child Growth Standards: (1) Severe Wasting – Percentage of children aged 0–59 months who are below minus three standard deviations from median weight-for-height; (2) Wasting – Moderate and severe: Percentage

of children aged 0–59 months who are below minus two standard deviations from median weight-for-height; (3) Overweight – Moderate and severe: Percentage of children aged 0–59 months who are above two standard deviations from median weight-for-height; (4) Stunting – Moderate and severe: Percentage of children aged 0–59 months who are below minus two standard deviations from median height-for-age; and (5) Underweight – Moderate and severe: Percentage of children aged 0–59 months who are below minus two standard deviations from median weight-for-age.

16 Source: Joint Malnutrition Estimates data jointly published by UNICEF, WHO and the World Bank. Retrieved from www.who.int/nutgrowthdb/estimates/en/; date of access: 3 December 2019.
17 Ibid.
18 Ibid.
19 Ibid.
20 Source: Lok Sabha Unstarred Question No. 2791, dated on 03.08.2018.
21 Shekar et al., 2016.

Bibliography

India Budget Portal, Government of India, 2019. *Union Budget Documents— Annual Financial Statement and Expenditure Budget* (Vol. II).

Meera, S., 2016. *An Investment Framework for Nutrition: Reaching the Global Targets for Stunting, Anemia, Breastfeeding, and Wasting*. World Bank.

Ministry of Statistics and Programme Implementation, Registrar General of India, GoI. Census of India 2011. New Delhi.

Ministry of Women and Child Development (MWCD), Government of India, 2019a. Demand No. 98. Retrieved from www.indiabudget.gov.in/budget/; date of access: 1 September 2019.

Ministry of Women and Child Development (MWCD), Government of India, 2019b. *Statement of Expenditure*. Retrieved from www.indiabudget.gov.in; date of access: 1 September 2019.

Reserve Bank of India, 2019. *State Finances: A Study of Budgets*. Retrieved from www.rbi.org.in/Scripts/AnnualPublications.aspx?head=State%20Finances%20:%20A%20Study%20of%20Budgets; date of access: 5 September 2019.

Shekar, M., Kakietek, J., Dayton Eberwein, J. and Walters, D., 2017. *An investment framework for nutrition: reaching the global targets for stunting, anemia, breastfeeding, and wasting*. The World Bank. Retrieved from http://documents.worldbank.org/curated/en/758331475269503930/pdf/108645-v2-PUBLIC-Investment-Framework-for-Nutrition.pdf; date of access: 16 January 2020.

7 The way forward

7.1 Key issues must be addressed

7.1.1 Let us together end the continued neglect of the young child

Despite some improvements in the state of the young child in recent years, this Report has noted that about 21 percent children under 6 years of age are malnourished, 36 percent are underweight and 38 percent do not receive full immunisation. An estimated 4.8 million children of the 26.9 million born every year have low birth weight, which is intricately linked with the nutrition status and health of the mother. Many are born with congenital defects and disabilities and many are vulnerable to infections that can be prevented. This situation of the young child is clearly untenable.

There are large variations both across and within states. The states of Bihar, UP, Jharkhand, MP, Chhattisgarh, Rajasthan and Assam have Young Child Indices below the country average and will need special attention till they catch up with the rest of the country, in addition to enhanced budget allocations. In addition to these states, Gujarat is the large state that ranks below the country average in respect of the Young Child Environment Index and needs to focus on improving the enabling factors that determine child outcomes.

There has to be a radical policy shift and an endorsement at the highest level of policy making as well as in the private domain in favour of the young child. The deprivations, exclusion, vulnerabilities, inaccessibility and how they impact the young child have also emerged as the fault lines of the COVID pandemic. The pandemic has had adverse impact on millions of impoverished households. And, within a household the young child is the most vulnerable. Hence, there is a more pressing imperative to make a sea change in our policy framework and development strategy. Failure to do so can result in untapped potential for physical and cognitive development, and value formation in the early years. Early childhood is a phase of life when significant growth takes place. All that is required is nurturing care – health, nutrition, protection, responsive parenting, together with intersections of maternal health, nutrition, care and protection to enable the youngest rights' holders to realise their full potential. The Report has noted that the right nutrition and care during the first 1,000 days between a woman's pregnancy and the child's second birthday has profound impact on the child's ability to grow, learn and rise out of poverty, and in the process shape society's long term stability and prosperity. Indeed, early childhood is a period which offers the highest returns on investment, leading to economic growth of the country.

The state of the young child in India is an indicator of the overall development of India. Several indicators of child well-being paint a grim picture and the available data demonstrates that India is nowhere near achieving many of the SDGs and their targets. Neonatal mortality, malnutrition and adverse child sex ratios are major concerns, even though India has witnessed economic growth, improved overall infrastructure, reduction in poverty levels and rising educational levels. **The time for change is now.**

7.1.2 The fight against income poverty and poor social conditions is equally critical

As an important determinant of child health indicators, poverty influences the availability, accessibility and utilisation of basic services. However, **the averages usually tend to subsume the most vulnerable and the marginalised, which is why inequities and inequalities are more pernicious than they appear.** Inconsistent performance across regions and states is reflected in the ranking and values in the Young Child Outcomes Index below the national average of eight states of Assam, Meghalaya, Rajasthan, Chhattisgarh, Madhya Pradesh, Jharkhand, Uttar Pradesh and Bihar, which perform poorly in YCEI as well, need special focus. Sub-optimal functioning of government systems, flagship programmes and schemes in many states subjects the very poor and marginalised to greater distress and further compounds inequality in wealth.

The vicious cycle of poverty has a compounding effect on the care and protection that a young child receives. Children from families which have better socio-economic capital generally have a higher probability of receiving warm, protective relationships. But only 14.7 percent of children under age 5 in India live in households in the richest quintile, while 25 percent live in households belonging to the poorest quintile. Unequal distribution of income, goods and services pushes children born into ST and SC households in the category of the most disadvantaged. They are less likely to access basic health services due to a toxic combination of poor social policies and programmes, unfair occupational opportunities and low and erratic incomes.

The young child growing up on streets or in urban slums and experiencing extreme poverty and unhealthy living arrangements is likely to miss out on the opportunities that will define her future. Children without parental care, children living in single-headed households, or in jails with their mothers, children living in armed conflict and children of sex workers mostly become invisible despite their vulnerabilities.

Gender discriminatory social norms have contributed to the neglect of the girl child, and the practice of female infanticide in some communities in conjunction with prenatal diagnostic technology has led to the lowest sex ratios since independence. The spectre of missing females has challenged policymakers, demographers, women and children's rights activists, public health experts, sociologists and economists. Further, the discriminatory norms are not restricted to gender alone. They work through other hierarchical forms as well, including caste, community, parental occupation, family income and illnesses, especially HIV.

Indeed, **threats to ECD tend to cluster together often in conjunction with poverty, social status, exclusion and gendered inequality.** Widespread neglect of the young child during their critical and formative years is compounded by multiplied effects as exposure to one risk leads to multiple other risks amidst varied crisis in the family.

7.1.3 Childcare is the most critical component

Human infants need care and protection from adults for their survival. The entire area of childcare has largely remained neglected across government programmes and schemes. **When the young child is seen from the lens of the family alone, especially as the responsibility of the woman to tend to and care for, it results in childcare being neglected at the policy level.** Infants and young children are looked after within and outside the household by a plethora of caregivers – family, domestic workers, neighbours, helpers at the AWCs, *balwadis*, crèches and day-care centres operated by private agencies and NGOs. The mushrooming of spontaneous and informal arrangements for childcare has resulted in children going to these institutions that are ill-equipped to deal with the emotional needs or provide the caring environment that is needed. Most stakeholders lack an understanding of care and development for the under 6 age group.

Developmental deprivation and under-nourishment result from leaving a child unattended, or in the care of an elder sibling, who is again burdened with responsibility at a young age. There is need to recognise that childcare, nurturing and protection, including childcare arrangements such as crèches and day-care centres need a fuller understanding of the needs of children. Its thrust has to be on an ecosystem which encourages gender and transformative parenting, inclusion and social justice and safety and well-being of the young child.

It is in this context that there is an urgent need to recognise the multi-faceted role of the childcare worker within and outside home. This would require fundamental improvement in the capacity and competency of workers and will require professionalisation of childcare services.

7.1.4 Disadvantaged children deserve urgent and extra attention

This would have to include children who fare poorly in terms of development indicators (e.g., extreme poor, young girls, Scheduled Caste and Scheduled Tribes), the marginalised (e.g., children with disabilities, children living in urban slums, homeless and street children) and the invisible child (e.g., children of migrants, children in the care of older children or with siblings on street, children in institutions and in single-headed households).

Despite multiple legislations, policy frameworks, campaigns and schemes, there continues to be a deficit in gender and socially transformative parenting of the young child. When parents are subjected to intersections of discrimination and disempowerment at various levels, they are not exposed to positive parenting practices, nor do they find the resources or the time and interest to spend on such parenting.

Over the years, increasing media visibility has given more traction to the issue of neglect and abuse of infants and young children. Varied markers of deprivation and disempowerment including poverty, gender, disabilities result in further vulnerability of the young child to neglect, violence, abuse and exploitation. Where disability exists, it is critical for these children to be able to access high quality early intervention services to assist them to reach their potential. However, in the current scenario, not only do services fail to respond effectively, they do not provide accessible and equitable support to such children.

7.1.5　ECCE has to be a universal entitlement, well-designed and effectively implemented

India has a long way to go before the goal of universal access to early childhood care and education can be realised. More investment in policy and planning and less in monitoring and evaluation and negligible investment in implementation have resulted in an environment where a comprehensive perspective to guide national efforts for good quality ECCE is yet to emerge. **Available ECCE services are unable to provide the level and quality of care and stimulation required for optimal cognitive development in the early years.**

The neglect of early childhood education has been a persisting critique of the ICDS. Differences along the rural-urban lines, social categories and wealth index impact participation in the AWCs and private pre-school education centres. Children from poor families, children with disabilities, children of migrants and street children are some groups that tend to be neglected. Unregulated pre-schools, catering to the popular demand of an aspirational society, pressurise children to read and write way ahead of their developmental readiness while the integrated elements of care, health, nutrition and love are neglected.

The draft National Education Policy 2019 recognises this deficit and has adopted a pragmatic approach of both strengthening the existing *anganwadi* centres as well as expansion of the existing pre-school arrangements, linking it to the school education continuum. Both these institutions will require huge investments in capacity building to ensure the *anganwadi* workers as well as pre-school teachers have the competencies required. Quality ECCE will also require the State to provide for adequate infrastructure, play and early simulation materials, intensive training of both the frontline teachers and workers as well as the supervisory staff and a remuneration commensurate with the role expectations.

7.1.6 *Governance issues and capacity deficit are major impediments to progress*

The evaluation of the ICDS and other child interventions has evidenced a huge governance and management deficit. There are also issues related to whether the primary responsibility with respect to both design and implementation, as well as funding, rests with the Central government or the state governments, or which ministry or department is best placed to take the lead on an issue that requires multi-sectoral response. The delegation of powers, and issues around duplication of services, require due attention. A perspective plan on increasing capacities is critical to improving the quality of services. Various complexities in the system of governance need to be addressed by political will at the highest level, which has to be premised on a recognition of the management gaps.

India has effectively demonstrated its ability to deliver limited services in a mission and time-bound manner (like eradication of polio in recent times through pulse polio campaign), but continuous and consistent service delivery has plagued the system. As a result, ongoing schemes are often taken for granted and remain neglected while new interventions and specific vertical missions linked to an issue take precedence. Furthermore, the inability to ensure ground-level convergence of health, education, nutrition, water and sanitation, protection and pre-school education services has seriously impaired programmes meant for children.

The inability to use financial resources effectively and efficiently is indicative of human resource deficit, which creates a vicious circle of underspending resulting in reduced allocations and so on. Fragmentation of responsibilities related to issues of the young child across laws, policies and programmes have prevented the emergence of a cohesive framework for action and limited the possible outcomes. Against this backdrop, childcare workers are untrained, overburdened and unsung.

Analysis of budgetary allocation and expenditure by various organisations has indicated consistent inadequacy of financial resources for interventions in the interests of the young child as well as under-utilisation of allocated resources. There has been plateauing or even decline in allocations for healthcare and education and provisions for child protection have been minimal.

Governance deficit is compounded by persistent discrimination against girls. It is symptomatic of a patriarchal societal set-up where sons are preferred over daughters, resulting in neglect of girls, declining sex ratio at birth and child sex ratios. Laws and strict enforcement of the letter of the law is indeed important but they alone cannot bring about lasting changes in entrenched prejudices and practices. It requires a transformation of the traditional style of parenting to one which is caring, nurturing and communicative. Civil society will need to lead social reform movements in the areas where they work and the State on its part needs to be proactive and supportive of such initiatives.

7.2 Towards a wholesome childhood for all: major recommendations

7.2.1 *Make ECD a national priority*

This Report highlights the rights of the child mandated by the Constitution, the country's commitment to the SDGs, and policy pronouncements of the government. The human rights approach, within which child rights are embedded, is the underlying principle which needs to be recognised and respected in both letter and spirit. **Prioritising and investing in ECD is an important component of the development strategy** and there is insurmountable evidence, as the earlier chapters highlight, of the huge returns on such investment at the individual, household and country levels. Early development, with its multi-dimensional nature, necessitates the coming together of multiple stakeholders, with varied expertise, to deliver the wide range of services within the gamut of ECD. Equitable, effective, efficient and synergistic delivery of services under ECD must be ensured to maximise the opportunities arising from such interventions.

It is also important to reiterate that many interconnected factors cutting across development sectors determine outcomes for the young child. Progress in all these domains is a prerequisite for young children to survive, thrive and play an equal role in transforming societies for better social, economic and political progress. National and state commitments need, therefore, to cut across all human development sectors – poverty alleviation, education, health, water supply and sanitation, labour, urban planning and food security. ECD has the potential to lay the foundation for achieving outcomes with regard to such other programmes, thereby necessitating more holistic planning frameworks.

The State must assume greater responsibility and create an enabling environment to ensure the well-being of the young child. The State's ECD policy must address the critical issues of such interventions being equitable and accessible to all children, across all intersecting domains.

7.2.2 *Quadruple the budgetary outlays for ECD*

As Chapter 6 notes, despite the primacy of the role of the State in providing a child-centred ecosystem, the budgetary commitments to existing programmes and other required interventions for the young child remain minimal. **The achievement of SDG goals, the holistic needs and entitlements** of the young child must translate into improved allocations to ECD. More children would be pushed to the margins of under-development and disempowerment if the capacity for delivering ECD services is hampered due to insufficient allocations. In the light of this understanding, Chapter 6 of this Report has proposed that the social sector budget needs to be enhanced from 2.6 percent to 4 percent of the GDP. This allocation for the redressal of the long neglect of the social sector would require an outlay of INR 6 trillion, thereby needing enhancement of the outlay from the current 14–16 percent to 25 percent. Within this, there would be adequate provisioning to fill all funding gaps, including the professionalisation of childcare services, as the child budget would be INR 1.25 trillion annually (20 percent of the social sector outlay). The returns on this social investment and child-centred programmes would exceed budgetary spends on any alternative government infrastructure or welfare programme.

Child development and welfare provisions, currently at 1 percent of the Union budget, needs to be enhanced to at least 3 percent. There must be a minimum allocation set out for providing a 'childcare ecosystem service' per child. This can be a national benchmark to be emulated by the states as well by aggregating all available resources to provide for children under 6 years of age. Additionally, more focus and due budgetary allocations would be needed for the inter-connected and related social sectors of public health, nutrition, water supply and sanitation and school education. Throughout the chapters, **this report demonstrates a strong case for increased allocations for ECD and for an urgent need to work towards securing stable funding so as to expand the reach and quality of the services.**

7.2.3 *Focus more on states and regions with poor child development indices*

India's diversity is marked by high variance across and within states with regard to performance on various child indicators in addition to socio-economic, cultural and topographical features. As the Young Child Indices in Chapter 1 show, eight states, including MP, Bihar, Rajasthan, Uttar Pradesh, Jharkhand, Chhattisgarh, Meghalaya and Assam fare poorly. Geographies within some states such Maharashtra, Gujarat, Karnataka, AP and Telangana may also need special focus as they have languished behind. **States and regions that have poor child development indicators need special provisions to enable them catch up with the rest of the country,** which ICDS does not provide as it treats all regions and states alike and budgets are provided based on the coverage of children.

Further, as Chapter 4 notes, even within the already vulnerable category of the young child, there is a need to bring to focus the more marginalised and disadvantaged groups, including the girl child, children living in difficult circumstances, children living in impoverished households and those in urban slums, and other invisibilised categories like children living in areas of armed conflict, children of sex workers, transgender children and children who suffer from diseases like HIV. **There must be specific interventions for each vulnerable category of the young child, otherwise they face the risk of lifelong consequences of deprivation.**

Along with higher budgetary support, these states also need support to improve their implementation capacity and address their governance deficit.

7.2.4 Comprehensive actions are needed to both expand and improve quality of ICDS services

A broader perspective on capacity development needs to guide efforts towards building a holistic and comprehensive child-centred ecosystem. As is evident from an analysis of ICDS across the chapters, **there is an urgent need to restructure and recalibrate the ICDS with a stated aim to reach the most marginalised.** The design and governance deficits addressed in the NNM need to be mainstreamed to cover the entire spectrum of services under the ICDS. There needs to be a complementary and convergent approach to the various service packages delivered under the ICDS so that holistic needs are met, and various entitlements of the young child do not get divided into sectors with no linkages. Importantly, early learning and care component that are missing from the ICDS need to be factored in and strengthened owing to their criticality for ECD.

The creation and strengthening of a cadre of childcare professionals, engagement with institutions of higher learning for research, training and other learning processes and improved management would require considerable investment in the social sector and for ECD but with commensurate outcomes.

Greater decentralisation in governance and implementation, and community engagement must be ensured through the more active formation of support committees with clearly demarcated accountability structures at all levels, starting from the *panchayats*. This will not only enable for an overall improvement in the design and delivery of services but also be able to address area-specific challenges and hold accountability at local levels.

7.2.5 Make crèche services and complementary childcare services the backbone of ECD

The inclusion of children under 3 years of age must be made in the ICDS. The only focus on this age group is in the aspect of immunisation while psychosocial and care-based needs tend to be ignored. This necessitates for well-equipped crèches to be established on a large scale, the required minimum standards for which have been listed out in Chapter 5. Not only do crèches have the potential to address the childcare deficit, but they will also enable women, especially those in the unorganised sector, to attend to work without neglecting the care of their young ones. These services will need a quantum enhancement of the role of *anganwadi* as well as ASHA workers as they will have to actively engage with each household to support them for their young child's health and nutrition needs. The childcare workers will have to play a lead role in bringing about gender and socially transformative change in parenting which otherwise remains untapped. In addition to enabling families for childcare, the State also needs to proactively engage in regulating the mushrooming of private pre-schools to ensure that minimum standards of quality are complied with.

Conversion of *anganwadis* into *anganwadi*-cum-crèches would result in an increased access to quality crèches for childcare. A phased process of conversion is recommended to provide holistic care, stimulation and protection services to children of women working in the unorganised sector with priority given to backward districts and urban slums with high presence of working mothers and poor child indicators. From the calculations in Chapter 6, INR 30.36 billion would be required annually to support 100,000 *anganwadi*-cum-crèches, which would benefit children belonging to poor urban and rural households and have multiplier beneficial impact on the economy.

7.2.6 Universalise quality ECCE as a right to education for the 3–6 age group

The Report strongly recommends that all children in the ages of 3 to 6 have a right to quality ECCE, irrespective of whether they are located at AWCs, pre-primary sections of government, private schools or any other pre-school centres. Quality ECCE programmes are central to the multi-dimensional needs of children under 6 years of age. They must also necessarily include other components including health and nutrition education, for holistic needs to be addressed, whether the children are based in *anganwadi* or private pre-schools. The underpinning of this right to quality ECCE must recognise the importance of the first 1,000 days of a child, and the holistic needs of young children at the age, that sets the stage for their optimal participation in ECCE services.

The ECCE has been the weakest link of the ICDS. The draft National Education Policy, 2019 has recognised the reality that pre-primary schools in the government space, at present, are minimal and therefore ECCE will have to be imparted at other locations, including *anganwadis*. This will require the ECCE component of ICDS to be strengthened, through intensive training of AWWs, development of appropriate curriculum and learning tools and appropriate training of pre-school teachers who can then deliver equitable quality ECCE for children in the 3–6 age group, across settings. This is possible only if the draft NEP 2019's recommendation to amend the Right to Education Act 2009 to include children in the ages of 3 to 6, is undertaken to make it a justiciable right for these children.

As Chapter 6 recommends, the overall budget and the budget for the training component of just the *anganwadi* workers need to increase significantly to cover training cost and material cost annually. The additional budget requirement for learning material and AWCs is estimated at INR 4.2 billion per annum, while for training the additional requirement is estimated at INR 10 billion per annum.

7.2.7 Each frontline worker providing childcare services is a professional and needs to be treated as one

Since the inception of the scheme, the ICDS has, de facto, treated *Anganwadi* Workers as part-time, 'honorary' workers. While the honorarium has been enhanced by the Centre and the states, *anganwadi* workers receive compensation well below the minimum wage in most states. Despite the centrality of the role of AWWs in the machinery meant to provide services to mothers and children, they have never got their due in terms of recognition, appreciation or remuneration. The role of the *anganwadi* worker extends well beyond the working hours of the *anganwadi*, as she is expected to reach out to each household, especially those where the young child is not attending the *anganwadi*. Households need counselling, information, education and support on a regular basis. AWWs, along with ASHA workers, have to be the fulcrum for community and household-level engagement.

Every child has the right to quality care. There is an urgent need for a professionally trained, officially recognised workforce. What is most important is to recognise the problems of the AWW, solve these at the supervisory level and recognise the good work done by her. Increasing the remuneration payable to her, creating decent working conditions for her, empowering her with funds to carry out localised activities, including minor purchases and repairs and ensuring timely transfers of funds to her will enable her to give of her best. Such workers must be recognised as professional cadre, their remuneration adequate, and there must be accreditation for quality. The need for enhanced remuneration is in line with the full-time professional role and the intensive community engagement envisaged for these workers. A sum of INR 167.76 billion would be required annually to pay the proposed monthly salary of INR 10,000 for about 1,400,000 sanctioned positions of AWW and INR 8,000 for about 900,000 sanctioned positions of ASHA workers

7.2.8 Urgently address rising incidence of child abuse and crimes against children

This Report has highlighted incidences of child abuse and crimes against children. The societal stigma and silences against such violence often result in partial reporting as well as policy inaction. Especially in cases of the girl child and sexual forms of violence, the issue goes unreported. The young child needs a protective and caring environment of social inclusion that is free from conflict. Therefore, **the first step must be the acknowledgement** and recognition of such violence and policy action in close collaboration with the civil society.

A support-group structure led by frontline workers who are properly trained is needed to reinforce parenting skills and closely monitor the child's well-being. Visiting worker visits are also required to observe and evaluate the progress of the child and the caregiving environment. Child abuse against girls also reflects cultural mindsets and needs strict enforcement of the law where major cases of abuse come to light. The Centre and the states need to actively engage with civil society organisations so that counselling sessions are coupled with punitive action to act as deterrents.

7.2.9 *The child database and monitoring systems need a fundamental revamp*

The next set of actions would be to take up the more important work on policy advocacy with the Centre/ states, civil society, the media, and the citizens of this country. As this Report has noted, right from the exercise of constructing child indices to attempting to visualise the most marginalised young child, there is a serious paucity of credible data that hampers any assessment of this nature and can also result in issues with identifying leakages and working on design and delivery systems. Publicly available databases must be created to record multi-dimensional data on children from the district level. As Chapter 6 notes, even for budgetary allocation, there is very little information in the public domain on the young child resulting in reliance on ministry budgets mostly. **This necessitates the collection and availability of disaggregated, credible state-level data so that the evidence-basis of policy and programme interventions is available.**

From ICDS monitoring systems reporting higher numbers than the actual number of participants to gross estimation of school enrolment data, there are multiple hindrances that are created. This Report recommends two ways to correct this:

1 Performance assessment of teachers, AWWs and ANMs and other government functionaries should be divorced from the numbers reported by her.
2 NSSO and NFHS will need to improve the frequency and extend their sampling surveys to cover critical child development indicators.

These exercises must use consistent methodology and the data must be made available in the public domain so as to enable policy correction as well as monitoring and documentation of successful interventions.

Overall, this Report calls for the young child to be treated as a rights' holder in her own right, and to be enabled through interventions by the State and other stakeholders to develop to their full potential.

Annexures

Annexure 1
Services provided under the ICDS

As one of the flagship programmes of the Government of India, the Integrated Child Development Services Scheme (ICDS) is the world's largest community based programme. It was launched on 2 October 1975 to cater to the needs of children under 6 years of age and pregnant and lactating mothers and work towards improving the health, nutrition and education indicators. The scheme was launched with the following aims:

*   improving the nutritional and health status of children in the 0–6 year age group
*   laying the foundation for proper psychological, physical and social development of the child
*   reducing incidence of mortality, morbidity, malnutrition and school dropout
*   achieving effective co-ordination of policy and implementation among the various departments to promote child development, and
*   enhancing the capability of the mother to look after the normal health and nutritional needs of the child through proper nutrition and health education.

The ICDS offers a package of six services keeping in mind the integrationist approach resulting in a larger impact and better outcomes. These services include supplementary nutrition, pre-school non-formal education, nutrition and health education, immunisation, health check-up and referral services. The target groups and service providers of these services are listed in Table A.1:

Table A.1 Target groups and service providers under ICDS

S. No	Service	Target group	Service provider
1.	Supplementary Nutrition	Children below 6 years, Pregnant and Lactating Mothers (P&LM)	*Anganwadi* Worker and *Anganwadi* Helper [MWCD]
2.	Immunisation*	Children below 6 years, Pregnant and Lactating Mothers (P&LM)	ANM/MO [Health system, MHFW]
3.	Health check-up*	Children below 6 years, Pregnant and Lactating Mothers (P&LM)	ANM/MO/AWW [Health system, MHFW]
4.	Referral Services	Children below 6 years, Pregnant and Lactating Mothers (P&LM)	AWW/ANM/MO [Health system, MHFW]
5.	Pre-school Education	Children 3–6 years	AWW [MWCD]
6.	Nutrition and Health Education	Women (15–45 years)	AWW/ANM/MO [Health system, MHFW & MWCD]

* AWW assists ANM in identifying the target group.

(Source: Ministry of Women and Child Development, Government of India Retrieved from https://icds-wcd.nic.in/icds.aspx Accessed 6/12/19)

Annexure 2
Technical note

Measuring well-being of the young child: outcomes and environment indices

1 Measuring development progress

Over the past few decades, measuring people's quality of life, or aspects of human development, has attained significance to track progress of people's well-being and autonomy. The Millennium Development Goals forged a consensus to counter human deprivation in developing countries by bringing together the global community to commit to eight goals, ranging from combating poverty and ill health to promoting gender equality and international cooperation for development, which were tracked using specific targets and indicators. Following the conclusion of the MDGs, the successor Sustainable Development Goals (SDGs) amplified global ambition manifold, universalising applicability to developed and developing countries, while focussing on the durability of development gains. Measuring SDG progress through identified indicators has become an important tool for countries to track and monitor change.

Apart from presenting dashboards of individual indicator values, aggregating a cluster of indicators that reflect varied dimensions of quality of life through indexing into a single number is a well-established tradition in development literature. While such aggregation has the obvious disadvantages of loss of detail and nuance, it also has the advantages of being able to present a summary picture, easy to communicate and compare across entities. Indexing, combined with a more disaggregated analysis, can draw upon the strengths of both. The Human Development Index (HDI), pioneered by UNDP, for example, includes the following components to measure progress –

- Health: By *Life expectancy at birth*
- Knowledge: By a combination of *Expected years of schooling* and *Mean years of schooling*
- Other opportunities for well-being and choices: By *Gross National Income per capita*.

There are a number of other indices capturing various aspects of development, for example, inequality-adjusted HDI, gender equality index, multidimensional poverty index, perceptions of corruption index, etc.

2 Existing child-related measures and indices

A number of studies have measured the condition of children specifically and constructed child indices using indicators of child well-being. These have been used to:

- measure the well-being of the child
- identify policy enablers
- facilitate comparisons across countries/regions and other key categories of interest, and
- track changes over time.

Not many have focussed on the young child directly. Owing to the specific development imperatives of children, especially young children, the impact of circumstances in which they grow and the care they receive become important. How the specific needs, vulnerabilities, opportunities, and outcomes of the young child are assessed, matter. From the National Family Health Survey 4 (2015–16),[1] the indicators most relevant to the physical well-being of the young child include Maternal and Child Health, Delivery Care, Child Immunisations and Vitamin A Supplementation, Treatment of Childhood Diseases, Child Feeding Practices and Nutritional Status, Anaemia among children and pregnant women.

In developing indices on child well-being, Moore et al. (2011) have developed a framework of family, neighbourhood and socio-demographic factors to construct a Positive and Negative Child Contextual Well-Being Index.[2] Jordan (1993)[3] came up with nine indicators to measure the quality of life of children including under 5 mortality rates, percentage of daily calorie requirements, male and female secondary enrolments rates, life expectancy, percentage of females in the work force, male and female literacy rates and GNP per capita.

Save the Children prepared a mirror of the HDI in 2008 that applies an "integrated index to evaluate the development of children about health, education and basic needs," replacing income with an indicator of nutrition.[4] The average of the variables – education, health and nutrition – is taken as the CDI. It used the indicators of under-5 mortality rate, percentage of primary age children not in school and under-weight prevalence among children under 5 for the index.

The *Kids Count Index* by the Annie E. Casey Foundation (2012)[5] proposed capturing four domains with four indicators under each. The four domains are Economic well-being, Education, Health, Family and Community. The Duke Centre for Child and Family Policy (2014)[6] came out with the Child and Youth Well-Being Index, including 28 key indicators, organised into seven Quality-of-Life/Well-Being Domains.

Based on a study of various NGO reports, Chang et al. (2015)[7] have come up with a Sustainable Child Development Index as the basis for an indicator framework, centralising the importance of child development for sustainable development, considering both the context and outcomes relevant for child development. In the context of the young child, the day-care arrangements could be considered instead of formal education.

To study variations in child development across regions in India, in terms of a child health index (survival, nutrition, immunisation, health expenditure), child development in education index (covering both child labour and education by calculating the percentage of school going children within a certain age group and dividing it by the percentage of child labour within the group) and child abuse index (percentage of children having reported physical, sexual, emotional abuse and neglect), Roy (2014)[8] has proposed a formula for a composite index constructed for each category of these child development indicators:

$$CI = \sum XI/N$$

where $XI = x_i/\bar{x}$
Where, x_i = State Level variable in i[th]-indicator
$\bar{x}$ = National Average in i[th]-indicator
N = Number of Indicators used at State Level

In the Indian context, Corrie (1995)[9] constructed the HDI keeping in mind the specific context and vulnerabilities of children, the Dalit child in this case, using "indicators from each of the three environments – material, physiological and social – critically influencing child survival and development, as well as an 'outcome' indicator of child survival and development" (Corrie 1995, p. 397). In their study, Dreze and Khera (2012)[10] extended their analysis of HDI to CDI in India. They present a Child Development Index which is a normalised variant of the 'Achievements of Babies and Children' (ABC) index.

While centralising the rights of the child, the HAQ Centre for Child Rights (2011),[11] came out with a composite child rights index with a view to look into all aspects of a child's well-being, covering 0–18 years old children in India. An exclusive focus on the young child remains a gap, even though it is acknowledged that development deficits among human beings below 3 years, and even earlier, they can contribute to longer term disadvantages in physical and cognitive development, which can be costly for the economy and society.

3 The two young child indices: capturing outcomes and environment

This Report seeks to build on the existing work on indexing to expand the range of measurement and aggregation for the young child in India. The aim here is to segregate indicators of child *outcomes* from *inputs*, and in particular, policy-relevant process inputs which influence the circumstances in which children grow and which could support positive change. Thus, measurement of the outcomes of well-being of the young child (outcome indicators) is distinguished from the policy and environment enablers that constitute the eco system in which the child is lives (process indicators).

Consequently, this Report proposes two indices – the outcome-indicators based **Young Child Outcomes Index (YCOI)** and the **Young Child Environment Index** (YCEI) that aim to capture the ecosystem and the circumstances in which the young child grows.

A dedicated technical group identified key components relevant for the young child's development, both outcomes and circumstances, and created a larger dashboard of relevant indicators under each component. From this data mart the most relevant indicators under each component were identified, constrained by satisfactory data availability and comparability across states in India. These have been aggregated into the Young Child Outcomes Index (YCOI) and the Young Child Environment Index (YCEI). The results are presented for the states in India.

Selection of indicators

In selecting the indicators for the two indices, the SDGs most relevant to the young child have also been considered. These include SDG 1 (End poverty in all its forms), SDG 2 (Ending hunger), SDG 3 (Ensure healthy lives), SDG 4 (Ensure inclusive and equitable quality education), SDG 5 (Achieve gender equality), SDG 6 (Ensure availability and sustainable management of water and sanitation for all) and SDG 8 (Promote sustained and inclusive economic growth).

Indicators for the YCOI components: Drawing from the literature, indicators for three major components have been considered in constructing the Young Child Outcomes Index, viz. health, nutrition and cognitive growth. For each of these three components the selection of the actual indicators was based on the following criteria – (1) credibility of the data source, (2) availability of time series data using the same methodology and (3) need to keep the number of indicators small and easy to comprehend.

For the health component the indicator selected is IMR, rather than the child mortality (0–5 years), as the Report recognises the critical importance of the initial months of the of the young child. In respect of nutrition, 'stunting' was used rather than nutrition status as measured by AWWs, both due to paucity as well as concerns regarding credibility of administrative data. Moreover, 'stunting' has been selected rather than 'wasting,' both because it is easier to comprehend and as NFHS data for 'wasting' showed high unexplained variance across states and over time periods. In respect of cognitive development, the challenge was to identify an appropriate measure. Given data limitations, the 'net primary school attendance rate' as periodically estimated by NSSO has been selected over enrolment data. An assessment of enrolment data shows that administrative data from state education departments leaves much to be desired. School based enrolment data and drop-out rates are at high variance in comparison to estimates of NSSO. There is a need to develop appropriate measure to capture activity-based learning at the *anganwadi* and pre-primary school levels to get a better measure of cognitive development at the 0–6 years age group.

Indicators for the YCEI components: For this process index the following components have been identified as critical – Poverty, Primary Health Care, Education, Gender Equity and Water Supply. For the poverty index, the poverty rate using the Tendulkar formula has been used. As a measure of the efficacy of the public health system the indicator selected is immunisation coverage. For the education index, female literacy rate was identified as the most relevant indicator. To compute the gender index, sex ratio is the selected indicator. For the Water Supply index, the percentage of households with protected water supply source has been used.

Construction of the indices was handicapped by serious data gaps in respect of what is available in public domain. This exercise brings to the fore the urgent need to bridge data gaps on critical indicators that measure young child well-being.

The Technical Group had also identified additional indicators to draw up a child safety index, for which the aggregate value of child murders, rapes, kidnaps and infanticide was used. While it was identified as relevant, the data drawn from the National Crime Research Bureau showed anomalies on account of non-registration and non-reporting of cases from a number of states, underlining the importance of better reporting as child safety is, both, a precondition for and an ingredient of child development. Reporting gaps affected data quality and the resulting index showed a negative association with respect to the composite Young Child Outcome Index. In respect of the remaining indicators, viz. Poverty, Primary Health Care, Education, Gender Equity and Water Supply, there was a positive correlation. Among the correlates, female literacy, immunisation and poverty showed higher associations.

The Group did not create a single composite index that combined the indicators used in the two indices – the YCOI and the YCEI – as it is of the view that mixing up process/input and outcome indicators could lead to difficulties in interpretation.

Indexing methodology

The data on selected indicators were normalised to make them unit free before aggregation using the standard Maximum–Minimum procedure. Maximum and minimum values have been drawn from global benchmarks. For converting component indicator values measured in different units into normalised values, the following formula was used:

Component Index = Value of indicator – Min Value/Max Value – Min Value.

In respect of weights, equal weights for each of the three component indices were applied. While this is ultimately arbitrary, there was no *a priori* reason to give greater (lesser) weight to one or the other component. This has been done in the literature based on the idea that all components are equally important. Equal weights also makes the formula simple, making the index easy to interpret.

It was ensured that all component indices were uni-directional – higher (lower) values meant better (worse) results. For example, a higher poverty share could not be directly aggregated with higher values of water supply. The individual Component Indices were then aggregated to calculate the composite Young Child Outcomes Index. Borrowing from the method used to calculate HDI, the indices have been multiplied together and their root taken to produce a geometric mean.

Hence, we have:

Young Child Outcomes Index = $\sqrt[3]{Health\ Index}$ X *Nutrition Index* X *Cognitive Development Index*

and

Young Child Environment Index = 5th root (*Primary Health Care Index* X *Education Index* X *Poverty Index* X *Gender Index* X *Water Supply Index*).

4 How states in India fare on the Young Child Outcomes: comparing the YCOI values

It was possible to construct the Young Child Outcomes Index for two time periods, 2005–2006 and 2015–2016. This not only facilitated inter-state comparisons but also provided an idea of change over time.

As may be seen from Table A.2.1, eight states have scores below the country average. These are Assam, Meghalaya, Rajasthan, Chhattisgarh, Madhya Pradesh, Jharkhand, Uttar Pradesh and Bihar. While each of these states have made progress between 2005–2006 and 2015–2016, they continue to be below the country average and need focussed attention.

5 How states in India fare on the circumstances in which young children develop: comparing the YCEI values

The YCEI has been constructed for 2015–2016 only due to limitations of data availability.

Apart from inter-state comparisons, the YCEI also shows that all the 8 states that have a below country average score on the Young Child Outcomes Index also fare poorly on the YCEI. This establishes that the six identified policy enablers – to alleviate poverty, strengthen primary health care,

Table A.2.1 The Young Child Outcomes Index, 2005–2006 and 2015–2016

Rank	State	Young Child Outcomes Index 2005–2006	Young Child Outcomes Index 2015–2016	Change
1	Kerala	0.796	0.858	0.062
2	Goa	0.757	0.817	0.060
3	Tripura	0.582	0.761	0.179
4	Tamil Nadu	0.659	0.731	0.071
5	Mizoram	0.632	0.719	0.088
6	Himachal Pradesh	0.601	0.719	0.118
7	Manipur	0.615	0.712	0.097
8	Punjab	0.581	0.708	0.126
9	Sikkim	0.581	0.700	0.119
10	Nagaland	0.562	0.699	0.137
11	Delhi	0.578	0.692	0.114
12	Maharashtra	0.528	0.679	0.151
13	West Bengal	0.503	0.665	0.163
14	Jammu & Kashmir	0.532	0.660	0.127
15	Telangana	0.536	0.659	0.123
16	Arunachal Pradesh	0.442	0.657	0.215
17	Haryana	0.501	0.643	0.142
18	Uttarakhand	0.524	0.642	0.118
19	Karnataka	0.513	0.634	0.121
20	Andhra Pradesh	0.523	0.624	0.101
21	Odisha	0.450	0.617	0.167
22	Gujarat	0.426	0.615	0.189
	INDIA	**0.443**	**0.585**	**0.142**
23	Assam	0.436	0.583	0.147
24	Meghalaya	0.369	0.562	0.193
25	Rajasthan	0.452	0.556	0.104
26	Chhattisgarh	0.366	0.555	0.189
27	Madhya Pradesh	0.397	0.526	0.129
28	Jharkhand	0.371	0.500	0.129
29	Uttar Pradesh	0.290	0.460	0.170
30	Bihar	0.298	0.452	0.155

improve education levels, augment safe water supply, ensure child safety and promote gender equity – all have a bearing on child well-being outcomes.

In addition to the 8 states, Gujarat, Nagaland, Manipur and Arunachal also have poor scores.

6 Interpreting the indices and making inter-state comparisons

Overall, one should be cautious in using the indices, given the challenges of data and loss of detail and nuance in aggregation. That said, the exercise did demonstrate that states with better young child circumstances tended to have better young child outcomes as well. Thus, there is an important role

Table A.2.2 The Young Child Environment Index, 2015–2016

Rank	State	Gender Index	Poverty Index	Health Index	Safe Water Supply Index	Education Index	Child Environment Index
1	Kerala	0.732	0.934	0.787	0.936	0.907	0.855
2	Goa	0.687	0.966	0.862	0.958	0.790	0.846
3	Sikkim	0.714	0.916	0.798	0.973	0.726	0.819
4	Punjab	0.601	0.914	0.870	0.990	0.667	0.794
5	Himachal Pradesh	0.671	0.918	0.637	0.943	0.728	0.769
6	West Bengal	0.721	0.725	0.814	0.939	0.665	0.767
7	Tamil Nadu	0.717	0.866	0.639	0.894	0.696	0.756
8	Delhi	0.624	0.889	0.600	0.775	0.780	0.726
9	Tripura	0.725	0.822	0.458	0.857	0.804	0.716
10	Mizoram	0.746	0.719	0.411	0.903	0.877	0.705
11	Jammu & Kashmir	0.616	0.882	0.704	0.879	0.512	0.703
12	Uttarakhand	0.647	0.866	0.496	0.920	0.659	0.700
13	Telangana	0.713	0.900	0.620	0.752	0.532	0.692
14	Karnataka	0.713	0.711	0.555	0.880	0.629	0.689
15	Haryana	0.583	0.868	0.550	0.907	0.614	0.689
16	Meghalaya	0.745	0.856	0.542	0.639	0.695	0.687
17	Maharashtra	0.644	0.767	0.480	0.904	0.715	0.687
18	Odisha	0.703	0.522	0.745	0.874	0.586	0.675
19	Andhra Pradesh	0.713	0.900	0.587	0.693	0.530	0.673
	INDIA	0.680	0.695	0.548	0.887	0.598	0.672
20	Gujarat	0.647	0.780	0.410	0.898	0.660	0.657
21	Chhattisgarh	0.738	0.404	0.719	0.900	0.540	0.636
22	Rajasthan	0.644	0.811	0.462	0.837	0.450	0.619
23	Bihar	0.702	0.504	0.544	0.980	0.460	0.613
24	Uttar Pradesh	0.662	0.574	0.418	0.960	0.526	0.604
25	Assam	0.729	0.532	0.370	0.818	0.620	0.592
26	Madhya Pradesh	0.677	0.538	0.448	0.828	0.535	0.591
27	Nagaland	0.714	0.743	0.235	0.782	0.729	0.589
28	Jharkhand	0.713	0.451	0.546	0.751	0.491	0.578
29	Manipur	0.703	0.452	0.593	0.344	0.690	0.537
30	Arunachal Pradesh	0.733	0.488	0.264	0.860	0.530	0.533

for policy and on-ground actions to improve the conditions in which children under 6 grow and develop.

The objective of this exercise is not to critique poor outcomes and/or circumstances but rather to motivate state actions where there are gaps and point to the links between circumstances that are amenable to policy and young child outcomes. In view of this, it is suggested that along with state rankings there is need to identify within each state, good outcomes and highlight them. Within a state district level comparative exercises could reveal more information regarding outcomes and circumstances. Districts that stand out could serve as good demonstration areas and yield useful lessons.

6 *Limitations and suggestions*

The identification of indicators and indexing has been limited by the extent of availability of relevant and credible disaggregated state level data. The evidence-basis of policy and programme interventions gets constrained in the absence of relevant data. Specifically, inter alia, the following data needs to be gathered on a regular basis:

1   Number of children by age groups – 0–3 years and 4–6 years actively participating and attending *anganwadi* centres. AWWs have a tendency of reporting higher numbers than the actual number of participants. The only way would be for NSSO to extend their sampling surveys of net attendance to the pre-primary/*anganwadi* level. With renewed focus on ECCE, the present participation of children at the pre-primary level weather at nursery schools, day care centres or at *anganwadis* needs to be captured.

2   NFHS data needs to capture malnutrition by grade – severe and moderate – and categorise this between those participating in ICDS centres and those who are not, to demonstrate the effectiveness or otherwise of ICDS interventions.

3   School enrolment data by age (gross and net) presently collected from state education departments appears to be grossly estimated by several state governments which explains the wide variance between school data and NSSO data. The Government of India needs to put in place a more reliable and credible system of capturing school enrolment and participation data.

4   In respect of both *anganwadi* as well as school data there is immediate need to separate performance assessment of *angawadi* and schoolteachers from data entered by the workers so that the present tendency of over-reporting participation and attendance rates is minimised.

5   Poverty rates need to be computed on a regular basis – disaggregated by state and separately for urban and rural areas. There is also need for using consistent methodology for poverty estimation.

6   There is need for a robust measure to assess child learning at the pre-primary level and the measure should be easy and practical to implement at the ground level so that data capture becomes feasible.

7   Data on child crimes does not appear credible at present. In many states, child crimes do not get reported which gives an incorrect picture on the performance of the state. This makes it difficult to draw up the child safety index which is a relevant indicator.

8   Budget allocation and expenditure incurred by states on various child-centred programmes is not available (and/or accessible) in public domain. This makes it difficult to use this as an indicator for usage in the child environment index.

Annexure 3
Sustainable development goals

Transforming our world: the 2030 agenda for sustainable development

Sustainable Development Goals and targets

The table presents the seventeen Sustainable Development Goals (SDGs) and the 169 targets. They were adopted at the United Nations Sustainable Development Summit (25–27 September 2015), a plenary session of the UN General Assembly.

There are two types of targets for each goal: (1) Monitoring targets are numbered by numerals; and (2) Means of Implementation targets are numbered by letters.

Note: *This table has been adapted based on the work at the Asian Development Bank drawing from the ICSU and UN websites.*
www.icsu.org/publications/reports-and-reviews/review-of-targets-for-the-sustainable-development-goals-the-science-perspective-2015/sdgs-report-supplement-goals-and-targets
https://sustainabledevelopment.un.org/sdgs
https://sustainabledevelopment.un.org/post2015/transformingourworld (Accessed 31 October 2019)

Goal 1 *End poverty in all its forms everywhere*	Goal 2 *End hunger, achieve food security and improved nutrition and promote sustainable agriculture*
1.1 by 2030, eradicate extreme poverty for all people everywhere, currently measured as people living on less than $1.25 a day 1.2 by 2030, reduce at least by half the proportion of men, women and children of all ages living in poverty, in all its dimensions according to national definitions 1.3 implement nationally appropriate social protection systems and measures for all, including floors, and by 2030 achieve substantial coverage of the poor and the vulnerable 1.4 by 2030, ensure that all men and women, in particular the poor and the vulnerable, have equal rights to economic resources, as well as access to basic services, ownership, and control over land and other forms of property, inheritance, natural resources, appropriate new technology, and financial services, including microfinance 1.5 by 2030, build the resilience of the poor and those in vulnerable situations, and reduce their exposure and vulnerability to climate-related extreme events and other economic, social and environmental shocks and disasters 1.a ensure significant mobilisation of resources from a variety of sources, including through enhanced development cooperation, in order to provide adequate and predictable means for developing countries, in particular LDCs, to implement programmes and policies to end poverty in all its dimensions 1.b create sound policy frameworks at the national, regional and international levels, based on pro-poor and gender-sensitive development strategies to support accelerated investments in poverty eradication actions	2.1 by 2030, end hunger and ensure access by all people, in particular the poor and people in vulnerable situations, including infants, to safe, nutritious and sufficient food all year round 2.2 by 2030, end all forms of malnutrition, including achieving by 2025 the internationally agreed targets on stunting and wasting in children under 5 years of age, and address the nutritional needs of adolescent girls, pregnant and lactating women, and older persons 2.3 by 2030, double the agricultural productivity and the incomes of small-scale food producers, in particular women, indigenous peoples, family farmers, pastoralists and fishers, including through secure and equal access to land, other productive resources and inputs, knowledge, financial services, markets, and opportunities for value addition and non-farm employment 2.4 by 2030, ensure sustainable food production systems and implement resilient agricultural practices that increase productivity and production, that help maintain ecosystems, that strengthen capacity for adaptation to climate change, extreme weather, drought, flooding and other disasters, and that progressively improve land and soil quality 2.5 by 2020, maintain the genetic diversity of seeds, cultivated plants, farmed and domesticated animals and their related wild species, including through soundly managed and diversified seed and plant banks at national, regional and international levels, and ensure access to and fair and equitable sharing of benefits arising from the utilisation of genetic resources and associated traditional knowledge as internationally agreed 2.a increase investment, including through enhanced international cooperation, in rural infrastructure, agricultural research and extension services, technology development, and plant and livestock gene banks in order to enhance agricultural productive capacity in developing countries, in particular least developed countries 2.b correct and prevent trade restrictions and distortions in world agricultural markets including through the parallel elimination of all forms of agricultural export subsidies and all export measures with equivalent effect, in accordance with the mandate of the Doha Development Round 2.c adopt measures to ensure the proper functioning of food commodity markets and their derivatives, and facilitate timely access to market information, including on food reserves, in order to help limit extreme food price volatility

Goal 3
Ensure healthy lives and promote well-being for all at all ages

3.1 by 2030, reduce the global maternal mortality ratio to less than 70 per 100,000 live births

3.2 by 2030, end preventable deaths of newborns and children under 5 years of age, with all countries aiming to reduce neonatal mortality to at least as low as 12 per 1,000 live births and under-5 mortality to at least as low as 25 per 1,000 live births

3.3 by 2030, end the epidemics of AIDS, tuberculosis, malaria, and neglected tropical diseases and combat hepatitis, water-borne diseases, and other communicable diseases

3.4 by 2030, reduce by one-third premature mortality from non-communicable diseases (NCDs) through prevention and treatment, and promote mental health and well-being

3.5 strengthen the prevention and treatment of substance abuse, including narcotic drug abuse and harmful use of alcohol

3.6 by 2020, halve the number of global deaths and injuries from road traffic accidents

3.7 by 2030, ensure universal access to sexual and reproductive health care services, including for family planning, information and education, and the integration of reproductive health into national strategies and programmes

3.8 achieve universal health coverage (UHC), including financial risk protection, access to quality essential health care services, and access to safe, effective, quality, and affordable essential medicines and vaccines for all

Goal 4
Ensure inclusive and equitable quality education and promote lifelong learning opportunities for all

4.1 by 2030, ensure that all girls and boys complete free, equitable and quality primary and secondary education leading to relevant and effective learning outcomes

4.2 by 2030, ensure that all girls and boys have access to quality early childhood development, care and pre-primary education so that they are ready for primary education

4.3 by 2030, ensure equal access for all women and men to affordable and quality technical, vocational and tertiary education, including university

4.4 by 2030, substantially increase the number of youth and adults who have relevant skills, including technical and vocational skills, for employment, decent jobs and entrepreneurship

4.5 by 2030, eliminate gender disparities in education and ensure equal access to all levels of education and vocational training for the vulnerable, including persons with disabilities, indigenous peoples, and children in vulnerable situations

4.6 by 2030, ensure that all youth and a substantial proportion of adults, both men and women, achieve literacy and numeracy

3.9 by 2030, substantially reduce the number of deaths and illnesses from hazardous chemicals and air, water, and soil pollution and contamination

3.a strengthen the implementation of the World Health Organization Framework Convention on Tobacco Control in all countries, as appropriate

3.b support the research and development of vaccines and medicines for the communicable and non-communicable diseases that primarily affect developing countries, provide access to affordable essential medicines and vaccines, in accordance with the Doha Declaration on the TRIPS Agreement and Public Health, which affirms the right of developing countries to use to the full the provisions in the Agreement on Trade-Related Aspects of Intellectual Property Rights regarding flexibilities to protect public health and, in particular, provide access to medicines for all

3.c substantially increase health financing and the recruitment, development, training and retention of the health workforce in developing countries, especially in LDCs and SIDS

3.d strengthen the capacity of all countries, in particular developing countries, for early warning, risk reduction, and management of national and global health risk

4.7 by 2030, ensure that all learners acquire the knowledge and skills needed to promote sustainable development, including, among others, through education for sustainable development and sustainable lifestyles, human rights, gender equality, promotion of a culture of peace and non-violence, global citizenship, and appreciation of cultural diversity and of culture's contribution to sustainable development

4.a build and upgrade education facilities that are child, disability and gender sensitive and provide safe, non-violent, inclusive and effective learning environments for all

4.b by 2020, substantially expand globally the number of scholarships available to developing countries in particular LDCs, SIDS and African countries for enrolment in higher education, including vocational training and ICT, technical, engineering and scientific programmes, in developed countries and other developing countries

4.c by 2030, substantially increase the supply of qualified teachers, including through international cooperation for teacher training in developing countries, especially LDCs and SIDS

Goal 5 *Achieve gender equality and empower all women and girls*	Goal 6 *Ensure availability and sustainable management of water and sanitation for all*
5.1 end all forms of discrimination against all women and girls everywhere	**6.1** by 2030, achieve universal and equitable access to safe and affordable drinking water for all
5.2 eliminate all forms of violence against all women and girls in the public and private spheres, including trafficking and sexual and other types of exploitation	**6.2** by 2030, achieve access to adequate and equitable sanitation and hygiene for all, and end open defecation, paying special attention to the needs of women and girls and those in vulnerable situations
5.3 eliminate all harmful practices, such as child, early and forced marriage and female genital mutilation	**6.3** by 2030, improve water quality by reducing pollution, eliminating dumping and minimising release of hazardous chemicals and materials, halving the proportion of untreated wastewater, and substantially increasing recycling and safe reuse globally
5.4 recognise and value unpaid care and domestic work through the provision of public services, infrastructure and social protection policies, and the promotion of shared responsibility within the household and the family as nationally appropriate	**6.4** by 2030, substantially increase water-use efficiency across all sectors and ensure sustainable withdrawals and supply of freshwater to address water scarcity, and substantially reduce the number of people suffering from water scarcity
5.5 ensure women's full and effective participation and equal opportunities for leadership at all levels of decision making in political, economic, and public life	**6.5** by 2030, implement integrated water resources management at all levels, including through transboundary cooperation as appropriate
5.6 ensure universal access to sexual and reproductive health and reproductive rights as agreed in accordance with the Programme of Action of the ICPD and the Beijing Platform for Action and the outcome documents of their review conferences	**6.6** by 2020, protect and restore water-related ecosystems, including mountains, forests, wetlands, rivers, aquifers and lakes
5.a undertake reforms to give women equal rights to economic resources, as well as access to ownership and control over land and other forms of property, financial services, inheritance and natural resources, in accordance with national laws	**6.a** by 2030, expand international cooperation and capacity-building support to developing countries in water and sanitation related activities and programmes, including water harvesting, desalination, water efficiency, wastewater treatment, recycling and reuse technologies
5.b enhance the use of enabling technology, in particular ICT, to promote the empowerment of women	**6.b** support and strengthen the participation of local communities in improving water and sanitation management
5.c adopt and strengthen sound policies and enforceable legislation for the promotion of gender equality and the empowerment of all women and girls at all levels	

Goal 7 Ensure access to affordable, reliable, and modern energy for all	Goal 8 Promote sustained, inclusive and sustainable economic growth, full and productive employment and decent work for all	Goal 9 build resilient infrastructure, promote inlcusive and sustainable industrialisation and foster innovation
7.1 by 2030, ensure universal access to affordable, reliable, and modern energy services	8.1 sustain per capita economic growth in accordance with national circumstances, and in particular at least 7 percent GDP growth per annum in the least-developed countries	9.1 develop quality, reliable, sustainable and resilient infrastructure, including regional and transborder infra- structure, to support economic development and human well-being, with a focus on affordable and equitable access for all
7.2 by 2030, increase substantially the share of renewable energy in the global energy mix	8.2 achieve higher levels of economic productivity through diversification, technological upgrading and innovation, including through a focus on high value added and labour-intensive sectors	9.2 promote inclusive and sustainable industrialisation, and by 2030, significantly raise industry's share of employment and GDP in line with national circumstances, and double its share in LDCs
7.3 by 2030, double the global rate of improvement in energy efficiency	8.3 promote development-oriented policies that support productive activities, decent job creation, entrepreneurship, creativity and innovation, and encourage the formalisation and growth of micro-, small- and medium-sized enterprises, including through access to financial services	9.3 increase the access of small-scale industrial and other enterprises, in particular developing countries, to financial services, including affordable credit, and their integration into value chains and markets
7.a by 2030, enhance international cooperation to facilitate access to clean energy research and technology, including renewable energy, energy efficiency and advanced and cleaner fossil fuel technology, and promote investment in energy infrastructure and clean energy technology	8.4 improve progressively through 2030, global resource efficiency in consumption and production, and endeavour to decouple economic growth from environmental degradation, in accordance with the 10-year framework of programmes on sustainable consumption and production, with developed countries taking the lead	9.4 by 2030, upgrade infrastructure and retrofit industries to make them sustainable, with increased resource-use efficiency and greater adoption of clean and environmentally sound technologies and industrial processes, with all countries taking action in accordance with their respective capabilities
	8.5 by 2030, achieve full and productive employment and decent work for all women and men, including for young people and persons with disabilities, and equal pay for work of equal value	9.5 enhance scientific research, upgrade the technological capabilities of industrial sectors in all countries, in particular developing countries, including by 2030, encouraging innovation and substantially increasing the number of R&D workers per one million people and public and private R&D spending
	8.6 by 2020, substantially reduce the proportion of youth not in employment, education or training	

(Continued)

(Continued)

Goal 7 *Ensure access to affordable, reliable, and sustainable and modern energy for all*	Goal 8 *Promote sustained, inclusive and sustainable economic growth, full and productive employment and decent work for all*	Goal 9 *build resilient infrastructure, promote inlcusive and sustainable industrialisation and foster innovation*
7.b by 2030, expand infrastructure and upgrade technology for supplying modern and sustainable energy services for all in developing countries, in particular LDCs and SIDS	**8.7** take immediate and effective measures to eradicate forced labour, end modern slavery and human trafficking and secure the prohibition and elimination of the worst forms of child labour, including recruitment and use of child soldiers, and by 2025 end child labour in all its forms **8.8** protect labour rights and promote safe and secure working environments for all workers, including migrant workers, in particular women migrants, and those in precarious employment **8.9** by 2030, devise and implement policies to promote sustainable tourism that creates jobs, and promotes local culture and products **8.10** strengthen the capacity of domestic financial institutions to encourage and expand access to banking, insurance and financial services for all **8.a** increase Aid for Trade support for developing countries, in particular LDCs, including through the Enhanced Integrated Framework for Trade-Related Technical Assistance to LDCs **8.b** by 2020, develop and operationalise a global strategy for youth employment and implement the Global Jobs Pact of the International Labour Organization	**9.a** facilitate sustainable and resilient infrastructure development in developing countries through enhanced financial, technological and technical support to African countries, LDCs, LLDCs and SIDS **9.b** support domestic technology development, research and innovation in developing countries including by ensuring a conducive policy environment for, inter alia, industrial diversification and value addition to commodities **9.c** significantly increase access to ICT and strive to provide universal and affordable access to the Internet in LDCs by 2020

Goal 10 Reduce inequality within and among countries	Goal 11 Make cities and human settlements inclusive, safe, resilient and sustainable	Goal 12 Ensure sustainable consumption and production patterns
10.1 by 2030, progressively achieve and sustain income growth of the bottom 40 percent of the population at a rate higher than the national average	11.1 by 2030, ensure access for all to adequate, safe and affordable housing and basic services, and upgrade slums	12.1 implement the 10-Year Framework of Programmes on sustainable consumption and production (10YFP), all countries taking action, with developed countries taking the lead, taking into account the development and capabilities of developing countries
10.2 by 2030, empower and promote the social, economic and political inclusion of all, irrespective of age, sex, disability, race, ethnicity, origin, religion or economic or other status	11.2 by 2030, provide access to safe, affordable, accessible and sustainable transport systems for all, improving road safety, notably by expanding public transport, with special attention to the needs of those in vulnerable situations, women, children, persons with disabilities and older persons	12.2 by 2030, achieve sustainable management and efficient use of natural resources
10.3 ensure equal opportunity and reduce inequalities of outcome, including by eliminating discriminatory laws, policies and practices, and promoting appropriate legislation, policies and actions in this regard	11.3 by 2030, enhance inclusive and sustainable urbanisation and capacity for participatory, integrated and sustainable human settlement planning and management in all countries	12.3 by 2030, halve per capita global food waste at the retail and consumer levels, and reduce food losses along production and supply chains, including post-harvest losses
10.4 adopt policies especially fiscal, wage, and social protection policies and progressively achieve greater equality	11.4 strengthen efforts to protect and safeguard the world's cultural and natural heritage	12.4 by 2020, achieve the environmentally sound management of chemicals and all wastes throughout their life cycle, in accordance with agreed international frameworks, and significantly reduce their release to air, water and soil in order to minimise their adverse impacts on human health and the environment
10.5 improve the regulation and monitoring of global financial markets and institutions and strengthen the implementation of such regulations	11.5 by 2030, significantly reduce the number of deaths and the number of people affected, and substantially decrease the direct economic losses relative to global GDP caused by disasters, including water-related disasters, with a focus on protecting the poor and people in vulnerable situations	12.5 by 2030, substantially reduce waste generation through prevention, reduction, recycling, and reuse
10.6 ensure enhanced representation and voice for developing countries in decision making in global international economic and financial institutions in order to deliver more effective, credible, accountable and legitimate institutions	11.6 by 2030, reduce the adverse per capita environmental impact of cities, including by paying special attention to air quality, and municipal and other waste management	12.6 encourage companies, especially large and transnational companies, to adopt sustainable practices and to integrate sustainability information into their reporting cycle
		12.7 promote public procurement practices that are sustainable, in accordance with national policies and priorities

(Continued)

(Continued)

Goal 10 *Reduce inequality within and among countries*	Goal 11 *Make cities and human settlements inclusive, safe, resilient and sustainable*	Goal 12 *Ensure sustainable consumption and production patterns*
10.7 facilitate orderly, safe, regular and responsible migration and mobility of people, including through the implementation of planned and well-managed migration policies	**11.7** by 2030, provide universal access to safe, inclusive and accessible, green and public spaces, in particular for women and children, older persons and persons with disabilities	**12.8** by 2030, ensure that people everywhere have the relevant information and awareness for sustainable development and lifestyles in harmony with nature
10.a implement the principle of special and differential treatment for developing countries, in particular least developed countries, in accordance with WTO agreements	**11.a** support positive economic, social and environmental links between urban, peri-urban and rural areas by strengthening national and regional development planning	**12.a** support developing countries to strengthen their scientific and technological capacity to move towards more sustainable patterns of consumption and production
10.b encourage ODA and financial flows, including foreign direct investment, to states where the need is greatest, in particular LDCs, African countries, SIDS, and LLDCs, in accordance with their national plans and programmes	**11.b** by 2020, substantially increase the number of cities and human settlements adopting and implementing integrated policies and plans towards inclusion, resource efficiency, mitigation and adaptation to climate change, resilience to disasters, and develop and implement, in line with the Sendai Framework for Disaster Risk Reduction 2015–2030 holistic disaster risk management at all levels	**12.b** develop and implement tools to monitor sustainable development impacts for sustainable tourism that creates jobs, promotes local culture and products
10.c by 2030, reduce to less than 3 percent the transaction costs of migrant remittances and eliminate remittance corridors with costs higher than 5 percent	**11.c** support least developed countries, including through financial and technical assistance, in building sustainable and resilient buildings utilising local materials	**12.c** rationalise inefficient fossil fuel subsidies that encourage wasteful consumption by removing market distortions, in accordance with national circumstances, including by restructuring taxation and phasing out those harmful subsidies, where they exist, to reflect their environmental impacts, taking fully into account the specific needs and conditions of developing countries and minimising the possible adverse impacts on their development in a manner that protects the poor and the affected communities

Goal 13 *Take urgent action to combat climate change and its impacts* *	*Goal 14* *Conserve and sustainably use the oceans, seas and marine resources for sustainable development*
* acknowledging that the UNFCCC is the primary international, intergovernmental forum for negotiating the global response to climate change.	14.1 by 2025, prevent and significantly reduce marine pollution of all kinds, in particular from land-based activities, including marine debris and nutrient pollution
13.1 strengthen resilience and adaptive capacity to climate-related hazards and natural disasters in all countries	14.2 by 2020, sustainably manage and protect marine and coastal ecosystems to avoid significant adverse impacts, including by strengthening their resilience, and take action for their restoration in order to achieve healthy and productive oceans
13.2 integrate climate change measures into national policies, strategies, and planning	14.3 minimise and address the impacts of ocean acidification, including through enhanced scientific cooperation at all levels
13.3 improve education, awareness-raising and human and institutional capacity on climate change mitigation, adaptation, impact reduction, and early warning	14.4 by 2020, effectively regulate harvesting, and end overfishing, illegal, unreported and unregulated fishing and destructive fishing practices and implement science-based management plans, to restore fish stocks in the shortest time feasible, at least to levels that can produce maximum sustainable yield as determined by their biological characteristics
13.a implement the commitment undertaken by developed-country parties to the UNFCCC to a goal of mobilising jointly USD100 billion annually by 2020 from all sources to address the needs of developing countries in the context of meaningful mitigation actions and transparency on implementation and fully operationalise the Green Climate Fund through its capitalisation as soon as possible	14.5 by 2020, conserve at least 10 percent of coastal and marine areas, consistent with national and international law and based on best available scientific information
	14.6 by 2020, prohibit certain forms of fisheries subsidies which contribute to overcapacity and overfishing, eliminate subsidies that contribute to I illegal, unreported and unregulated fishing and refrain from introducing new such subsidies, recognising that appropriate and effective special and differential treatment for developing and least developed countries should be an integral part of the World Trade Organization fisheries subsidies negotiation *
	14.7 by 2030 increase the economic benefits to Small Island Developing States and least developed countries from the sustainable use of marine resources, including through sustainable management of fisheries, aquaculture and tourism
13.b Promote mechanisms for raising capacity for effective climate change-related planning and management in LDCs, including focussing on women, youth, and local and marginalised communities	14.a increase scientific knowledge, develop research capacities and transfer marine technology taking into account the Intergovernmental Oceanographic Commission Criteria and Guidelines on the Transfer of Marine Technology, in order to improve ocean health and to enhance the contribution of marine biodiversity to the development of developing countries, in particular Small Island Developing States and least developed countries
	14.b provide access of small-scale artisanal fishers to marine resources and markets
	14.c enhance the conservation and sustainable use of oceans and their resources by implementing international law as reflected in UNCLOS, which provides the legal framework for the conservation and sustainable use of oceans and their resources, as recalled in paragraph 158 of The Future We Want

Goal 15
Protect, restore and promote sustainable use of terrestrial ecosystems, sustainably manage forests, combat desertification, and halt and reverse land degradation and halt biodiversity loss

15.1 by 2020, ensure the conservation, restoration and sustainable use of terrestrial and inland freshwater ecosystems and their services, in particular forests, wetlands, mountains and drylands, in line with obligations under international agreements

15.2 by 2020, promote the implementation of sustainable management of all types of forests, halt deforestation, restore degraded forests, and substantially increase afforestation and reforestation globally

15.3 by 2030, combat desertification, restore degraded land and soil, including land affected by desertification, drought and floods, and strive to achieve a land degradation-neutral world

15.4 by 2030, ensure the conservation of mountain ecosystems, including their biodiversity, in order to enhance their capacity to provide benefits that are essential for sustainable development

15.5 take urgent and significant action to reduce degradation of natural habitats, halt the loss of biodiversity, and, by 2020, protect and prevent the extinction of threatened species

15.6 ensure fair and equitable sharing of the benefits arising from the utilisation of genetic resources, and promote appropriate access to such resources

15.7 take urgent action to end poaching and trafficking of protected species of flora and fauna, and address both demand and supply of illegal wildlife products

15.8 by 2020, introduce measures to prevent the introduction and significantly reduce the impact of invasive alien species on land and water ecosystems, and control or eradicate the priority species

15.9 by 2020, integrate ecosystems and biodiversity values into national and local planning, development processes and poverty reduction strategies, and accounts

15.a mobilise and significantly increase financial resources from all sources financial resources to conserve and sustainably use biodiversity and ecosystems

15.b mobilise significant resources from all sources and at all levels to finance sustainable forest management, and provide adequate incentives to developing countries to advance such management, including for conservation and reforestation

15.c enhance global support for efforts to combat poaching and trafficking of protected species, including by increasing the capacity of local communities to pursue sustainable livelihood opportunities

Goal 16
Promote peaceful and inclusive societies for sustainable development, provide access to justice for all and build effective, accountable and inclusive institutions at all levels

16.1 significantly reduce all forms of violence and related death rates everywhere

16.2 end abuse, exploitation, trafficking and all forms of violence against and torture of children

16.3 promote the rule of law at the national and international levels, and ensure equal access to justice for all

16.4 by 2030, significantly reduce illicit financial and arms flows, strengthen the recovery and return of stolen assets, and combat all forms of organised crime

16.5 substantially reduce corruption and bribery in all their forms

16.6 develop effective, accountable and transparent institutions at all levels

16.7 ensure responsive, inclusive, participatory and representative decision making at all levels

16.8 broaden and strengthen the participation of developing countries in the institutions of global governance

16.9 by 2030, provide legal identity for all, including birth registration

16.10 ensure public access to information and protect fundamental freedoms, in accordance with national legislation and international agreements

16.a strengthen relevant national institutions, including through international cooperation, for building capacity at all levels, in particular in developing countries, to prevent violence and combat terrorism and crime

16.b promote and enforce non-discriminatory laws and policies for sustainable development

Goal 17
Strengthen the means of implementation and revitalise the global partnership for sustainable development

Finance

17.1 strengthen domestic resource mobilisation, including through international support to developing countries to improve domestic capacity for tax and other revenue collection

17.2 developed countries to implement fully their ODA commitments, including the commitment by many developed countries to achieve the target of 0.7 percent of ODA/GNI to developing countries and 0.15–0.20 percent t of ODA/GNI to LDCs; ODA providers are encouraged to consider setting a target to provide at least 0.20 percent of ODA/GNI to LDCs

17.3 mobilise additional financial resources for developing countries from multiple sources

17.4 assist developing countries in attaining long- term debt sustainability through coordinated policies aimed at fostering debt financing, debt relief and debt restructuring, as appropriate, and address the external debt of highly indebted poor countries (HIPC) to reduce debt distress

17.5 adopt and implement investment promotion regimes for LDCs

Technology

17.6 enhance North-South, South-South and triangular regional and international cooperation on and access to science, technology and innovation, and enhance knowledge sharing on mutually agreed terms, including through improved coordination among existing mechanisms, in particular at the UN level, and through a global technology facilitation mechanism when agreed

17.7 promote the development, transfer, dissemination and diffusion of environmentally sound technologies to developing countries on favourable terms, including on concessional and preferential terms, as mutually agreed

17.8 fully operationalise the technology bank and STI (Science, Technology and Innovation) capacity-building mechanism for LDCs by 2017, and enhance the use of enabling technology, in particular ICT

Capacity building

17.9 enhance international support for implementing effective and targeted capacity-building in developing countries to support national plans to implement all sustainable development goals, including through North- South, South-South, and triangular cooperation

Trade

17.10 promote a universal, rules-based, open, non- discriminatory and equitable multilateral trading system under the WTO, including through the conclusion of negotiations under its Doha Development Agenda *Data, monitoring and accountability*

(Continued)

(Continued)

Goal 17
Strengthen the means of implementation and revitalise the global partnership for sustainable development

17.11 Significantly increase the exports of developing countries, in particular with a view to doubling the LDC share of global exports by 2020

17.12 realise timely implementation of duty-free, and quota-free market access on a lasting basis for all least developed countries consistent with WTO decisions, including by ensuring that preferential rules of origin applicable to imports from LDCs are transparent and simple, and contribute to facilitating market access

Systemic issues
Policy and institutional coherence

17.13 enhance global macroeconomic stability, including through policy coordination and policy coherence

17.14 enhance policy coherence for sustainable development

17.15 respect each country's policy space and leadership to establish and implement policies for poverty eradication and sustainable development

Multi-stakeholder partnerships

17.16 enhance the global partnership for sustainable development, complemented by multi-stakeholder partnerships that mobilise and share knowledge, expertise, technology and financial resources, to support the achievement of the sustainable development goals in all countries, in particular developing countries

17.17 encourage and promote effective public, public- private, and civil society partnerships, building on the experience and resourcing strategies of partnerships

Data, monitoring and accountability

17.18 by 2020, enhance capacity-building support to developing countries, including for LDCs and SIDS, to increase significantly the availability of high-quality, timely and reliable data disaggregated by income, gender, age, race, ethnicity, migratory status, disability, geographic location and other characteristics relevant in national contexts

17.19 by 2030, build on existing initiatives to develop measurements of progress on sustainable development that complement GDP, and support statistical capacity-building in developing countries

Annexure 4

Extracts from draft national education policy, 2019

Chapter 1, early childhood care and education

What does quality ECCE entail? During the ages prior to 3 years, quality ECCE includes the health and nutrition of both the mother and the child but also crucially includes cognitive and emotional stimulation of the infant through talking, playing, moving, listening to music and sounds, and stimulating all the other senses particularly sight and touch. Exposure to languages, numbers, and simple problem-solving is also considered important during this period.

From 3 to 6 years of age, ECCE includes continued healthcare and nutrition, but also crucially self-help skills (such as "getting ready on one's own"), motor skills, cleanliness, the handling of separation anxiety, being comfortable around one's peers, moral development (such as knowing the difference between "right" and "wrong"), physical development through movement and exercise, expressing and communicating thoughts and feelings to parents and others.

 . . . Therefore, it is important that children of ages 3–8 have access to a flexible, multifaceted, multilevel, play-based, activity-based, and discovery-based education. It also becomes natural then to view this period, from up to three years of pre-school (ages 3–6) to the end of Grade 2 (age 8), as a single pedagogical unit called the "Foundational Stage". It is necessary, therefore, to develop and establish such an integrated foundational curricular and pedagogical framework, and corresponding teacher preparation, for this critical Foundational Stage of a child's development.

 . . . At the current time, most early childhood education is delivered in the form of Anganwadis and private pre-schools, with a very small proportion coming from pre-schools run by NGOs and other organisations. Where well supported, the Anganwadi system of pre-primary education, under the aegis of the Integrated Child Development Services (ICDS), has worked with great success in many parts of India, especially with respect to healthcare for mothers and infants. These centres have truly helped support parents and build communities; they have served to provide critical nutrition and health awareness, immunisation, basic health check-ups, and referrals and connections to local public health systems, thus preparing crores of children for healthy development and therefore far more productive lives. However, while providing some essential cognitive stimulation, play, and day care, most Anganwadis have remained relatively light on the educational aspects of ECCE . . .

. . . Meanwhile, private and other pre-schools have largely functioned as downward extensions of primary school. Though providing better infrastructure and learning supplies for children, they consist primarily of formal teaching and rote memorisation, with high Pupil Teacher Ratios (PTRs) and limited developmentally appropriate play-based and activity-based learning; they too generally contain teachers untrained in early childhood education. They generally are very limited on the health aspects, and do not usually cater to younger children in the age range of 0–4 years.

The Policy therefore focuses on developing an excellent curricular and pedagogical framework for early childhood education by NCERT in accordance with the previous guidelines, which would be delivered through a significantly expanded and strengthened system of early childhood educational institutions, consisting of Anganwadis, pre-primary schools/sections co-located with existing primary schools, and stand-alone pre-schools, all of which will employ workers/teachers specially trained in the curriculum and pedagogy of ECCE. The numerous rich traditions of India over millennia in ECCE, involving art, stories, poetry, songs, gatherings of relatives, and more, that exist throughout India must also be incorporated in the curricular and pedagogical framework of ECCE to impart a sense of local relevance, enjoyment, excitement, culture, and sense of identity and community.

To reinforce the public system's commitment to provide quality early childhood care and education to all children before the age of 6, the Policy suggests that ECCE be included as an integral part of the RTE Act. The 86th Amendment of the Constitution in 2002 in fact provided an unambiguous commitment for universalisation of ECCE by directing the "State to provide ECCE to all children until they complete the age of six years". Section 11 of the RTE Act also already discussed the possible public provision of early childhood education:

The mandate of the NCERT will be expanded to include the development of a Curricular and Pedagogical Framework for Early Childhood Education..

. . . The new Curricular and Pedagogical Framework for Early Childhood Education will be delivered to children up to the age of 6 via a four pronged approach: a. Strengthening and expansion of the Anganwadi system to include a robust education component . . . b. Co-locating Angawadis with primary schools: When possible, co-locating Anganwadis with existing primary schools will provide further benefits to parents and children, both from the comprehensive services provided by the Anganwadi and the improved opportunity for children to learn in a cohesive educational environment with their siblings and peers at primary schools. . . . Alternatively, up to three years of quality pre-school for ages 3–6 will be added to existing or new primary schools. Such composite schools will also be supported by a package of health, nutrition, and growth-monitoring services, especially for the pre-school students. The care and educational requirements of 0–3 year olds in the region would continue to be handled by neighborhood Anganwadis in such cases. d. Building stand-alone pre-schools: High quality stand-alone pre-schools will be built in areas where existing Anganwadis and primary schools are not able to take on the educational requirements of children in the age range of 3–6 years. Such pre-schools would again be supported by the health, nutrition, and growth-monitoring services as required for children in this age range. All four of the mentioned approaches will be implemented in accordance with local needs and feasibility of geography and infrastructure. Overall, the goal will be to ensure that every child of 0–6 years has free and easy access to quality ECCE. . . .

Due to the equalising nature of ECCE, special attention and high priority will be given to those districts or locations that are particularly socio-economically disadvantaged.

. . . All aspects of early childhood education will come under the purview of the Ministry of Human Resource Development (MHRD), in order to ensure continuity of curriculum and pedagogy from preprimary school to primary school, and to ensure due attention nationwide to the foundational aspects of education.

. . . Anganwadis, pre-schools, and primary schools will all have high quality physical infrastructure that is conducive to learning.

(Source: Draft NEP 2019, https://mhrd.gov.in/sites/upload_files/mhrd/files/Draft_NEP_2019_EN_Revised.pdf Accessed 6/12/19)

Annexure 5

List of laws, policies and programmes mentioned in the Report

Table A.5.1 Laws, policies and programmes

Laws
Prenatal Diagnostic Techniques (PNDT) Act, 1994
Juvenile Justice (care and protection of children) Act, 2000 – Amended in 2006, 2011, 2015
Pre-conception and Prenatal Diagnostic Techniques (Regulation and Prevention of Misuse) Act, 2004
Commission for Protection of Child Rights Act, 2005
Right to Free and Compulsory Education (RtE) Act, 2009
Protection of Children from Sexual Offences (POCSO) Act, 2012
National Food Security Act (NFSA), 2013

Policies
National Policy for Children, 1974
National Policy on Education, 1986
National Nutrition Policy, 1993
National Early Childhood Care and Education (ECCE) Policy, 2013
National Policy for Children, 2013
National Curriculum Framework and Quality Standards, 2014

Programmes/Schemes/Charter
Integrated Child Development Scheme (ICDS), 1975
National Maternity Benefit Scheme, 1995
National Plan of Action on Nutrition, 1995
National Charter for Children, 2003
National Plan of Action for Children, 2005
National Crèche Scheme, 2006 – Earlier called Rajiv Gandhi National Crèche Scheme
Twelfth National Five Year Plan, 2012
Swachh Bharat Abhiyan, 2014
Beti Bachao, Beti Padhao Yojana, 2015
National Plan of Action for Children, 2016
National Nutrition Mission, 2017
National Nutrition Strategy, 2017
Integrated Child Protection Scheme (ICPS), 2006 – Implemented from 2009

International Commitments
United Nations Convention on the Rights of the Child, 1989
Sustainable Development Goals, 2015

Table A.5.2 Legislations relating to Crèches

- Maternity Benefit (Amendment) Act, 2017
- Statutory Crèches under Labour Laws:
  1. Factories Act, 1948
  2. Plantations Labour Act, 1951
  3. Mines Act, 1952
  4. *Beedi* and Cigar Workers (Conditions of Employment) Act, 1966
  5. Contract Labour Regulation and Abolition Act, 1970
  6. Interstate Migrant Workmen (Regulation of Employment and Conditions of Service) Act, 1979
  7. Building and Other Construction Workers (Regulation of Employment and Conditions of Service) Act, 1996
  8. Mahatma Gandhi National Rural Employment Guarantee Act, 2005

Annexure 6
Statistical tables

Table A.6.1 Human Development Index: how India compares

S. No	Indicators	2005		2010		2015		2017	
	Country	HDI Rank	HDI Value	HDI Rank	HDI Value	HDI Rank	HDI Value	HDI Rank	HDI Value
1.	**India**	**128**	**0.619**	**119**	**0.519**	**131**	**0.624**	**130**	**0.640**
2.	Bangladesh	140	0.547	129	0.469	139	0.579	136	0.608
3.	Brazil	70	0.800	73	0.699	79	0.754	79	0.759
4.	China	81	0.777	89	0.663	90	0.738	86	0.752
5.	Indonesia	107	0.728	108	0.600	113	0.689	116	0.694
6.	Malaysia	63	0.811	57	0.744	59	0.789	57	0.802
7.	Maldives	100	0.741	107	0.602	105	0.701	101	0.717
8.	Pakistan	136	0.551	125	0.490	147	0.550	150	0.562
9.	Philippines	90	0.771	97	0.638	116	0.682	113	0.699
10.	Sri Lanka	99	0.743	91	0.658	73	0.766	76	0.770
11.	Thailand	78	0.781	92	0.654	87	0.740	83	0.755
12.	Vietnam	105	0.733	113	0.572	115	0.683	116	0.694

Human Development Index (HDI): a composite index measuring average achievement in three basic dimensions of human development – a long and healthy life, knowledge and a decent standard of living.

Source: UNDP Human Development Data (1990–2017)

Table A.6.2 Key indicators: how India compares

S. No	Indicators	Population under age five (millions)				Life Expectancy at Birth		
	Country	2005	2010	2015	2017	2005	2010	2015
1.	**India**	**129.6**	**128.5**	**121.4**	**119.8**	**64.6**	**66.6**	**68.3**
2.	Bangladesh	16.7	15.8	15.3	15.2	67.9	70.2	72.2
3.	Brazil	16.4	15.2	14.9	14.8	72.0	73.8	75.3
4.	China	79.3	82.6	85.9	85.1	74.0	75.2	76.1
5.	Indonesia	22.7	23.8	24.6	24.7	67.2	68.2	69.0
6.	Malaysia	2.5	2.4	2.6	2.6	73.5	74.2	75.1

Table A.6.2 (Continued)

S. No	Indicators	Population under age five (millions)				Life Expectancy at Birth		
	Country	2005	2010	2015	2017	2005	2010	2015
7.	Maldives	NA	NA	NA	NA	74.2	76.1	77.0
8.	Pakistan	20.1	22.5	24.7	25.1	63.8	65.1	66.3
9.	Philippines	11.4	11.0	11.4	11.6	67.8	68.3	69.0
10.	Sri Lanka	1.7	1.8	1.6	1.6	73.9	74.4	75.1
11.	Thailand	4.2	4.0	3.8	3.7	72.1	73.9	75.1
12.	Vietnam	6.8	7.3	7.8	7.7	74.3	75.1	76.1

NA: Not Available/Not Applicable

Population under age 5: de facto population in a country, area or region aged less than 5 years old as of 1 July.

Life Expectancy at Birth: number of years a newborn infant could expect to live if prevailing patterns of age-specific mortality rates at the time of birth stay the same throughout the infant's life.

Source: UNDESA, 2017

Table A.6.3 Key indicators: how India compares

S. No	Indicators	Infant mortality rate (per 1000 live births)			U5MR (per 1000 live births)		
	Country	2005	2010	2015	2005	2010	2015
1.	**India**	**55.7**	**45.5**	**36.2**	**74.4**	**58.8**	**45.2**
2.	Bangladesh	50.6	39.1	29.7	66.5	49.4	36.3
3.	Brazil	23.1	17.7	14.0	26.1	19.8	15.7
4.	China	20.3	13.5	9.2	24.0	15.7	10.7
5.	Indonesia	33.5	27.5	22.9	41.5	33.3	27.3
6.	Malaysia	7.0	6.8	7.0	8.1	7.9	8.2
7.	Maldives	19.2	11.3	7.7	22.6	13.2	9.0
8.	Pakistan	80.3	73.6	65.7	101.6	92.1	81.0
9.	Philippines	27.5	24.9	22.1	35.8	31.9	28.0
10.	Sri Lanka	12.3	9.7	8.3	14.3	11.2	9.6
11.	Thailand	15.6	12.8	10.8	18.2	14.9	12.6
12.	Vietnam	20.2	18.6	17.6	25.3	23.3	22.0

IMR: probability of dying between birth and age 1 year, expressed per 1,000 live births.

U5MR (per 1,000 live births): probability of dying between birth and exactly age 5, expressed per 1,000 live births.

Source: UN Inter-agency Group for Child Mortality Estimation 2017

Table A.6.4 Key indicators: how India compares

S. No	Indicators Country	Mean years of schooling				GER Pre Primary		
		2005	2010	2015	2017	2005	2010	2015
1.	**India**	**4.8**	**5.4**	**6.3**	**6.4**	**6**	**7**	**12**
2.	Bangladesh	4.5	4.9	5.2	5.8	11	13	31
3.	Brazil	6.3	6.9	7.6	7.8	NA	NA	NA
4.	China	6.9	7.3	7.7	7.8	NA	55	80
5.	Indonesia	7.4	7.4	7.9	8.0	31	41	NA
6.	Malaysia	7.6	9.8	10.2	10.2	62	80	94
7.	Maldives	3.5	4.9	6.3	6.3	75	NA	108
8.	Pakistan	4.5	4.7	5.1	5.2	51	NA	72
9.	Philippines	8.7	8.9	9.3	9.3	37	NA	100
10.	Sri Lanka	10.4	10.8	10.9	10.9	NA	NA	93
11.	Thailand	7.0	7.7	7.6	7.6	NA	NA	68
12.	Vietnam	6.4	7.5	8.0	8.2	59	71	83

NA: Not Available/ Not Applicable

Mean Years of Schooling: average number of years of education received by people ages 25 and older, converted from education attainment levels using official durations of each level.

Gross Enrollment Ratio Pre Primary (% of pre-school age children): total enrolment in a given level of education (pre-primary in this case), regardless of age, expressed as a percentage of the official school-age population for the same level of education.

Source: UNESCO Institute for Statistics, 2018

Table A.6.5 Key indicators: how India compares

S. No	Indicators Country	GDP per capita (2011 PPP $)			Labour force participation % (ages 15 and older)			Female labour force participation % (ages 15 and older)		
		2005	2010	2015	2005	2010	2015	2005	2010	2015
1.	**India**	**3179**	**4405**	**5757**	**60.6**	**55.3**	**54.0**	**36.8**	**28.6**	**27.3**
2.	Bangladesh	1930	2443	3133	57.6	57.0	56.5	28.0	30.0	32.4
3.	Brazil	12299	14538	14703	67.0	65.8	63.8	55.4	54.6	53.4
4.	China	5719	9526	13570	73.4	71.0	69.7	66.8	63.8	62.4
5.	Indonesia	6825	8433	10368	67.5	67.9	65.8	49.9	51.9	48.9
6.	Malaysia	18577	21107	25002	61.1	60.3	64.3	44.0	43.5	50.3
7.	Maldives	9274	12006	13705	63.9	66.1	66.2	50.4	50.1	44.5
8.	Pakistan	4013	4284	4696	52.6	51.6	53.2	19.3	21.7	23.9
9.	Philippines	4779	5597	6875	62.1	62.4	62.4	47.7	48.6	49.4
10.	Sri Lanka	6476	8530	11080	56.3	54.7	53.9	36.9	34.8	34.9
11.	Thailand	11525	13487	15252	73.4	72.4	69.1	65.7	64.5	61.0
12.	Vietnam	3406	4408	5555	76.8	76.9	78.5	72.5	72.5	73.4

GDP Per Capita: GDP in a particular period divided by the total population in the same period.

Labour Force Participation: Percentage of a country's working-age population that engages actively in the labour market, either by working or looking for work. It provides an indication of the relative size of the supply of labour available to engage in the production of goods and services.

Female Labour Force Participation: Proportion of the working-age female population (ages 15 and older) that engages in the labour market, either by working or actively looking for work, expressed as a percentage of the working-age population.

Source: International Labour Organization Database, 2018

Table A.6.6 Child population in India (0–6 years): number and proportion by sex

S. No	State/UT	2001				2011			
		Number of children	Percentage			Number of children	Percentage		
			Total	Male	Female		Total	Male	Female
	INDIA	163,819,614	15.93	15.97	15.88	15,87,89,287	13.12	13.30	12.93
1.	Andaman and Nicobar	44,781	12.57	11.86	11.15	39,497	10.44	9.93	10.92
2.	Andhra Pradesh	10,171,857	13.35	13.46	13.23	86,42,686	10.21	10.46	9.95
3.	Arunachal Pradesh	205,871	18.7	18.08	19.5	2,02,759	14.66	14.36	15.0
4.	Assam	4,498,075	16.87	16.62	17.15	45,11,307	14.47	14.45	14.50
5.	Bihar	16,806,063	20.25	20.01	20.51	1,85,82,229	17.90	17.75	18.07
6.	Chandigarh	115,613	12.84	12.36	13.45	1,17,953	11.18	10.89	11.54
7.	Chhattisgarh	3,554,916	17.06	17.19	16.94	35,84,028	14.03	14.23	13.84
8.	Dadra and Nagar Haveli	40,199	18.23	16.69	20.13	49,196	14.35	13.24	15.78
9.	Daman and Diu	20,578	13.01	11.55	15.06	25,880	10.65	9.03	13.28
10.	Delhi	2,016,849	14.56	14.19	15.01	19,70,510	11.76	11.76	11.76
11.	Goa	145,968	10.83	10.96	10.69	1,39,495	9.57	9.81	9.32
12.	Gujarat	7,532,404	14.87	15.16	14.54	74,94,176	12.41	12.62	12.18
13.	Haryana	3,335,537	15.77	16.14	15.36	32,97,724	13.01	13.34	12.62
14.	Himachal Pradesh	793,137	13.05	13.55	12.53	7,63,864	11.14	11.53	10.74
15.	Jammu and Kashmir	1,485,803	14.65	14.28	15.06	20,08,642	16.01	16.21	15.77
16.	Jharkhand	4,956,827	18.40	18.16	18.64	52,37,582	15.89	15.92	15.85
17.	Karnataka	7,182,100	13.59	13.72	13.45	68,55,801	11.21	11.36	11.07
18.	Kerala	3,793,146	11.91	12.51	11.35	33,22,247	9.95	10.59	9.36
19.	Lakshadweep	9,091	14.99	14.91	15.08	7,088	11.0	11.22	10.77
20.	Madhya Pradesh	10,782,214	17.87	17.75	18.0	1,05,48,295	14.53	14.67	14.38
21.	Maharashtra	13,671,126	14.11	14.08	14.04	1,28,48,375	11.43	11.69	11.16

(Continued)

Table A.6.6 (Continued)

S. No	State/UT	2001				2011			
		Number of children	Percentage			Number of children	Percentage		
			Total	Male	Female		Total	Male	Female
	INDIA	163,819,614	15.93	15.97	15.88	15,87,89,287	13.12	13.30	12.93
22.	Manipur	308,585	14.23	14.35	14.10	3,53,237	12.98	13.34	12.61
23.	Meghalaya	467,979	20.18	20.17	20.19	5,55,822	18.75	18.91	18.60
24.	Mizoram	143,734	16.18	15.94	16.43	1,65,536	15.17	15.20	15.14
25.	Nagaland	289,678	14.56	14.09	15.08	2,85,981	14.44	14.34	14.54
26.	Odisha	5,358,810	14.56	14.71	14.41	50,35,650	12.0	12.28	11.73
27.	Puducherry	117,159	12.02	12.23	11.82	1,27,610	10.25	10.64	9.89
28.	Punjab	3,171,829	13.02	13.58	12.38	29,41,570	10.62	10.89	10.32
29.	Rajasthan	10,651,002	18.85	18.97	18.72	1,05,04,916	15.31	15.67	14.92
30.	Sikkim	78,195	14.46	13.81	15.20	61,077	10.05	9.77	10.37
31.	Tamil Nadu	7,235,160	11.59	11.86	11.32	68,94,821	9.56	9.80	9.32
32.	Telangana	NA	NA	NA	NA	NA	NA	NA	NA
33.	Tripura	436,446	13.64	13.52	13.77	4,44,055	12.10	12.15	12.04
34.	Uttar Pradesh	31,624,628	19.03	18.85	19.22	2,97,28,235	14.90	14.97	14.82
35.	Uttarakhand	1,360,032	16.02	16.48	15.54	13,28,844	13.14	13.67	12.58
36.	West Bengal	11,414,222	14.24	14.05	14.44	1,01,12,599	11.07	11.05	11.09

NA: Not Available/ Not Applicable

Telangana was formed by dividing Andhra Pradesh in 2014, hence the census figures are not available.

Source: Census of India, 2001, 2011

Table A.6.7 Sex ratio (0–6 population)

S. No	India	1991	2001	2011	2015–16 (NFHS 4)
	India	945	927	919	916
	State/UT				
1.	Andaman and Nicobar	973	957	968	NA
2.	Andhra Pradesh	975	961	939	874
3.	Arunachal Pradesh	982	964	972	936
4.	Assam	975	965	962	923
5.	Bihar	953	942	935	939
6.	Chandigarh	899	845	880	NA
7.	Chhattisgarh	984	975	969	977
8.	Dadra and Nagar Haveli	1013	979	926	NA
9.	Daman and Diu	958	926	904	NA
10.	Delhi	915	868	871	NA
11.	Goa	964	938	942	897
12.	Gujarat	928	883	890	884
13.	Haryana	879	819	834	838
14.	Himachal Pradesh	951	896	909	915
15.	Jammu and Kashmir	NA	941	862	917
16.	Jharkhand	979	965	948	920
17.	Karnataka	960	946	948	937
18.	Kerala	958	960	964	1020
19.	Lakshadweep	941	959	911	NA
20.	Madhya Pradesh	941	932	918	918
21.	Maharashtra	946	913	894	918
22.	Manipur	974	957	936	985
23.	Meghalaya	986	973	970	991
24.	Mizoram	969	964	970	961
25.	Nagaland	993	964	943	955
26.	Odisha	967	953	941	934
27.	Puducherry	963	967	967	NA
28.	Punjab	875	798	846	852
29.	Rajasthan	916	909	888	887
30.	Sikkim	965	963	957	907
31.	Tamil Nadu	948	942	943	939
32.	Telangana	NA	NA	NA	907
33.	Tripura	967	966	957	987
34.	Uttar Pradesh	927	916	902	903
35.	Uttarakhand	948	908	890	918
36.	West Bengal	967	960	956	939

NA: Not Available/ Not Applicable

Census 1991 was not conducted in Jammu and Kashmir.

Sex ratio: number of females per thousand males.

Source: Census of India, 1991, 2001, 2011, NFHS 4 for 2015–2016

Table A.6.8 Stunting and wasting in children under 5

Indicators		Stunting in children under 5			Wasting in children under 5		
		1998–1999*	2005–2006	2015–2016	1998–1999*	2005–2006	2015–2016
S. No	INDIA	45.5	48.0	38.4	15.5	19.8	21.0
	STATE/UT						
1.	Andaman and Nicobar	NA	NA	23.3		NA	18.9
2.	Andhra Pradesh	38.6	38.4	31.4	9.1	14.9	17.2
3.	Arunachal Pradesh	26.5	43.3	29.4	7.9	15.3	17.3
4.	Assam	50.2	46.5	36.4	13.3	13.7	17.0
5.	Bihar	53.7	55.6	48.3	21.0	27.1	20.8
6.	Chandigarh	NA	NA	28.7	NA	NA	10.9
7.	Chhattisgarh	NA	52.9	37.6	NA	19.5	23.1
8.	Dadra and Nagar Haveli	NA	NA	41.7	NA	NA	27.6
9.	Daman and Diu	NA	NA	23.4	NA	NA	24.1
10.	Delhi	36.8	42.2	32.3	12.5	15.4	17.1
11.	Goa	18.1	25.6	20.1	13.1	14.1	21.9
12.	Gujarat	43.6	51.7	38.5	16.2	18.7	26.4
13.	Haryana	50.0	45.7	34.0	5.3	19.1	21.2
14.	Himachal Pradesh	41.3	38.6	26.3	16.9	19.3	13.7
15.	Jammu and Kashmir	38.8	35.0	27.4	11.8	14.8	12.1
16.	Jharkhand	NA	49.8	45.3	NA	32.3	29.0
17.	Karnataka	36.6	43.7	36.2	20.0	17.6	26.1
18.	Kerala	21.9	24.5	19.7	11.1	15.9	15.7
19.	Lakshadweep	NA	NA	27.0	NA	NA	13.8
20.	Madhya Pradesh	51.0	50.0	42.0	19.8	35.0	25.8
21.	Maharashtra	39.9	46.3	34.4	21.2	16.5	25.6
22.	Manipur	31.3	35.6	28.9	8.2	9.0	6.8
23.	Meghalaya	44.9	55.1	43.8	13.3	30.7	15.3
24.	Mizoram	34.6	39.8	28.0	10.2	9.0	6.1
25.	Nagaland	33.0	38.8	28.6	10.4	13.3	11.2
26.	Odisha	44.0	45.0	34.1	24.3	19.6	20.4
27.	Puducherry	NA	NA	23.7	NA	NA	23.6
28.	Punjab	39.2	36.7	25.7	7.1	9.2	15.6
29.	Rajasthan	52.0	43.7	39.1	11.7	20.4	23.0
30.	Sikkim	31.7	38.3	29.6	4.8	9.7	14.2
31.	Tamil Nadu	29.4	30.9	27.1	19.9	22.2	19.7
32.	Telangana	NA	NA	28.1	NA	NA	18.0
33.	Tripura	NA	35.7	24.3	NA	24.6	16.8
34.	Uttar Pradesh	55.5	56.8	46.3	11.1	14.8	17.9
35.	Uttarakhand	NA	44.4	33.5	NA	18.8	19.5
36.	West Bengal	41.5	44.6	32.5	13.6	16.9	20.3

*NFHS 2 (1998–1999) covers population under 3 years of age for stunting and wasting

NA: Not Available

Chhattisgarh, Jharkhand and Uttarakhand were formed in 2000, hence NFHS 2 data is not available for them.

Stunting (Height-for-age %): children who are more than two standard deviations below the median of the reference population in terms of height-for-age are considered short for their age or stunted.

Wasting (Weight-for-height): children who are more than two standard deviations below the median of the reference population in terms of weight-for-height are considered too thin or wasted.

Source: National Family Health Survey 2 (1998–1999), NFHS 3 (2005–2006), NFHS 4 (2015–2016)

Table A.6.9 Under 5 mortality and infant mortality rate

Indicators		Under 5 mortality rate			Infant mortality rate		
		1998–1999	2005–2006	2015–2016	1998–1999	2005–2006	2015–2016
S. No	India	94.9	74	50	67.6	57	41
	STATE/UT						
1.	Andaman and Nicobar	NA	NA	13	NA	NA	10
2.	Andhra Pradesh	85.5	NA	41	65.8	NA	35
3.	Arunachal Pradesh	98.1	88	33	63.1	61	23
4.	Assam	89.5	85	57	69.5	66	48
5.	Bihar	105.1	85	58	72.9	62	48
6.	Chandigarh	NA	NA	NA	NA	NA	NA
7.	Chhattisgarh	NA	90	64	NA	71	54
8.	Dadra and Nagar Haveli	NA	NA	(42)	NA	NA	33
9.	Daman and Diu	NA	NA	(34)	NA	NA	34
10.	Delhi	55.4	47	47	46.8	40	31
11.	Goa	46.8	20	(13)	36.7	15	13
12.	Gujarat	85.1	61	43	62.6	50	34
13.	Haryana	76.8	52	41	56.8	42	33
14.	Himachal Pradesh	42.4	42	38	34.4	36	34
15.	Jammu and Kashmir	80.1	51	38	65.0	45	32
16.	Jharkhand	NA	93	54	NA	69	44
17.	Karnataka	69.8	55	32	51.5	43	27
18.	Kerala	18.8	16	07	16.3	15	6
19.	Lakshadweep	NA	NA	(23)	NA	NA	27
20.	Madhya Pradesh	137.6	94	65	86.1	70	51
21.	Maharashtra	58.1	47	29	43.7	38	24
22.	Manipur	56.1	42	26	37.0	30	22
23.	Meghalaya	122.0	70	40	89.0	45	30
24.	Mizoram	54.7	53	46	37.0	34	40
25.	Nagaland	63.8	65	37	42.1	38	30
26.	Odisha	104.4	91	49	81.0	65	40
27.	Puducherry	NA	NA	16	NA	NA	16
28.	Punjab	72.1	52	33	57.1	42	29
29.	Rajasthan	114.9	85	51	80.4	65	41
30.	Sikkim	71.0	40	32	43.9	34	30
31.	Tamil Nadu	63.3	36	27	48.2	30	20
32.	Telangana	NA	NA	34	NA	NA	28
33.	Tripura	NA	59	33	NA	51	27
34.	Uttar Pradesh	122.5	96	78	86.7	73	64
35.	Uttarakhand	NA	57	47	NA	42	40
36.	West Bengal	67.6	60	32	48.7	48	28

NA: Not Available/Not Applicable

(): based on 25–49 unweighted cases.

Under 5 Mortality Rate: number of deaths of children under 5 years of age per 1000 live births for the five years preceding the survey.

Infant Mortality Rate: number of deaths of children under 1 year age per 1000 live births for the five years preceding the survey.

Source: National Family Health Survey 2 (1998–1999), NFHS 3 (2005–2006), NFHS 4 (2015–2016)

Table A.6.10 Percentage of underweight children

Indicator		Children under 5 years who are underweight	
		2005–2006	*2015–2016*
S. No	*India*	*42.5*	*35.8*
	STATE/UT		
1.	Andaman and Nicobar	NA	21.6
2.	Andhra Pradesh	29.8*	31.9
3.	Arunachal Pradesh	32.5	19.4
4.	Assam	36.4	29.8
5.	Bihar	55.9	43.9
6.	Chandigarh	NA	24.5
7.	Chhattisgarh	47.1	37.7
8.	Dadra and Nagar Haveli	NA	38.9
9.	Daman and Diu	NA	26.7
10.	Delhi	26.1	27.0
11.	Goa	25.0	23.8
12.	Gujarat	44.6	39.3
13.	Haryana	39.6	29.4
14.	Himachal Pradesh	36.5	21.2
15.	Jammu and Kashmir	25.6	16.6
16.	Jharkhand	56.5	47.8
17.	Karnataka	37.6	35.2
18.	Kerala	22.9	16.1
19.	Lakshadweep	NA	23.6
20.	Madhya Pradesh	60.0	42.8
21.	Maharashtra	37.0	36.0
22.	Manipur	22.2	13.8
23.	Meghalaya	48.8	28.9
24.	Mizoram	19.9	12.0
25.	Nagaland	25.2	16.7
26.	Odisha	40.7	34.4
27.	Puducherry	NA	22.7
28.	Punjab	24.9	21.6
29.	Rajasthan	39.9	36.7
30.	Sikkim	19.7	14.2
31.	Tamil Nadu	29.8	23.8
32.	Telangana	NA	28.4
33.	Tripura	39.6	24.1
34.	Uttar Pradesh	42.4	39.5
35.	Uttarakhand	38.0	26.6
36.	West Bengal	38.7	31.6

NA: Not available/Not Applicable

*For children under 3 years.

Underweight children: children under 5 years who are underweight (weight-for-age) based on the WHO standard of below-2 Standard Deviation.

Source: NFHS 3 (2005–2006), NFHS 4 (2015–2016)

Table A.6.11 Immunisation

Indicator		Percentage of children (12–23 months) fully immunised		
		1998–1999	*2005–2006*	*2015–2016*
S. No	*India*	42	43.5	62
	STATE/UT			
1.	Andaman and Nicobar	NA	NA	73.2
2.	Andhra Pradesh	58.7	46.0	65.3
3.	Arunachal Pradesh	20.5	28.4	38.2
4.	Assam	17.0	31.4	47.1
5.	Bihar	11.0	32.8	61.7
6.	Chandigarh	NA	NA	(79.5)
7.	Chhattisgarh	NA	48.7	76.4
8.	Dadra and Nagar Haveli	NA	NA	43.2
9.	Daman and Diu	NA	NA	66.3
10.	Delhi	69.8	63.2	66.4
11.	Goa	82.6	78.6	88.4
12.	Gujarat	53.0	45.2	50.4
13.	Haryana	62.7	65.3	62.2
14.	Himachal Pradesh	83.4	74.2	69.5
15.	Jammu and Kashmir	56.7	66.7	75.1
16.	Jharkhand	NA	34.2	61.9
17.	Karnataka	60.0	55.0	62.6
18.	Kerala	79.7	75.3	82.1
19.	Lakshadweep	NA	NA	86.9
20.	Madhya Pradesh	22.4	40.3	53.6
21.	Maharashtra	78.4	58.8	56.3
22.	Manipur	42.3	46.8	65.8
23.	Meghalaya	14.3	32.9	61.5
24.	Mizoram	59.6	46.5	50.5
25.	Nagaland	14.1	21.0	35.7
26.	Odisha	43.7	51.8	78.6
27.	Puducherry	NA	NA	91.3
28.	Punjab	72.1	60.1	89.1
29.	Rajasthan	17.3	26.5	54.8
30.	Sikkim	47.4	69.6	83.0
31.	Tamil Nadu	88.8	80.9	69.7
32.	Telangana	NA	NA	68.1
33.	Tripura	NA	49.7	54.5
34.	Uttar Pradesh	21.2	23.0	51.1
35.	Uttarakhand	NA	60.0	57.7
36.	West Bengal	43.8	64.3	84.4

NA: Not Available/Not Applicable

(): based on 25–49 unweighted cases.

Full Immunisation: percentage of children age 12–23 months fully immunised (BCG, measles and three doses each of polio and DPT) (%)

Source: NFHS 3 (2005–2006), NFHS 4 (2015–2016)

Table A.6.12 Breastfeeding

Indicators		Children under 3 Breastfed within one hour of birth (%)*			Children under 6 months exclusively breastfed (%)*	
		1998–1999	2005–2006	2015–2016	2005–2006	2015–2016
S. No	India	16.0	23.4	41.6	46.4	54.9
	STATE/UT					
1.	Andaman and Nicobar	NA	NA	41.9	NA	66.8
2.	Andhra Pradesh	10.3	22.4	40.0	62.7	70.2
3.	Arunachal Pradesh	49.0	55.0	58.6	60.0	57.0
4.	Assam	44.7	50.7	64.4	63.1	63.5
5.	Bihar	5.4	4.0	34.9	28.0	53.4
6.	Chandigarh	NA	NA	33.5	NA	NA
7.	Chhattisgarh	13.9	24.6	47.1	82.0	77.2
8.	Dadra and Nagar Haveli	NA	NA	47.8	NA	(72.7)
9.	Daman and Diu	NA	NA	55.8	NA	(52.3)
10.	Delhi	23.8	19.3	28.0	34.5	49.6
11.	Goa	34.4	59.7	73.3	17.7	(60.9)
12.	Gujarat	10.1	27.1	49.9	47.8	55.8
13.	Haryana	11.7	22.3	42.4	16.9	50.3
14.	Himachal Pradesh	20.7	43.4	41.1	27.2	67.2
15.	Jammu and Kashmir	20.8	31.9	46.0	42.3	65.4
16.	Jharkhand	9.0	10.9	33.1	57.8	64.8
17.	Karnataka	18.5	35.6	56.3	58.6	54.2
18.	Kerala	42.9	55.4	64.3	56.2	53.3
19.	Lakshadweep	NA	NA	57.7	NA	(54.8)
20.	Madhya Pradesh	8.9	14.9	34.4	21.6	58.2
21.	Maharashtra	22.8	51.8	57.5	53.0	56.6
22.	Manipur	27.0	57.2	65.4	62.1	73.6
23.	Meghalaya	26.7	58.6	60.6	26.3	35.8
24.	Mizoram	54.0	65.5	70.3	46.1	61.1
25.	Nagaland	24.5	51.4	53.1	29.5	44.3
26.	Odisha	24.9	54.4	68.5	50.8	65.6
27.	Puducherry	NA	NA	64.6	NA	47.6
28.	Punjab	6.1	10.3	30.7	35.7	53.0
29.	Rajasthan	4.8	13.3	28.4	33.2	58.2
30.	Sikkim	31.4	43.3	66.5	37.2	54.6
31.	Tamil Nadu	50.3	55.2	54.7	34.1	48.3
32.	Telangana	NA	NA	36.9	NA	67.0
33.	Tripura	31.8	33.1	44.4	36.1	70.7
34.	Uttar Pradesh	5.7	7.2	25.2	51.3	41.6
35.	Uttarakhand	24.1	32.9	27.8	31.2	51.2
36.	West Bengal	25.0	23.7	47.4	58.6	52.3

NA: Not Available/Not Applicable

(): based on 25–49 unweighted cases

* Based on the WHO standard, covering the last two births in the three years before the survey to ever-married women.

Source: National Family Health Survey 2 (1998–1999), NFHS 3 (2005–2006), NFHS 4 (2015–2016)

Table A.6.13 Life expectancy

Indicator	Life expectancy at birth by sex											
S. No	1998–2002			2002–06			2006–10			2010–14		
India	Total	Male	Female	Total	Male	Female	Total	Male	Female	Total	Male	Female
	62.5	62.0	63.0	63.4	62.6	64.2	66.1	64.6	67.7	67.9	66.4	69.6
STATE/UT												
1. Andaman and Nicobar	NA	NA	NA	NA	NA	NA	NA	NA	NA	NA	NA	NA
2. Andhra Pradesh	63.5	62.0	65.0	64.2	62.9	65.5	65.8	63.5	68.2	68.5	66.3	70.8
3. Arunachal Pradesh	NA	NA	NA	NA	NA	NA	NA	NA	NA	NA	NA	NA
4. Assam	58.0	58.0	58.0	58.9	58.6	59.3	61.9	61.0	63.2	63.9	62.7	65.5
5. Bihar	60.5	61.0	60.0	61.3	62.2	60.4	65.8	65.5	66.2	68.1	67.8	68.4
6. Chandigarh	NA	NA	NA	NA	NA	NA	NA	NA	NA	NA	NA	NA
7. Chhattisgarh	NA	NA	NA	NA	NA	NA	NA	NA	NA	64.8	63.3	66.3
8. Dadra and Nagar Haveli	NA	NA	NA	NA	NA	NA	NA	NA	NA	NA	NA	NA
9. Daman and Diu	NA	NA	NA	NA	NA	NA	NA	NA	NA	NA	NA	NA
10. Delhi	NA	NA	NA	NA	NA	NA	NA	NA	NA	73.2	72.0	74.7
11. Goa	NA	NA	NA	NA	NA	NA	NA	NA	NA	NA	NA	NA
12. Gujarat	63.0	62.0	64.0	64.0	62.9	65.2	66.8	64.9	69.0	68.7	66.6	71.0
13. Haryana	65.0	65.0	65.0	66.1	65.9	66.3	67.0	67.0	69.5	68.6	66.3	71.3
14. Himachal Pradesh	66.0	66.0	66.0	66.9	66.5	67.3	70.0	67.7	72.4	71.6	69.3	74.1
15. Jammu and Kashmir	NA	NA	NA	NA	NA	NA	70.1	69.2	71.1	72.6	70.9	74.9
16. Jharkhand	NA	NA	NA	NA	NA	NA	NA	NA	NA	66.6	66.2	66.9
17. Karnataka	64.5	63	66	65.3	63.6	67.1	67.2	64.9	69.7	68.8	66.9	70.8
18. Kerala	73.5	71	76	73.8	71.4	76.3	74.2	71.5	76.9	74.9	72.0	77.8
19. Lakshadweep	NA	NA	NA	NA	NA	NA	NA	NA	NA	NA	NA	NA
20. Madhya Pradesh	57.0	57.0	57.0	58.0	58.1	57.9	62.4	61.1	63.8	64.2	62.5	66.0
21. Maharashtra	66.0	65.0	67.0	67.2	66.0	68.4	69.9	67.9	71.9	71.6	69.9	73.6

(Continued)

Table A.6.13 (Continued)

Indicator	Life expectancy at birth by sex											
	1998–2002			2002–06			2006–10			2010–14		
S. No	Total	Male	Female	Total	Male	Female	Total	Male	Female	Total	Male	Female
India	62.5	62.0	63.0	63.4	62.6	64.2	66.1	64.6	67.7	67.9	66.4	69.6
STATE/UT												
22. Manipur	NA	NA	NA	NA	NA	NA	NA	NA	NA	NA	NA	NA
23. Meghalaya	NA	NA	NA	NA	NA	NA	NA	NA	NA	NA	NA	NA
24. Mizoram	NA	NA	NA	NA	NA	NA	NA	NA	NA	NA	NA	NA
25. Nagaland	NA	NA	NA	NA	NA	NA	NA	NA	NA	NA	NA	NA
26. Odisha	58.5	58.0	59.0	59.5	59.5	59.6	63.0	62.2	63.9	65.8	64.7	67.1
27. Puducherry	NA	NA	NA	NA	NA	NA	NA	NA	NA	NA	NA	NA
28. Punjab	68.5	67.0	70.0	69.4	68.4	70.4	69.3	67.4	71.6	71.6	69.7	73.8
29. Rajasthan	61.5	61.0	62.0	61.9	61.5	62.3	66.5	64.7	68.3	67.7	65.5	70.2
30. Sikkim	NA	NA	NA	NA	NA	NA	NA	NA	NA	NA	NA	NA
31. Tamil Nadu	65.0	64.0	66.0	66.2	65.0	67.4	68.9	67.1	70.9	70.6	68.6	72.7
32. Telangana	NA	NA	NA	NA	NA	NA	NA	NA	NA	NA	NA	NA
33. Tripura	NA	NA	NA	NA	NA	NA	NA	NA	NA	NA	NA	NA
34. Uttar Pradesh	59.0	59.0	59.0	59.9	60.3	59.5	62.7	61.8	63.7	64.1	62.9	65.4
35. Uttarakhand	NA	NA	NA	NA	NA	NA	NA	NA	NA	71.7	69.1	74.5
36. West Bengal	64.0	63.0	65.0	64.9	64.1	65.8	69.0	67.4	71.0	70.2	68.9	71.6

NA: Not Available/Not Applicable

Life expectancy: average number of years a newborn is expected to live if current mortality rates continue to apply.

Source: NITI Aayog, 2017, from Sample Registration System Statistics

Table A.6.14 Gross enrolment ratio

Indicators	GER primary			GER upper primary		
	2005–2006	2010–2011	2015–2016	2005–2006	2010–2011	2015–2016
S. No STATE/UT						
1. Andaman and Nicobar	70.83	81.6	88.93	73.75	85.7	84.14
2. Andhra Pradesh	96.84	107.0	84.48	74.32	83.9	81.33
3. Arunachal Pradesh	153.94	246.0	126.76	72.54	115.2	130.13
4. Assam	96.65	136.1	106.11	37.73	90.0	93.05
5. Bihar	92.44	143.6	107.67	30.42	59.8	107.89
6. Chandigarh	72.55	93.9	81.44	66.20	88.5	95.53
7. Chhattisgarh	131.48	125.8	100.02	90.77	95.7	102.33
8. Dadra and Nagar Haveli	123.73	163.1	82.53	46.47	125.5	90.96
9. Daman and Diu	85.70	97.0	82.03	73.43	83.2	79.15
10. Delhi	89.57	119.9	110.71	85.94	99.9	128.12
11. Goa	54.12	66.1	102.57	38.74	67.2	98.74
12. Gujarat	100.30	110.2	97.24	49.91	69.2	95.73
13. Haryana	57.90	95.7	91.41	41.45	79.3	92.39
14. Himachal Pradesh	110.53	111.3	98.80	109.27	115.9	104.36
15. Jammu and Kashmir	94.40	119.4	85.98	71.55	108.0	70.20
16. Jharkhand	123.58	155.8	109.22	37.21	84.4	102.73
17. Karnataka	93.58	108.6	102.98	56.54	71.5	93.37
18. Kerala	76.16	77.3	95.44	77.14	87.9	95.39
19. Lakshadweep	87.39	90.9	73.80	80.04	99.2	83.26
20. Madhya Pradesh	129.76	136.6	94.47	71.28	102.1	94.02
21. Maharashtra	96.82	105.3	97.74	80.74	92.3	99.24
22. Manipur	132.10	182.9	130.85	64.57	93.2	129.89
23. Meghalaya	132.83	238.7	140.90	42.62	94.8	135.89
24. Mizoram	155.76	213.4	122.99	88.84	99.6	134.78
25. Nagaland	133.13	157.5	99.50	76.35	89.7	102.28
26. Odisha	117.38	124.6	103.73	49.43	90.2	94.26
27. Puducherry	79.54	102.2	84.79	72.27	106.9	87.04
28. Punjab	65.34	112.2	101.70	54.96	100.9	98.38
29. Rajasthan	112.72	116.1	100.43	63.60	76.9	91.34
30. Sikkim	138.0	181.0	102.87	76.38	98.0	150.61
31. Tamil Nadu	118.58	118.3	103.89	106.46	120.6	94.03
32. Telangana	NA	NA	103.02	NA	NA	89.41
33. Tripura	133.40	134.3	107.96	84.23	97.4	127.97
34. Uttar Pradesh	107.27	105.2	92.15	41.96	59.6	75.08
35. Uttarakhand	97.0	110.2	99.29	63.38	96.1	86.89
36. West Bengal	104.45	136.9	103.68	66.17	92.4	105.0

NA: Not Available/Not Applicable

Gross Enrolment Ratio: total enrolment in a particular stage of school education, regardless of age, expressed as a percentage of the official age-group of the Population which corresponds to the given stage of school education in a given school year. The GER shows the general level of participation per stage of school education.

Source: District Information System for Education State Report Cards, 2006, 2011, 2016

Table A.6.15 Net enrolment ratio

Indicators	NER primary			NER upper primary		
	2005–2006	2010–2011	2015–2016	2005–2006	2010–2011	2015–2016
S. No STATE/UT						
1. Andaman and Nicobar	55.37	70.9	77.69	44.21	62.0	65.91
2. Andhra Pradesh	75.28	85.70	72.10	53.02	62.0	63.37
3. Arunachal Pradesh	110.58	NA	NA	49.31	87.1	NA
4. Assam	88.84	NA	99.60	35.01	74.9	77.83
5. Bihar	84.13	NA	NA	26.46	52.7	96.88
6. Chandigarh	59.31	77.6	72.23	48.45	64.0	74.64
7. Chhattisgarh	NA	NA	91.69	57.99	67.8	82.10
8. Dadra and Nagar Haveli	93.82	NA	76.92	30.61	93.1	69.18
9. Daman and Diu	70.11	80.5	71.42	52.85	62.4	62.45
10. Delhi	65.81	96.3	93.36	61.63	72.9	98.08
11. Goa	48.17	58.4	95.66	26.95	51.1	84.78
12. Gujarat	78.89	85.7	82.46	36.64	48.8	73.35
13. Haryana	38.08	75.7	73.76	20.29	57.9	69.36
14. Himachal Pradesh	87.29	90.2	82.10	75.29	82.5	80.46
15. Jammu and Kashmir	75.86	95.3	72.39	52.49	80.8	56.04
16. Jharkhand	63.66	NA	97.21	18.41	69.7	89.12
17. Karnataka	83.97	99.8	96.40	48.46	61.7	79.37
18. Kerala	63.90	66.3	85.65	58.53	68.8	79.94
19. Lakshadweep	69.33	78.2	73.28	57.04	73.1	68.20
20. Madhya Pradesh	94.22	NA	79.83	46.86	71.5	72.31
21. Maharashtra	79.32	88.3	85.79	57.09	69.8	78.49
22. Manipur	102.27	NA	NA	50.70	84.4	NA
23. Meghalaya	94.01	NA	96.86	27.82	59.2	72.87
24. Mizoram	117.66	NA	99.0	67.43	74.5	92.52
25. Nagaland	110.38	NA	83.20	59.08	69.3	80.89
26. Odisha	94.05	99.4	90.51	30.01	64.4	72.0
27. Puducherry	56.66	86.0	69.30	49.01	80.2	63.96
28. Punjab	51.78	89.4	84.10	37.68	71.8	89.24
29. Rajasthan	81.52	87.3	79.20	44.66	55.0	67.18
30. Sikkim	94.54	NA	75.47	39.52	42.8	82.57
31. Tamil Nadu	93.92	98.2	90.90	77.27	90.9	77.05
32. Telangana	NA	NA	80.64	NA	NA	68.45
33. Tripura	121.0	NA	97.99	63.92	83.5	NA
34. Uttar Pradesh	97.74	94.2	83.07	33.52	47.1	60.53
35. Uttarakhand	83.32	88.9	84.42	47.35	70.4	66.24
36. West Bengal	82.76	NA	94.02	48.65	67.7	81.30

NA: Not Available/Not Applicable

Net Enrolment Ratio: total number of pupils enrolled in a particular stage of school education who are of the corresponding official age group expressed as a percentage of the official age-group of the population in a given school year.

Source: District Information System for Education State Report Cards, 2006, 2011, 2016

Table A.6.16 Dropout rate

Indicator		Average dropout rate at primary level (I–V)		
		2006–2007	*2010–2011*	*2015–2016*
S. No	*STATE/UT*			
1.	Andaman and Nicobar	NA	3.5	0.51
2.	Andhra Pradesh	5.4	5.4	6.72
3.	Arunachal Pradesh	16.9	18.7	10.82
4.	Assam	9.3	8.6	15.36
5.	Bihar	9.3	6.4	NA
6.	Chandigarh	NA	NA	NA
7.	Chhattisgarh	10.5	5.4	2.91
8.	Dadra and Nagar Haveli	NA	2.0	1.47
9.	Daman and Diu	7.8	6.3	1.11
10.	Delhi	NA	NA	NA
11.	Goa	1.1	1.0	0.73
12.	Gujarat	5.7	4.3	0.89
13.	Haryana	11.9	6.2	5.61
14.	Himachal Pradesh	1.9	NA	0.64
15.	Jammu and Kashmir	5.3	5.3	6.79
16.	Jharkhand	8.1	10.5	5.48
17.	Karnataka	6.7	3.6	2.02
18.	Kerala	1.8	NA	NA
19.	Lakshadweep	NA	2.4	NA
20.	Madhya Pradesh	5.3	8.6	6.59
21.	Maharashtra	6.1	2.1	1.26
22.	Manipur	20.2	9.1	9.66
23.	Meghalaya	18.8	12.7	9.46
24.	Mizoram	5.5	12.0	10.10
25.	Nagaland	3.1	5.2	5.61
26.	Odisha	21.0	6.1	2.86
27.	Puducherry	NA	0.4	0.37
28.	Punjab	2.3	1.8	3.05
29.	Rajasthan	13.7	10.8	5.02
30.	Sikkim	8.3	7.1	2.27
31.	Tamil Nadu	1.5	1.2	NA
32.	Telangana	NA	NA	2.08
33.	Tripura	7.3	11.9	1.28
34.	Uttar Pradesh	12.3	11.1	8.58
35.	Uttarakhand	8.8	5.8	4.04
36.	West Bengal	9.4	6.5	1.47

NA: Not Available/Not Applicable

Dropout Rate: proportion of pupils from a cohort enrolled in a given stage at a given school year who are no longer enroled in the following school year.

Source: District Information System for Education State Report Cards, 2007, 2011, 2016

Table A.6.17 Female literacy rate

Indicator		Total literacy rate among females					
		2001			2011		
		Total	Rural	Urban	Total	Rural	Urban
S. No	INDIA	53.67	46.13	72.86	65.46	58.75	79.92
	STATE/UT						
1.	Andaman and Nicobar	75.24	72.26	81.47	81.84	79.58	85.79
2.	Andhra Pradesh	50.43	43.50	68.74	59.74	52.05	75.02
3.	Arunachal Pradesh	43.53	36.94	69.49	59.57	53.78	79.04
4.	Assam	54.61	50.70	80.24	67.27	64.09	85.71
5.	Bihar	33.12	29.61	62.59	53.33	50.82	72.36
6.	Chandigarh	76.47	66.37	77.40	81.38	74.17	81.55
7.	Chhattisgarh	51.85	46.99	71.11	60.59	55.40	77.65
8.	Dadra and Nagar Haveli	40.23	30.83	74.54	65.93	51.36	84.86
9.	Daman and Diu	65.61	59.33	73.41	79.59	71.97	82.94
10.	Delhi	74.71	67.39	75.22	80.93	74.03	81.10
11.	Goa	75.37	71.92	78.98	81.84	76.84	84.96
12.	Gujarat	57.80	47.84	74.50	70.73	62.41	82.08
13.	Haryana	55.73	49.27	71.34	66.77	60.97	77.51
14.	Himachal Pradesh	67.42	65.68	85.03	76.60	75.33	88.66
15.	Jammu and Kashmir	43.00	36.74	61.98	58.01	53.36	70.19
16.	Jharkhand	38.87	29.89	69.96	56.21	49.75	76.17
17.	Karnataka	56.87	48.01	74.12	68.13	59,60	81.71
18.	Kerala	87.72	86.69	90.62	91.98	90.74	93.33
19.	Lakshadweep	80.47	78.27	83.13	88.25	88.66	88.13
20.	Madhya Pradesh	50.29	42.76	70.47	60.02	53.20	77.39
21.	Maharashtra	67.03	58.40	79.09	75.48	67.38	85.44
22.	Manipur	60.53	56.95	70.01	73.17	69.95	80.21
23.	Meghalaya	59.61	53.24	83.50	73.78	69.45	89.49
24.	Mizoram	86.75	77.26	95.80	89.40	80.04	97.54
25.	Nagaland	61.46	57.52	81.42	76.69	72.01	88.10
26.	Odisha	50.51	46.66	72.87	64.36	61.10	80.70
27.	Puducherry	73.90	64.38	78.57	81.22	73.82	84.60
28.	Punjab	63.36	57.72	74.49	71.34	66.47	79.62
29.	Rajasthan	43.85	37.33	64.67	52.66	46.25	71.53
30.	Sikkim	60.40	58.01	79.16	76.43	73.42	85.19
31.	Tamil Nadu	64.43	55.28	75.99	73.86	65.52	82.67
32.	Telangana	NA	NA	NA	NA	NA	NA
33.	Tripura	64.91	60.50	85.03	83.15	80.06	91.38
34.	Uttar Pradesh	42.22	36.90	61.73	59.26	55.61	71.68
35.	Uttarakhand	59.63	54.70	74.77	70.70	66.70	80.02
36.	West Bengal	59.61	53.16	75.74	71.16	66.08	81.70

NA: Not Available/Not Applicable

Female Literacy Rate: the ratio of total literate female population aged 7 and above to the total female population expressed as a percentage.

Source: Census of India, 2001, 2011

Table A.6.18 Number and percentage of population below poverty line

Indicator		Population below poverty line (based on Tendulkar method on mixed reference period)					
		2004–2005		2009–2010		2011–2012	
		Number (in thousands)	Percentage	Number (in thousands)	Percentage	Number (in thousands)	Percentage
S. No	INDIA	407220	37.20	354680	29.80	269783	21.92
	STATE/UT						
1.	Andaman and Nicobar	10	3.0	NA	0.40	4	1.0
2.	Andhra Pradesh	23510	29.60	17660	21.10	7878	9.20
3.	Arunachal Pradesh	380	31.40	350	25.90	491	34.67
4.	Assam	9770	34.40	11640	37.90	10127	31.98
5.	Bihar	49380	54.40	54350	53.50	35815	33.74
6.	Chandigarh	110	11.60	100	9.20	235	21.81
7.	Chhattisgarh	11150	49.40	12190	48.70	10411	39.93
8.	Dadra and Nagar Haveli	130	49.30	130	39.10	143	39.31
9.	Daman and Diu	20	8.80	80	33.30	26	9.86
10.	Delhi	1930	13.0	2330	14.20	1696	9.91
11.	Goa	340	24.90	130	8.70	75	5.09
12.	Gujarat	17140	31.60	13620	23.0	10223	16.63
13.	Haryana	5460	24.10	5000	20.10	2883	11.16
14.	Himachal Pradesh	1460	22.90	640	9.50	559	8.06
15.	Jammu and Kashmir	1450	13.10	1150	9.40	1327	10.35
16.	Jharkhand	13210	45.30	12620	39.10	12433	36.96
17.	Karnataka	18650	33.30	14230	23.60	12976	20.91
18.	Kerala	6200	19.60	3960	12.0	2395	7.05
19.	Lakshadweep	NA	6.40	NA	6.80	2	2.77
20.	Madhya Pradesh	31570	48.60	26180	36.70	23406	31.65
21.	Maharashtra	39240	38.20	27080	24.50	19792	17.35
22.	Manipur	900	37.90	1250	47.10	1022	36.89
23.	Meghalaya	410	16.10	490	17.10	361	11.87
24.	Mizoram	150	15.40	230	21.10	227	20.40
25.	Nagaland	170	8.80	410	20.90	376	18.88
26.	Odisha	22160	57.20	15320	37.0	13853	32.59
27.	Puducherry	150	14.20	10	1.20	124	9.69
28.	Punjab	5360	20.90	4350	15.90	2318	8.26
29.	Rajasthan	20980	34.40	16700	24.80	10292	14.71
30.	Sikkim	170	30.90	80	13.10	51	8.19
31.	Tamil Nadu	19410	29.40	12180	17.10	8263	11.28
32.	Telangana	NA	NA	NA	NA	NA	NA
33.	Tripura	1340	40.0	630	17.40	524	14.05
34.	Uttar Pradesh	73070	40.90	73790	37.70	59819	29.43
35.	Uttarakhand	2970	32.70	1790	18.0	1160	11.26
36.	West Bengal	28830	34.20	24030	26.70	18498	19.98

NA: Not Available/Not Applicable

Population as on 1 March 2012 has been used for estimating number of persons below poverty line (2011 Census population extrapolated).

Poverty line of Tamil Nadu has been used for Andaman and Nicobar Island.

Urban Poverty Line of Punjab has been used for both rural and urban areas of Chandigarh.

Poverty Line of Maharashtra has been used for Dadra and Nagar Haveli.

Poverty line of Goa has been used for Daman and Diu.

Poverty Line of Kerala has been used for Lakshadweep.

Tendulkar Method: its methodology is based on an exogenously determined poverty line expressed in terms of per capita consumption expenditure in a month and the class distribution of NSS (National Sample Survey) consumer expenditure data of the National Sample Survey Office (NSSO). The poverty ratio (percentage of people living below the poverty line) is obtained by counting the persons lying below the poverty line from the class distribution of persons.

Source: Reserve Bank of India, 2015

Table A.6.19 Net state domestic product

Indicator	Per capita NSDP at constant prices (in Rupees)			
	1998–1999 (Base 1993–1994)	2005–2006 (Base 2004–2005)	2015–2016 (Base 2011–2012)	2016–2017 (Base 2011–2012)
S. No All India NNP	9650	26015	77803	82269
STATE/UT				
1. Andaman and Nicobar	14502	41645	107873	NA
2. Andhra Pradesh	9144	27179	86118	95566
3. Arunachal Pradesh	8712	26870	100387	NA
4. Assam	5684	17050	48465	NA
5. Bihar	3210	7588	24572	26693
6. Chandigarh	26718	78167	195448	NA
7. Chhattisgarh	6873	18530	67185	71214
8. Dadra and Nagar Haveli	NA	NA	NA	NA
9. Daman and Diu	NA	NA	NA	NA
10. Delhi	23762	69128	226583	240318
11. Goa	25364	80844	267329	NA
12. Gujarat	13735	36102	122502	NA
13. Haryana	12728	40627	133591	143211
14. Himachal Pradesh	10131	35806	114478	121843
15. Jammu and Kashmir	7296	22406	60171	NA
16. Jharkhand	7754	17406	50817	54201
17. Karnataka	10549	29295	113506	120403
18. Kerala	9819	35492	119763	NA
19. Lakshadweep	NA	NA	NA	NA
20. Madhya Pradesh	7621	15927	46783	51852
21. Maharashtra	14199	40671	121514	NA
22. Manipur	6401	19341	45652	NA
23. Meghalaya	8507	24278	59949	NA
24. Mizoram		25826	91985	NA
25. Nagaland	9118	33072	61363	NA
26. Odisha	5471	18194	57616	61678
27. Puducherry	19279	60046	127284	135110
28. Punjab	14334	34096	99372	103726
29. Rajasthan	8754	19445	66342	NA
30. Sikkim	9914	29008	193569	205112
31. Tamil Nadu	11592	34126	111454	118915
32. Telangana		27921	108788	118684
33. Tripura	7396	25688	NA	NA
34. Uttar Pradesh	5432	13445	36883	39028
35. Uttarakhand	7385	27781	126562	NA
36. West Bengal	8814	23808	NA	NA

NA: Not Available/Not Applicable

Net State Domestic Product: Net State Domestic Product (NSDP) is defined as a measure, in monetary terms, of the volume of all goods and services produced within the boundaries of the state during a given period of time after deducting the wear and tear or depreciation, accounted without duplication. The data describes the average annual growth rates in per capita NSDP at constant prices of the base year.

Source: Reserve Bank of India Publication 2019 based on Central Statistics Office data

Table A.6.20 Gross state domestic product

Indicator		Gross state domestic product at constant prices (in Rupees Crores)			
		1998–1999 (Base 1993–1994)	2005–2006 (Base 2004–2005)	2015–2016 (Base 2011–2012)	2017–2018 (Base 2011–2012)
S. No	All India GDP	NA	3253073	11369493	13179857
	STATE/UT				
1.	Andaman and Nicobar	NA	1907	5092	NA
2.	Andhra Pradesh	114937	141977	498606	612794
3.	Arunachal Pradesh	1515	3584	14167	16314
4.	Assam	25558	55214	191109	
5.	Bihar	39033	76466	295622	361504
6.	Chandigarh	NA	9413	25051	
7.	Chhattisgarh	NA	49408	191020	218539
8.	Dadra and Nagar Haveli	NA	NA	NA	NA
9.	Daman and Diu	NA	NA	NA	NA
10.	Delhi	47484	110406	475623	554908
11.	Goa	6075	13672	46091	NA
12.	Gujarat	105305	233776	894465	NA
13.	Haryana	43646	104608	399646	NA
14.	Himachal Pradesh	10696	26107	96274	109748
15.	Jammu and Kashmir	11415	28883	96978	NA
16.	Jharkhand	87841	57848	174881	203358
17.	Karnataka	56204	184277	831449	987832
18.	Kerala	69216	131294	448473	NA
19.	Lakshadweep	NA	NA	NA	NA
20.	Madhya Pradesh	24061	118919	818856	500151
21.	Maharashtra	209699	470929	1660387	1959920
22.	Manipur	2430	5459	16424	17548
23.	Meghalaya	2939	7078	20638	23257
24.	Mizoram	1246	2869	12324	17620
25.	Nagaland	2385	6436	14660	
26.	Odisha	35581	82145	292792	346294
27.	Puducherry	2982	7188	19060	22048
28.	Punjab	55736	102556	330052	375890
29.	Rajasthan	73180	136285	563567	634033
30.	Sikkim	787	1909	14370	16390
31.	Tamil Nadu	118209	249567	967562	1090802
32.	Telangana	NA	104233	464542	565101
33.	Tripura	3814	9422	27787	32253
34.	Uttar Pradesh	153853	277818	907700	1042113
35.	Uttarakhand	9946	28340	152699	172849
36.	West Bengal	115516	221789	609545	718054

NA: Not Available/Not Applicable

Gross State Domestic Product (GSDP) is defined as a measure, in monetary terms, of the volume of all goods and services produced within the boundaries of the state during a given period of time, accounted without duplication. Data describes average annual growth rates in per capita GSDP at constant price.

Source: NITI Aayog, 2019 based on Central Statistics Office data

Table A.6.21 Households by sanitation and drinking water facilities

Indicators		Households with improved drinking water source*				Households with improved sanitation facility**			
		NFHS 3	NFHS 4			NFHS 3	NFHS 4		
S. No		Total	Urban	Rural	Total	Total	Urban	Rural	Total
	India	87.6	91.1	81.3	89.9	29.1	70.3	36.7	48.4
	STATE/UT								
1.	Andaman and Nicobar	NA	100	89.9	94.3	NA	87.4	64.4	74.3
2.	Andhra Pradesh	NA	70.7	73.6	72.7	NA	77.4	43.1	53.6
3.	Arunachal Pradesh	85.0	94.7	85.0	84.5	39.6	73.3	57.1	61.3
4.	Assam	72.5	89.1	82.9	83.8	30.7	62.2	45.1	47.7
5.	Bihar	96.1	97.8	98.2	98.2	14.6	54.9	20.7	25.2
6.	Chandigarh	NA	99.5	NA	99.5	NA	84.4	NA	82.9
7.	Chhattisgarh	77.9	97.3	89.2	91.1	14.6	64.4	22.6	32.7
8.	Dadra and Nagar Haveli	NA	80.2	74.7	77.5	NA	58.2	11.7	35.4
9.	Daman and Diu	NA	89.8	88.0	89.4	NA	58.2	68.5	60.4
10.	Delhi	90.5	80.1	69.7	80.0	62.6	73.2	87.7	73.3
11.	Goa	79.9	97.8	93.7	96.3	60.9	76.8	80.8	78.3
12.	Gujarat	89.2	92.7	89.4	90.9	44.2	85.3	47.0	64.3
13.	Haryana	95.6	88.0	94.3	91.7	40.0	81.7	77.4	79.2
14.	Himachal Pradesh	88.4	94.4	94.9	94.9	37.2	79.1	69.6	70.7
15.	Jammu and Kashmir	80.8	97.9	85.0	89.2	24.5	66.2	45.9	52.5
16.	Jharkhand	57.0	88.6	74.0	77.8	15.1	59.0	12.4	24.4
17.	Karnataka	86.1	89.9	88.9	89.3	33.5	77.3	42.6	57.8
18.	Kerala	69.1	95.7	93.0	94.3	90.5	98.7	97.5	98.1
19.	Lakshadweep	NA	91.1	93.0	91.5	NA	99.4	98.6	99.2
20.	Madhya Pradesh	74.2	96.8	79.5	84.7	18.7	66.6	19.4	33.7

21. Maharashtra	92.7	97.7	85.6	91.5	31.6	59.8	44.2	51.9
22. Manipur	52.1	47.1	38.0	41.6	30.2	47.8	51.3	49.9
23. Meghalaya	63.1	85.2	62.9	67.9	37.6	67.9	58.1	60.3
24. Mizoram	85.0	94.1	87.7	91.4	75.5	90.9	73.3	83.3
25. Nagaland	62.8	79.9	80.9	80.6	46.5	68.2	78.8	75.1
26. Odisha	78.4	95.3	87.5	88.8	15.3	61.0	23.0	29.4
27. Puducherry	NA	94.4	99.0	95.8	NA	76.0	45.7	66.5
28. Punjab	99.4	99.3	99.0	99.1	50.5	85.0	79.1	81.5
29. Rajasthan	81.8	91.7	83.3	85.5	19.3	72.5	35.6	45.0
30. Sikkim	77.6	99.3	96.8	97.6	60.7	76.0	94.2	88.2
31. Tamil Nadu	91.4	86.9	94.5	90.6	22.4	69.7	34.0	52.2
32. Telangana	NA	80.7	75.6	77.9	NA	64.5	38.9	50.5
33. Tripura	76.1	97.7	82.8	87.3	51.5	65.1	59.6	61.3
34. Uttar Pradesh	93.7	92.6	97.8	96.4	20.6	68.4	23.2	35.0
35. Uttarakhand	87.4	98.9	89.5	92.9	44.4	73.3	59.6	64.5
36. West Bengal	93.7	93.5	95.1	94.6	34.7	62.0	45.5	50.9

NA: Not Available/Not Applicable

* Piped water into dwelling/yard/plot, public tap/standpipe, tube well or borehole, protected dug well, protected spring, rainwater or community RO plant.
** Flush to piped sewer system, flush to septic tank, flush to pit latrine, ventilated improved pit (VIP)/biogas latrine, pit latrine with slab, twin pit/composting toilet, which is not shared with any other household.

Source: NFHS 3 (2005–2006), NFHS 4 (2015–2016)

Table A.6.22 Children in slums

Indicators		Number of children (0–6 years) living in slums							
		2001				2011			
S. No	India	Number	Percentage	Male	Female	Number	Percentage	Male	Female
	India	7576856	14.5	3944105	3632751	8082743	12.3	4204451	3878292
	STATE/UT								
1.	Andaman and Nicobar	1991	12.3	1013	978	1588	11.2	788	800
2.	Andhra Pradesh	829914	13.2	423304	406610	1149779	11.3	593145	556634
3.	Arunachal Pradesh	NA	NA	NA	NA	2226	14.3	1102	1124
4.	Assam	11699	13.3	6024	5675	22229	11.3	11378	10851
5.	Bihar	152886	18.7	78409	74477	208383	16.8	107994	100389
6.	Chandigarh	22395	20.9	11681	10714	14720	15.5	7697	7023
7.	Chhattisgarh	169340	15.4	86903	82437	254080	13.4	130178	123902
8.	Dadra and Nagar Haveli	NA	NA	NA	NA	NA	NA	NA	NA
9.	Daman and Diu	NA	NA	NA	NA	NA	NA	NA	NA
10.	Delhi	334949	16.5	174527	160422	229029	12.8	119508	109521
11.	Goa	2816	15.3	1499	1317	3240	12.3	1691	1549
12.	Gujarat	311506	15.8	165024	146482	240589	14.3	126331	114258
13.	Haryana	260745	15.5	27200	25635	225889	13.6	122124	103765
14.	Himachal Pradesh	NA	NA	NA	NA	6509	10.6	3493	3016
15.	Jammu and Kashmir	41912	11.2	22252	19660	94204	14.2	50649	43555
16.	Jharkhand	52835	15.5	27200	25635	53465	14.3	27703	25762
17.	Karnataka	345614	14.8	177480	168134	418295	12.7	212928	205367
18.	Kerala	9933	13.3	5096	4837	20327	10.1	10271	10056
19.	Lakshadweep	NA	NA	NA	NA	NA	NA	NA	NA
20.	Madhya Pradesh	601655	15.9	314122	287533	771999	13.6	403360	368639
21.	Maharashtra	1696429	14.2	879038	817391	1428850	12.1	743603	685247

22. Manipur	NA	NA	NA	NA	NA	NA	NA	NA
23. Meghalaya	13782	12.6	6938	6844	8241	14.4	4162	4079
24. Mizoram	NA	NA	NA	NA	10430	13.3	5292	5138
25. Nagaland	NA	NA	NA	NA	11114	13.5	5569	5545
26. Odisha	153189	14.1	78365	74824	188962	12.1	97551	91411
27. Puducherry	12680	13.8	6378	6302	16002	11.1	8222	7780
28. Punjab	198100	13.4	108734	89366	176257	12.1	94781	81476
29. Rajasthan	277822	17.8	145898	131924	307035	14.8	161872	145163
30. Sikkim	NA	NA	NA	NA	3229	10.3	1621	1608
31. Tamil Nadu	511095	12.1	261252	249843	614969	10.6	314363	300606
32. Telangana	NA	NA	NA	NA	NA	NA	NA	NA
33. Tripura	4957	10.4	2562	2395	14755	10.6	7467	7288
34. Uttar Pradesh	972144	16.9	516349	455795	863392	13.8	457036	406356
35. Uttarakhand	57543	16.4	30171	27372	66176	13.6	35131	31045
36. West Bengal	528925	11.3	271725	257200	656780	10.2	337441	319339

NA: Not Available/Not Applicable

Children in Slums: number of children in the age group 0–6 years living in slums and percentage of 0–6 age group slum population in the total slum population in the state.

Source: Census of India, 2001, 2011

Table A.6.23 Total cognisable crimes

Indicator	Cases reported under total cognizable crimes (IPC) and percentage contribution to all india total					
	2005		2010		2016	
	Cases reported	% contribution	Cases reported	% contribution	Cases reported	% contribution
S. No India	1822602	100	2224831	100	2975711	100
STATE/UT						
1. Andaman and Nicobar	682	0.0	980	0.0	802	0.0
2. Andhra Pradesh	157123	8.6	181438	8.2	106744	3.6
3. Arunachal Pradesh	2304	0.1	2439	0.1	2534	0.1
4. Assam	42006	2.3	61668	2.8	102250	3.4
5. Bihar	97850	5.4	127453	5.7	164163	5.5
6. Chandigarh	3133	0.2	3373	0.2	2996	0.1
7. Chhattisgarh	43633	2.4	54958	2.5	55029	1.8
8. Dadra and Nagar Haveli	432	0.0	378	0.0	244	0.0
9. Daman and Diu	243	0.0	203	0.0	271	0.0
10. Delhi	56065	3.1	51292	2.3	209519	7.0
11. Goa	2119	0.1	3293	0.1	2692	0.1
12. Gujarat	113414	6.2	116439	5.2	147122	4.9
13. Haryana	42664	2.3	59120	2.7	88527	3.0
14. Himachal Pradesh	12345	0.7	13049	0.6	13386	0.4
15. Jammu and Kashmir	20115	1.1	23223	1.0	24501	0.8
16. Jharkhand	35175	1.9	38889	1.7	40710	1.4
17. Karnataka	117580	6.5	142322	6.4	148402	5.0
18. Kerala	104350	5.7	148313	6.7	260097	8.7
19. Lakshadweep	42	0.0	42	0.0	36	0.0
20. Madhya Pradesh	189172	10.4	214269	9.6	264418	8.9
21. Maharashtra	187027	10.3	208168	9.4	261714	8.8
22. Manipur	2913	0.2	2715	0.1	3170	0.1
23. Meghalaya	1880	0.1	2505	0.1	3366	0.1
24. Mizoram	2156	0.1	2174	0.1	2425	0.1
25. Nagaland	1049	0.1	1059	0.0	1376	0.0
26. Odisha	51685	2.8	56459	2.5	81460	2.7
27. Puducherry	4575	0.3	3935	0.2	4086	0.1
28. Punjab	27136	1.5	36648	1.6	40007	1.3
29. Rajasthan	140917	7.7	162957	7.3	180398	6.1
30. Sikkim	552	0.0	552	0.0	809	0.0
31. Tamil Nadu	162360	8.9	185678	8.3	179896	6.0
32. Telangana	NA	NA	NA	NA	108991	3.7
33. Tripura	3356	0.2	5805	0.3	3933	0.1
34. Uttar Pradesh	122108	6.7	174179	7.8	282171	9.5
35. Uttarakhand	8803	0.4	9240	0.4	10867	0.4
36. West Bengal	66406	3.6	129616	5.8	176569	5.9

NA: Not Available/Not Applicable

Cognisable Crimes: number of crimes reported under Indian Penal Code (IPC) crimes and Special and Local Laws (SLL) crimes.

Source: National Crime Records Bureau Statistics, 2005, 2010, 2016

Table A.6.24 Cases reported of crimes against children (0–6 years) for 2016

Indicators		Victims of murder			Kidnapping and abduction			Victims of rape
		Male	Female	Total	Male	Female	Total	Total
S. No	India	249	242	491	882	1014	1896	520
	STATE/UT							
1.	Andaman and Nicobar	1	0	1	1	3	4	1
2.	Andhra Pradesh	14	15	29	23	44	67	17
3.	Arunachal Pradesh	0	0	0	0	1	1	3
4.	Assam	1	1	2	7	1	8	0
5.	Bihar	1	2	3	6	1	7	0
6.	Chandigarh	0	1	1	1	2	3	2
7.	Chhattisgarh	8	9	17	99	153	252	33
8.	Dadra and Nagar Haveli	0	0	0	0	0	0	0
9.	Daman and Diu	0	0	0	0	0	0	0
10.	Delhi	5	6	11	175	153	328	55
11.	Goa	0	1	1	10	8	18	2
12.	Gujarat	30	23	53	23	28	51	10
13.	Haryana	9	4	13	10	30	40	32
14.	Himachal Pradesh	0	1	1	2	2	4	6
15.	Jammu and Kashmir	2	0	2	0	1	1	2
16.	Jharkhand	1	2	3	1	44	45	0
17.	Karnataka	26	27	53	21	30	51	39
18.	Kerala	13	10	23	3	6	9	42
19.	Lakshadweep	0	0	0	0	0	0	0
20.	Madhya Pradesh	15	17	32	71	59	130	39
21.	Maharashtra	46	48	94	174	160	334	107
22.	Manipur	0	0	0	1	0	1	1
23.	Meghalaya	1	0	1	7	5	12	12
24.	Mizoram	1	0	0	2	0	2	1
25.	Nagaland	0	0	0	0	2	2	2
26.	Odisha	4	2	6	4	17	21	5
27.	Puducherry	0	0	0	0	0	0	0
28.	Punjab	5	3	8	20	10	30	15
29.	Rajasthan	11	3	14	40	33	73	6
30.	Sikkim	0	0	0	0	0	0	0
31.	Tamil Nadu	17	24	41	11	12	23	0
32.	Telangana	4	11	15	37	112	149	25
33.	Tripura	0	1	1	1	0	1	5
34.	Uttar Pradesh	26	23	49	93	42	135	56
35.	Uttarakhand	1	0	1	18	16	34	2
36.	West Bengal	8	8	16	21	39	60	0

Source: National Crime Records Bureau Statistics, 2016

Table A.6.25 Number of cases reported of crimes against children (0–18 years)

Indicators	Incidence of infanticide			Incidence of foeticide			Incidence of murder			Incidence of rape		
S. No *India*	2005	2010	2015	2005	2010	2015	2005	2010	2015	2005	2010	2015
India	108	100	91	86	111	97	1219	1408	1758	4026	5484	10854
STATE/UT												
1. Andaman and Nicobar	0	0	0	0	3	0	1	1	1	2	15	26
2. Andhra Pradesh	1	6	4	1	1	0	56	63	44	315	446	489
3. Arunachal Pradesh	0	0	0	0	0	0	0	0	6	10	12	34
4. Assam	1	0	1	1	0	0	12	10	16	90	39	43
5. Bihar	1	2	0	0	0	0	25	200	97	8	144	116
6. Chandigarh	0	0	4	0	0	0	3	1	1	21	16	41
7. Chhattisgarh	9	1	4	21	9	11	28	51	66	382	382	317
8. Dadra and Nagar Haveli	0	0	0	0	0	0	1	0	2	0	3	2
9. Daman and Diu	0	0	0	0	0	0	1	0	1	1	1	0
10. Delhi	0	0	3	3	7	3	34	29	54	235	304	927
11. Goa	1	1	0	0	0	0	4	1	3	15	23	50
12. Gujarat	2	0	1	4	10	1	74	66	81	90	102	57
13. Haryana	0	7	5	8	2	14	38	22	50	131	107	261
14. Himachal Pradesh	0	1	2	1	0	1	6	5	7	58	72	139
15. Jammu and Kashmir	0	0	1	0	1	0	4	1	6	22	8	28
16. Jharkhand	0	3	0	0	0	0	33	1	8	4	0	24
17. Karnataka	5	2	0	7	4	1	42	43	108	48	108	0
18. Kerala	0	1	4	1	0	1	45	41	39	140	208	720
19. Lakshadweep	0	0	0	0	0	0	0	0	0	0	0	0
20. Madhya Pradesh	28	20	25	12	18	17	122	124	124	870	1182	1568
21. Maharashtra	3	3	7	4	5	11	189	211	207	634	747	2231
22. Manipur	0	0	0	0	0	0	3	2	5	4	11	13

No.	State/UT												
23.	Meghalaya	1	0	0	0	0	0	8	2	5	51	91	38
24.	Mizoram	0	0	0	0	0	0	0	1	3	0	42	30
25.	Nagaland	0	0	0	0	0	0	0	0	2	0	3	8
26.	Odisha	1	0	0	0	0	0	9	9	20	28	74	1052
27.	Puducherry	0	0	0	0	0	0	0	0	0	3	3	0
28.	Punjab	9	8	3	12	15	10	17	37	45	51	144	462
29.	Rajasthan	1	7	18	10	18	13	56	75	59	246	369	728
30.	Sikkim	1	0	1	1	0	0	0	3	0	14	14	1
31.	Tamil Nadu	1	7	0	0	0	2	53	73	87	115	203	0
32.	Telangana	NA	NA	NA	NA	NA	NA	NA	NA	72	NA	NA	705
33.	Tripura	0	0	2	0	0	2	1	2	4	20	107	98
34.	Uttar Pradesh	44	31	9	0	18	12	346	315	474	394	451	594
35.	Uttarakhand	0	0	0	0	0	0	6	3	8	18	10	52
36.	West Bengal	0	0	0	0	0	0	2	16	53	6	73	0

NA: Not Available/Not Applicable

Source: National Crime Records Bureau Statistics, 2005, 2010, 2015

Table A.6.26 Crime rate against children (0–18 years)

Indicators		Rate of infanticide			Rate of murder			Rate of rape			Rate of foeticide		
S. No	India	2005	2010	2015	2005	2010	2015	2005	2010	2015	2005	2010	2015
	India	0.0	0.0	0.0	0.1	0.1	0.4	0.4	0.5	2.4	0.0	0.0	0.0
	STATE/UT												
1.	Andaman and Nicobar	0.0	0.0	0.0	0.3	0.2	0.7	0.5	3.5	19.1	0.0	0.7	0.0
2.	Andhra Pradesh	0.0	0.0	0.0	0.1	0.1	0.3	0.4	0.5	3.1	0.0	0.0	0.0
3.	Arunachal Pradesh	0.0	0.0	0.0	0.0	0.0	1.3	0.9	1.0	7.3	0.0	0.0	0.0
4.	Assam	0.0	0.0	0.0	0.0	0.0	0.1	0.3	0.1	0.4	0.0	0.0	0.0
5.	Bihar	0.0	0.0	0.0	0.0	0.2	0.2	0.0	0.1	0.3	0.0	0.0	0.0
6.	Chandigarh	0.0	0.0	0.0	0.3	0.1	0.3	2.1	1.4	10.3	0.0	0.0	0.1
7.	Chhattisgarh	0.0	0.0	0.0	0.1	0.2	0.7	1.7	1.6	3.2	0.1	0.0	0.0
8.	Dadra and Nagar Haveli	0.0	0.0	0.0	0.4	0.0	1.6	0.0	1.1	1.6	0.0	0.0	0.0
9.	Daman and Diu	0.0	0.0	0.0	0.6	0.0	1.1	0.6	0.5	0.0	0.0	0.0	0.1
10.	Delhi	0.0	0.0	0.1	0.2	0.2	1.0	1.5	1.7	16.6	0.0	0.0	0.0
11.	Goa	0.0	0.1	0.0	0.3	0.1	0.6	1.0	1.3	9.6	0.0	0.0	0.0
12.	Gujarat	0.0	0.0	0.0	0.1	0.1	0.4	0.2	0.2	0.3	0.0	0.0	0.0
13.	Haryana	0.0	0.0	0.1	0.2	0.1	0.5	0.6	0.4	2.8	0.0	0.0	0.0
14.	Himachal Pradesh	0.0	0.0	0.1	0.1	0.1	0.3	0.9	1.1	6.4	0.0	0.0	0.0
15.	Jammu and Kashmir	0.0	0.0	0.0	0.0	0.0	0.1	0.0	0.1	0.6	0.0	0.0	0.0
16.	Jharkhand	0.0	0.0	0.0	0.1	0.0	0.1	0.1	0.0	0.2	0.0	0.0	0.0
17.	Karnataka	0.0	0.0	0.0	0.1	0.1	0.6	0.1	0.2	0.0	0.0	0.0	0.0
18.	Kerala	0.0	0.0	0.0	0.1	0.1	0.4	0.4	0.6	7.7	0.0	0.0	0.0
19.	Lakshadweep	0.0	0.0	0.0	0.0	0.0	0.0	0.0	0.0	0.0	0.0	0.0	0.0
20.	Madhya Pradesh	0.0	0.0	0.1	0.2	0.2	0.4	1.3	1.6	5.2	0.0	0.0	0.0
21.	Maharashtra	0.0	0.0	0.0	0.2	0.2	0.5	0.6	0.7	5.9	0.0	0.0	0.0
22.	Manipur	0.0	0.0	0.0	0.1	0.1	0.5	0.2	0.4	1.3	0.0	0.0	0.0
23.	Meghalaya	0.0	0.0	0.0	0.3	0.1	0.5	2.1	3.5	3.8	0.0	0.0	0.0

24.	Mizoram	0.0	0.0	0.0	0.1	0.8	0.0	4.2	8.1	0.0	0.0
25.	Nagaland	0.0	0.0	0.0	0.0	0.3	0.0	0.1	1.2	0.0	0.0
26.	Odisha	0.0	0.0	0.0	0.0	0.1	0.1	0.2	7.5	0.0	0.0
27.	Puducherry	0.0	0.0	0.0	0.0	0.0	0.3	0.3	0.0	0.0	0.0
28.	Punjab	0.0	0.0	0.1	0.1	0.5	0.2	0.5	5.3	0.0	0.1
29.	Rajasthan	0.0	0.0	0.1	0.1	0.2	0.4	0.5	2.6	0.1	0.0
30.	Sikkim	0.2	0.0	0.0	0.5	0.0	2.4	2.3	0.5	0.2	0.0
31.	Tamil Nadu	0.0	0.1	0.1	0.1	0.4	0.2	0.3	0.0	0.0	0.0
32.	Telangana*	NA	NA	NA	NA	0.6	NA	NA	6.3	NA	NA
33.	Tripura	0.0	0.0	0.0	0.1	0.3	0.6	3.0	7.9	0.0	0.1
34.	Uttar Pradesh	0.0	0.2	0.2	0.2	0.5	0.2	0.2	0.7	0.0	0.0
35.	Uttarakhand	0.0	0.1	0.1	0.0	0.2	0.2	0.1	1.4	0.0	0.0
36.	West Bengal	0.0	0.0	0.0	0.0	0.2	0.0	0.1	0.0	0.0	0.0

NA: Not Available/Not Applicable

Population Source: Registrar General of India estimated population of 2005, 2010, 2015, based on 2001 and 2011 Censuses.

*Adjusted mid-year projected population for 2015, due to absence of population figures of newly created states, namely Andhra Pradesh and Telangana carved out from erstwhile 'Andhra Pradesh.'

Crime Rate: number of cases reported/mid-year projected population in lakhs.

Source: National Crime Records Bureau Statistics, 2005, 2010, 2015

Table A.6.27 Crimes against women

| Indicator | | Cases reported of crimes against women | | | | | | | | |
| | | Rape | | | Kidnapping and abduction | | | Cruelty by husbands and relatives | | |
S. No		2005	2010	2015	2005	2010	2015	2005	2010	2015
	India	18359	22172	34651	15750	29795	59277	58319	94041	113403
	STATE/UT									
1.	Andaman and Nicobar	4	24	36	1	8	21	5	9	14
2.	Andhra Pradesh	935	1362	1027	995	1531	684	8696	12080	6121
3.	Arunachal Pradesh	35	47	71	39	46	128	9	12	66
4.	Assam	1238	1721	1733	1456	2767	5039	2206	5410	11255
5.	Bihar	1147	795	1041	929	2569	5158	1574	2271	3792
6.	Chandigarh	33	31	72	45	28	165	75	41	126
7.	Chhattisgarh	990	1012	1560	184	279	1354	732	861	620
8.	Dadra and Nagar Haveli	5	3	8	9	10	9	5	3	2
9.	Daman and Diu	2	1	5	2	2	13	3	3	3
10.	Delhi	658	507	2199	1106	1740	4301	1324	1404	3521
11.	Goa	20	36	86	12	18	70	11	17	19
12.	Gujarat	324	408	503	916	1290	1569	4090	5600	4133
13.	Haryana	461	720	1070	344	714	2336	2075	2720	3525
14.	Himachal Pradesh	141	160	244	102	162	239	228	275	226
15.	Jammu and Kashmir	201	245	296	658	840	1071	76	211	400
16.	Jharkhand	753	773	1053	283	696	930	590	650	1654
17.	Karnataka	343	586	589	312	586	1611	1883	3441	2732
18.	Kerala	478	634	1256	129	184	192	3283	4797	3668
19.	Lakshadweep	0	0	0	0	0	0	0	0	2
20.	Madhya Pradesh	2921	3135	4391	604	1030	4547	2989	3756	5281

21.	Maharashtra	1545	1599	4144	851	1124	5096	6233	7434	7640
22.	Manipur	25	34	46	69	107	94	20	18	39
23.	Meghalaya	63	149	93	19	37	58	3	24	44
24.	Mizoram	37	92	58	0	0	8	0	3	9
25.	Nagaland	17	16	35	9	6	30	0	1	4
26.	Odisha	799	1025	2251	547	912	2587	1671	2067	3605
27.	Puducherry	6	3	3	3	14	14	6	7	4
28.	Punjab	398	546	886	329	576	1253	729	1163	1583
29.	Rajasthan	993	1571	3644	1549	2477	4167	5997	11145	14383
30.	Sikkim	18	18	5	2	6	21	4	3	2
31.	Tamil Nadu	571	686	421	783	1464	1335	1650	1570	1900
32.	Telangana	NA	NA	1105	NA	NA	648	NA	NA	7329
33.	Tripura	162	238	213	43	91	120	439	937	501
34.	Uttar Pradesh	1217	1563	3025	2256	5468	10135	4505	7978	8660
35.	Uttarakhand	133	121	283	125	249	336	272	334	407
36.	West Bengal	1686	2311	1199	1039	2764	3938	6936	17796	20163

NA: Not Available/Not Applicable

Source: National Crime Records Bureau Statistics, 2005, 2010, 2015

Table A.6.28 Trend of social sector expenditure* to total disbursement in states

State	2001–02	2002–03	2003–04	2004–05	2005–06	2006–07	2007–08	2008–09	2009–10	2010–11	2011–12	2012–13	2013–14	2014–15	2015–16	2016–17 (RE)	2017–18 (BE)
1. Andhra Pradesh	35.0	32.5	33.3	29.3	30.8	32.9	32.7	38.9	35.6	38.9	39.2	38.2	39.3	41.2	49.3	51.1	48.2
2. Bihar	38.9	36.4	36.7	30.5	38.4	41.0	43.8	43.9	41.8	38.2	40.0	44.4	43.4	44.8	46.9	48.7	49.7
3. Chhattisgarh	43.3	41.3	36.2	37.7	44.2	47.6	46.2	50.1	54.2	50.2	51.6	48.7	53.4	50.2	52.2	56.6	51.5
4. Goa	23.1	26.1	28.4	31.4	30.9	31.8	31.6	32.2	32.5	33.5	33.1	34.0	35.8	35.2	35.1	35.4	37.8
5. Gujarat	35.2	30.4	27.3	29.0	32.1	33.4	34.9	35.0	38.4	39.9	38.2	38.7	40.0	40.5	42.2	40.2	37.7
6. Haryana	34.3	26.6	18.6	24.2	32.0	28.5	33.3	37.2	41.0	39.6	40.9	40.8	37.0	39.3	31.1	38.6	43.0
7. Jharkhand	47.0	50.0	44.4	44.1	45.9	47.0	43.5	47.8	44.2	46.4	41.2	39.6	39.0	44.3	40.2	51.7	47.3
8. Karnataka	34.8	31.4	28.4	28.5	33.4	32.7	36.7	37.8	39.9	39.9	37.8	39.2	37.6	40.0	41.7	41.8	40.7
9. Kerala	37.6	37.4	30.0	36.2	35.6	31.0	31.4	33.4	33.6	33.4	34.8	34.9	34.5	35.7	36.3	35.9	36.5
10. Madhya Pradesh	35.4	37.7	28.4	24.7	32.5	35.3	35.7	36.7	35.2	39.0	33.6	40.0	39.8	39.7	44.6	40.7	43.2
11. Maharashtra	36.4	33.3	30.9	28.1	35.3	37.3	37.0	36.8	40.3	41.4	41.1	42.6	41.9	42.7	41.6	43.6	44.7
12. Odisha	34.2	31.7	28.0	28.9	34.2	31.7	35.9	41.6	41.0	42.3	42.9	41.6	44.2	44.6	45.8	45.9	45.3
13. Punjab	23.8	17.2	17.3	17.8	19.8	17.9	18.8	23.8	22.7	22.5	27.1	28.2	27.5	29.1	25.9	45.7	29.0
14. Rajasthan	40.7	37.3	35.7	34.1	40.1	39.5	38.9	45.2	44.3	42.4	42.6	41.5	44.5	47.1	36.7	42.4	42.3
15. Tamil Nadu	37.0	32.0	34.3	32.6	36.9	33.1	35.9	39.7	40.3	40.2	38.3	38.5	41.1	39.9	41.5	34.4	36.1
16. Telangana	–	–	–	–	–	–	–	–	–	–	–	–	–	39.2	43.6	43.4	44.3

17. Uttar Pradesh	32.2	31.1	18.7	28.6	33.7	32.1	34.4	37.8	39.0	37.7	38.8	38.8	38.1	36.6	36.3	39.5	37.0
18. West Bengal	34.1	30.5	23.4	29.1	28.2	31.9	34.7	31.9	40.7	41.9	42.5	42.1	42.0	46.5	48.0	49.0	47.5
19. Arunachal Pradesh	32.5	30.9	28.3	31.2	30.4	30.2	31.1	29.9	33.7	28.1	32.4	30.5	32.8	34.6	27.8	30.5	38.8
20. Assam	35.5	36.2	35.0	32.4	36.8	38.7	40.0	38.7	36.7	39.5	37.0	36.5	39.0	45.1	48.2	47.4	45.3
21. Himachal Pradesh	33.7	29.8	29.0	29.0	32.7	33.0	35.2	36.6	35.0	37.3	34.6	34.3	37.1	37.5	36.6	39.6	38.7
22. Jammu and Kashmir	28.8	28.8	28.3	27.9	29.9	31.3	30.0	29.9	30.6	29.1	29.3	28.7	29.7	32.2	34.6	36.6	29.9
23. Manipur	26.0	26.0	26.0	33.6	34.2	28.7	31.7	32.9	32.5	31.6	29.4	29.3	29.4	35.3	33.9	37.9	36.5
24. Meghalaya	40.5	35.9	36.2	35.8	38.2	37.6	37.5	35.7	36.6	36.7	39.4	37.7	39.9	43.3	40.7	41.7	45.9
25. Mizoram	40.7	40.0	35.7	35.6	33.3	34.8	36.7	40.1	41.5	38.6	36.6	39.7	40.8	43.3	44.0	37.2	37.4
26. Nagaland	26.9	29.6	27.0	27.6	28.6	29.6	29.5	28.3	25.9	28.3	24.9	27.4	29.8	31.0	29.8	36.9	35.0
27. Sikkim	16.5	16.3	27.5	22.2	23.3	24.3	23.5	27.4	28.8	30.9	36.8	35.4	37.8	36.7	35.6	39.7	36.7
28. Tripura	39.3	38.4	34.8	37.6	34.0	36.5	36.5	37.2	37.9	38.4	41.7	40.9	41.6	47.9	49.4	50.2	46.9
29. Uttarakhand	40.0	35.2	32.7	36.6	36.3	37.9	37.4	38.4	42.3	42.5	45.5	41.5	43.6	47.9	45.6	45.4	43.4
30. NCT Delhi	34.6	34.2	29.6	33.1	41.0	39.6	40.5	43.8	42.2	42.4	50.0	48.8	45.3	51.9	50.1	52.9	55.1
31. Puducherry	-	-	-	-	36.7	34.7	35.8	35.9	38.1	38.3	45.9	39.6	37.1	40.4	41.8	39.6	40.1

RE: Revised Estimates. BE: Budget Estimates.

* includes expenditure on social services, rural development and food storage and warehousing under revenue expenditure, capital outlay and loans and advances by the state governments.

■ Indicates expenditure below 30 percent.

Indicates expenditure between 30 and 49 percent.

Indicates expenditure above 50 percent.

Source: Budget documents of the state governments, CAG for 2015–2016, in respect of Jammu and Kashmir

Annexure 7
Technical background paper contributions

Table A.7.1 TBP titles and authors

S. No.	Name of the author(s)	Title of the paper
1.	Mridula Bajaj	*Childcare and Childcare Worker: Challenges, Prospects and Way Forward*
2.	Dr Nandita Chaudhary Shraddha Kapoor Punya Pillai	*Early learning and holistic development: Challenges, prospects and way forward*
3.	Ranjani K. Murthy	*Gender and Social Inclusion in Parenting of the Young Child in India*
4.	Dr Renu Singh Dr Ranjana Kesarwani	*The Disadvantaged Young Child in India*
5.	Venkatesan Ramani	*Physical well-being of the Young Child in India: Challenges, Prospects and Way Forward.*
6.	Vimala Ramachandran	*From the Womb to Primary School: Challenges, Policies and Prospects for the Young Child in India.*

Annexure notes

1 Ministry of Health and Family Welfare India, 2016. *National Family Health Survey 4, 2015–16.*

2 Moore, K. A. et al., 2011. Children's Developmental Contexts: An Index Based on Data of Individual Children. *Child Trends Research Brief.* Vol 2011. No 11, pp. 1–9.

3 Jordon, T. E., 1993. Estimating the Quality of Life for Children Around the World (NICQL '92'). *Social Indicators Research.* Vol 30, pp. 17–38.

4 Save the Children Fund, 2008. *The Child Development Index—Holding Governments to Account Children's Wellbeing.* London.

5 The Annie E. Casey Foundation, 2012. *2012 KIDS COUNT Data Book: State Trends in Child Well-Being.* The Annie E. Casey Foundation, Baltimore.

6 Duke Centre for Child and Family Policy, 2014. *Child and Youth Well-Being Index Report.* Retrieved from https://childandfamilypolicy.duke.edu/wp-content/uploads/2014/12/Child-Well-Being-Report.pdf; date of access: 16 April 2018.

7 Chang, Y. et al., 2015. Assessing Child Development: A Critical Review and the Sustainable Child Development Index (SCDI). *Sustainability.* Vol 7, pp. 4973–4996.

8 Roy, C., 2014. *Child Rights & Child Development in India: A Regional Analysis.* MPRA Paper No. 52784. Retrieved from https://mpra.ub.uni-muenchen.de/52784/1/MPRA_paper_52784.pdf; date of access: 18 April 2018.

9 Corrie, B. P., 1995. A Human Development Index for the Dalit Child in India. *Social Indicators Research.* Vol 34. No 3, pp. 395–409.

10 Drèze, J. and R. Khera, 2012. Regional Patterns of Human and Child Deprivation in India. Vol xlvii. No 39, pp. 42–49.

11 Thukral, E. G. and P. Thukral, 2011. *India: Child Rights Index.* HAQ: Centre for Child Rights, New Delhi.

Glossary of terms

Accredited Social Health Activist (ASHA) Trained community-based health activist instituted by the Ministry of Health and Family Welfare (MoHFW) under the National Rural Nutrition Mission.

Anaemia A medical condition wherein there are less than required amount of red blood cells or haemoglobin.

***Anganwadi* Helper (AWH)** A person who supports the AWW delivering ICDS centre's services.

***Anganwadi* Worker (AWW)** A person who runs the *Anganwadi* and facilitates distribution of its services.

Anganwadi/*Anganwadi* Centre (AWC)/ICDS Centre Government of India-run childcare centres mandated under the ICDS for facilitating the holistic needs of children between 3 and 6 years of age, along with providing facilities such as immunisation, supplementary nutrition, etc., for children under 3 and pregnant and lactating women.

Antenatal Care (ANC) Care provided to pregnant women by skilled health professionals in order to reduce risks of morbidity and mortality of the mother and child, both, before and after birth.

Auxiliary Nurse Midwife (ANM) Often the first person of contact between the community and health service providers, working at the grassroots level. ANM acts as a resource person with ASHA on trainings regarding, child and maternal healthcare, family planning, etc.

***Beti Bachao Beti Padhao* Scheme** Aimed at uplifting female sex ratio through empowerment of girls.

Body mass index (BMI) A simple index of weight-for-height that is commonly used to classify underweight, overweight and obese adults. It is defined as the weight in kilograms divided by the square of the height in meters (kg/m^2). (BMI < 18.5 = underweight; BMI ≥ 25.0 = overweight; and BMI ≥ 30.0 = obesity).

Child mortality The probability of dying between the first and the fifth birthdays.

Child Sex Ratio Number of females born per 1000 males for the population aged 6 years or under.

Civil Society Organization (CSO)   People/organisations operating the community in a manner that is unlike government or businesses.

Early Childhood Care and Education (ECCE)   Establishing a strong foundation of human life by ensuring comprehensive development of the child's physical, cognitive, social and emotional needs.

Early Childhood Development (ECD)   According to the World Bank's Nurturing Care Framework, ECD refers to the cognitive, linguistics, physical as well as socio-emotional development from the period of conception to 8 years of a human being.

Early Childhood   UNESCO defines it as the period from birth to eight years, characterised by outstanding rate of growth, wherein brain development is most rapid. According to UNICEF, this period ranges from conception to 8 years of age.

Expected years of schooling   The number of years a child of school entrance age is expected to spend at school or university, including years spent repeating one or more classes.

Female Literacy Rate   The female literacy rate is the ratio of the total literate female population aged 6 years and above to the total female population in the same age group and is expressed as a percentage.

GDP Per Capita   The aggregate of production (GDP) divided by the size of the population.

Gross Domestic Product   An aggregate measure of production equal to the sum of the gross values added of all resident institutional units engaged in production.

Gross Enrolment Ratio   The number of students enrolled in a given level of education, regardless of age, expressed as percentage of the official school-age population corresponding to the same level of education.

Infant Mortality Rate (IMR)   The probability of dying between birth and the age of 1 year per 1000 live births.

Infanticide   Killing of a child within a year of birth.

Institutional Delivery   Facility-based (hospitals, trained health professional, etc.) births to reduce neonatal and maternal mortality.

Integrated Child Development Scheme (ICDS)   A government programme established for children in the age group of 0–6, adolescent girls, pregnant women and lactating mothers, involving dissemination of non-formal pre-school education and discontinuing the unfortunate cycle of malnutrition, morbidity, affected learning capacity and mortality.

Life expectancy at birth   The number of years a newborn could expect to live if prevailing patterns of mortality at the time of its birth were to stay the same throughout its life.

Low Birth Weight   When the weight at birth is less than 2.5 kgs.

Malnutrition prevalence – weight for age (% children under 5)   Percentage of children under 5 whose weight for age is more than two standard deviations below the median reference standard for their age, as established by the World Health Organization.

Maternal Mortality Ratio (per 100,000 live births)   The number of women who die during pregnancy (before a child is born) and childbirth, per 100,000 live births.

Mean years of schooling   An average of number of years of schooling attained by population aged 25 or more.

Millennium Development Goals   These were eight goals endorsed by 191 UN member states; eradication of extreme poverty, achieving universal primary school, promoting gender equality and empowerment of women, reducing child mortality, improving maternal health, combatting HIV/AIDS, malaria and other diseases, ensuring environmental sustainability and developing a global partnership for development.

National Nutrition Mission (NNM)   Implemented by the Ministry of Women and Child Development in order to tackle the nutrition related issues of children under the age of 6 years, adolescent girls and pregnant and lactating women.

Neonatal mortality (NMR)   The probability of dying in the first month of life.

Net Enrolment Ratio   The total number of students in the theoretical age group for a given level of education enroled in that level, expressed as a percentage of the total population in that age group.

Open defecation   Open defecation refers to the practice whereby people go out in fields, bushes, forests, open bodies of water or other open spaces rather than using the toilet to defecate.

Panchayati Raj Institutions (PRI)   Unit of local self-governance at the rural level established under the 73rd Constitutional Amendment Act, 1992.

Perinatal mortality   The probability of a foetal death (stillbirth) or an early neonatal death.

Poshan Abhiyaan   *Poshan Abhiyaan* is India's flagship programme to improve nutritional outcomes of children, adolescents, pregnant women and lactating mothers by leveraging technology, a targeted approach and convergence.

Post neonatal mortality (PNMR)   The probability of dying after the first month of life but before the first birthday.

Postnatal Care (PNC)   Care provided to mothers and their newborn children by skilled health professionals, during the first six weeks after birth.

Preterm Child   Preterm refers to a baby born before 37 weeks of pregnancy have been completed. Normally, a pregnancy lasts about 40 weeks.

Public Distribution System (PDS)   A system to facilitate dissemination of food grains and essential commodities to people below the poverty line to ensure their access to these items at affordable rates. Implemented under the National Food Security Act (NFSA), 2013.

Public Policy   A strategic course undertaken by the government to address a problem and ensure public welfare. It is often not a definitive process.

Sex ratio at birth   The number of boys born alive per 100 girls born alive.

Social Audit   A review of official documents and records by the people who are direct recipients of that particular service.

Statutes   Law which is expressed in writing and has been passed by a legislative body.

Stillbirths   Stillbirth is when a baby dies in the womb after 20 weeks of pregnancy. Most stillbirths happen before a woman goes into labour, but a small number happen during labour and birth.

Stunting – height for age (% children under 5)   Percentage of children under 5 whose height for age is more than two standard deviations below the median for the international reference, as established by the World Health Organization, population aged 0 to 59 months.

Supplementary Nutrition Program   The Supplementary Nutrition is one of the six services provided under the Integrated Child Development Services (ICDS) Scheme which is primarily designed to bridge the gap between the Recommended Dietary Allowance (FDA) and the Average Daily Intake (ADI).

Surrogate parenthood   When a woman agrees to carry a child to term for another individual, who then becomes the legal parent of the child at birth, it is called surrogate parenthood.

Sustainable Development Goals (SDGs)   Building upon the Millennium Development Goals, since January 2016, SDGs are a call for action towards issues such as poverty, climate change, education, economic inequality, peace, etc. These 17 goals are to be achieved by 2030.

Sustainable development   Sustainable development is development that meets the needs of the present without compromising the ability of future generations to meet their own needs.

Swachh Bharat Mission   A campaign started in October 2014 that aims towards making India cleaner through various awareness-building mechanisms and infrastructural revisions.

Take home rations   Supplementary Nutrition Programme (SNP) is one of the core components of ICDS. Balbhog (Energy Dense Micronutrient Fortified Extruded Blended Food) is provided as Take Home Ration (THR) to children 7 months to 3 years (seven packets to normal weight and ten packets to severe underweight).

Under-5 mortality (U5MR)   The probability of dying before the fifth birthday.

Urbanisation   Urbanisation is an increase in the number of people living in towns and cities. Urbanisation occurs mainly because people move from rural areas to urban areas, and it results in growth in the size of the urban population and the extent of urban areas.

Wasting – weight for height) (% children under 5)   Percentage of children under 5 whose weight for height is more than two standard deviations below the median for the international reference, as established by the World Health Organization, population aged 0 to 59 months.

Contributors

Mridula Bajaj, an MSc in Child Development from University of Delhi, India, is a specialist in Child Development with more than three decades of experience in programming, research and training. She has worked as the Executive Director of Mobile Creches for more than twenty years. She is currently the Vice Chairperson of Oxfam India Board. She has also been a Member of the Steering Committee for the 10th Five Year Plan and has served on the Expert Committee to evaluate proposals and field inspection under experimental and innovative education projects by the Ministry of Human Resource Development, Department of Education. She has done extensive work in the area of empowerment of women and child development.

Nandita Chaudhary is a consultant and collaborator for projects, programmes and publications on Child Development, Family Studies and Cultural Psychology with specific reference to Indian communities. She blogs at Masala Chai: Musings about little people (https://masalachai-musings.com/). She has taught at Lady Irwin College, University of Delhi, India. She has been a Fulbright Scholar and Senior Fellow of the Indian Council for Social Science Research, India.

Ranjana Kesarwani has been associated with Young Lives India since 2018 as Research Associate. Prior to joining Young Lives, she worked as a research officer at Save the Children, Research Fellow at the Public Health Foundation of India, and as a data analyst for the Annual Health Survey. She is skilled in statistical analysis, advanced multivariate and multilevel analysis, sampling, research design, data management, monitoring and evaluation of programmes and policies and handling large-scale sample surveys. Her interest areas are maternal and child health, social determinants of health, mortality analysis and small area estimation.

Ranjani Murthy brings to the table about twenty-four years of experience in evaluation, mainstreaming, research and training/toolkit development on gender and development; with a focus on issues of agriculture, food security, poverty reduction, health, disaster-risk-reduction and SDGs.

Her work on gender and child rights has been with UNICEF (India and Nepal), Save the Children and CCFC (India and Bangladesh), including on SDGs. Her primary clients include UN organisations, national governments and NGOs. She is also on the editorial board of the journal *Gender and Development*.

Vimala Ramachandran has been working on elementary education, girls' education, women's empowerment and the intersections between health, nutrition and education, especially with respect to children. She was involved in the conceptualisation of Mahila Samakhya (Education for Women's Equality) and served as the first National Project Director from 1988–1993 in Ministry of Human Resource Development, Government of India. She established the Educational Resource Unit (now known as ERU Consultants Private Limited) in 1998 as a network of researchers and practitioners working on education. From 2011 to mid-2015, she was National Fellow and Professor of Teacher Management and Development in NUEPA, India.

Venkatesan Ramani is a retired IAS officer of the Maharashtra cadre, with degrees in economics and law. He has served in various capacities in the Governments of India and Maharashtra between 1980 and 2010. His last official assignment was as Director General of the Maharashtra State Nutrition Mission, which he helped set up in 2005. The Mission's work in child malnutrition reduction saw significant reduction in stunting rates of under-2 children. He continues to work in this area with governments, corporates and nonprofits. His blogsite *The Gadfly Column* analyses current happenings in India and elsewhere.

Renu Singh has over twenty-six years of experience in school management, teacher education, policy analysis and research both in India and abroad. Currently she is working as Country Director for Young Lives, University of Oxford, on a fifteen-year longitudinal research study on childhood poverty. A trained Montessorian, special educator and educational psychologist, she has managed a pre-school in Dubai, held the position of Director, School of Rehabilitation Sciences, University of Delhi, India, Director AADI (formerly Spastic Society of Northern India) and has been a member of the Senior Management Team of Save the Children, India.

Core team members

Anuradha K. Rajivan served in the Asian Development Bank as Adviser, Strategy and Policy Department, Manila, before retiring, and was the ADB-wide focal point on Sustainable Development Goals. Her work included financing for development, as well as guiding joint outputs under the UN-ADB partnership on the SDGs. Prior to the ADB, Anuradha served as UNDP's Practice Leader on Inclusive Growth and Poverty Reduction in Asia Pacific and led the regional Human Development Reports series. She is a former IAS officer of the Tamil Nadu cadre and has a PhD in Economics. Her early professional work and research on pre-school ages seeded a long-term interest in child and human development issues.

Sanjay Kaul is the Chairman, National Collateral Management Services Limited. He is a former Indian Administrative Service officer. Before joining NCML, he was the Director and CEO of the NCDEX Institute of Commodity Markets and Research, New Delhi, India, and he has worked as the Joint Secretary, Department of Food and Public Distribution, Government of India. He has worked extensively with policymakers, project leaders, international agencies and government ministries and also led multi-sectoral development projects and teams. He is a postgraduate in Economics from the University of Delhi, India.

V.S. Sambandan is Chief Administrative Officer, The Hindu Centre for Politics and Public Policy. He holds a PhD in Economics from the University of Madras, India, and an MBA from Bournemouth University, UK. During his journalism career he has reported and written extensively on economic and social issues and served as *The Hindu's* foreign correspondent in Sri Lanka for six years during the Sri Lankan separatist conflict. His areas of interests include economic and social policy, politics and political communication and political economy. He is a member of the Board of Studies for Economics, University of Madras, and Academic Council Member of the Dwaraka Doss Goverdhan Doss Vaishnav College (Autonomous), Chennai, India.

Sumitra Mishra is a postgraduate in special education for persons with disabilities. She has over twenty years of work experience ranging from grassroots direct practice in rural, urban poor and urban contexts to working with the most excluded and disenfranchised – persons with disabilities, victims of trafficking and survivors of violence, especially women, girls and children. Her work has encompassed, programme development and partnerships, strategic programming, policy advocacy and influence, fundraising and communications and organisation development.

Samreen Mushtaq holds a PhD from the Department of Political Science, Jamia Millia Islamia, New Delhi, India. She was awarded a Doctoral Fellowship by the Indian Council of Social Science Research (2015–17). She worked as Research Assistant Consultant with The Hindu Centre for Politics and Public Policy (April 2018–March 2019). Her research interests include gender, violence and human rights. Her writings have appeared in the *Economic and Political Weekly*, *Open Democracy*, *Contemporary South Asia*, *Al Jazeera*, *The Caravan*, *Indian Express* and *The Hindu Centre*, among others.

Neelam Singh is an independent international consultant with extensive work experience of situation analysis, policy research and knowledge management related to children's rights, gender and rights based development for international organisations, governments and national non-governmental organisations. She has a multidisciplinary background with master's in political science from the University of Delhi, a postgraduate diploma in journalism for developing countries from the Indian Institute of Mass Communications and an MPhil in development studies from the Institute of Development Studies, Sussex, UK.

List of participants in roundtable consultation

In an attempt to bring together social researchers and policy influencers to get firsthand comments and insights with regard to this Report, Mobile Creches organised a roundtable at the India International Centre, New Delhi, on Saturday, 13 October 2018.

Invitees	Designation and Organisation
Akhila Sivadas	Executive Director, *Centre for Advocacy and Research*
Ambika Pandit	Senior Assistant Editor, *Times of India*
Amrita Jain	Chairperson, *Mobile Creches*
Anjali Gokhale	Manager, *Forbes Marshall Foundation*
Anjela Taneja	Technical Director – Education, *CARE India*
Chirashree Ghosh	Sr. Manager – Advocacy, *Mobile Creches*
Devika Singh	Member, *Alliance for Right to ECD*
Dhanpal	Research Team Member, *HAQ – Centre for Child Rights*
Dhvani Mehta	Senior Resident Fellow, *Vidhi Centre for Legal Policy*
Dr Anuradha K. Rajivan	*Former IAS, Researcher*
Dr Niranjan Aradhya VP	Fellow & Programme Head (Right to Education), *National Law School of India University*
Ranjani Murthy	*Gender and Child Rights Consultant*
Dr Venita Kaul	Professor Emerita Education, *Ambedkar University Delhi, Former CECED*
Enakshi Ganguly	Co-Director, HAQ – *Centre for Child Rights*
Geeta Verma	Team Leader, Girls' Education Program, *CARE India*
Madhumita Pujari	Chairperson and Founder, *Sai's Angel Foundation*
Madhusudan Rao	*TATA Trusts*
Meha Tiwari	Program Officer, *HCL Foundation*
Mirai Chaterjee	Director – Social Security, *Self Employed Women's Association*
Mridula Bajaj	Vice Chairperson, *Oxfam India Board*
Nidhi Pundhir	Director – CSR, *HCL Foundation*
Padmini ji	Trustee, *Child Rights Trust*
Prianka Rao	Senior Resident Fellow, *Vidhi Centre for Legal Policy*
Prof. Amita Dhanda	Professor, *NALSAR Hyderabad*
Dr Punya Pillai	Assistant Professor, *Human Development and Childhood Studies*

Invitees	Designation and Organisation
Radhika Sharma	Program Officer – Advocacy, *Mobile Creches*
Prof. Rekha Sharma Sen	Professor, *Indira Gandhi National Open University*
Dr Renu Singh	Country Director, *Young Lives*
Rita Brara	Professor Emerita, Department of Sociology, *University of Delhi*
Rushda Majeed	Representative India, *Bernard van Leer Foundation*
Dr V.S. Sambandan	Chief Administrative Officer, *The Hindu Centre for Politics and Public Policy*
Dr Samreen Mushtaq	Research Assistant, *The Hindu Centre for Politics and Public Policy*
Sanjay Kaul	CEO, *National Collateral Management Services Limited*
Shreya Shrivastava	Research Fellow, *Vidhi Centre for Legal Policy*
Sumitra Mishra	Executive Director, *Mobile Creches*
Sunisha Ahuja	Education Specialist ECE, *UNICEF*
Varsha Sharma	Head – Advocacy and Knowledge Management, *Mobile Creches*
Vimala Ramachandran	Director, *ERU Consultants Private Limited*
Zakiya Kurrien	*Centre for Learning Resources*

Partners

Bernard van Leer Foundation (BvLF): BvLF is an independent foundation working worldwide to inspire and inform large scale action to improve the health and well-being of babies, toddlers and the people who care for them. They provide financial support and expertise to partners in government, civil society and business to help test and scale effective services for young children and families.

The Hindu Centre for Politics and Public Policy: The Hindu Centre endeavours to promote a vision of nationhood firmly anchored to the rights of all Indian citizens. The Centre's explorations include the manner in which certain concepts like secularism and social justice have become such contentious items of political discourse. As a public policy resource, the Centre's goal is to enlighten the Indian public and to increase their awareness of their political and social choices.

TATA Trusts: TATA Trusts have played a pioneering role in transforming traditional ideas of charity and introducing the concept of philanthropy to make a real difference to communities, in the areas of healthcare and nutrition, water and sanitation, energy, education, rural livelihoods, natural resource management, urban poverty alleviation, enhancing civil society and governance, media, arts, crafts and culture; and diversified employment.

HCL Foundation: As the corporate social responsibility arm of HCL, it is a gold standard not for profit organisation that matches the national and international development standards and brings about lasting positive impact in the lives of people through long term sustainable programmes implemented in full engagement with HCL's own employees and partners.

National Collateral Management Limited (NCML): The National Collateral Management Services Limited (NCML) is India's leading organisation, providing a bouquet of commodity based services under a single umbrella. Since its incorporation in 2004, NCML has empowered a multitude of stakeholders in the commodity value chain in managing their risks.

Index